# CRASH COURSE
# Respiratory System
## SECOND EDITION

Series editor
**Daniel Horton-Szar**
BSc (Hons) MBBS (Hons)
GP Registrar
Northgate Medical Practice
Canterbury
Kent

Faculty advisor
**Dr Ian Adcock**
PhD
National Heart and Lung Institute
Royal Brompton Hospital
Dovehouse Street
London

# Respiratory System

## SECOND EDITION

# Pippa McGowan

BA (Hons)
4th year medical student
University of Edinburgh Medical School
Teviot Place
Edinburgh

First edition authors
**Angus Jeffries, Andrew Turley**

 Mosby

Edinburgh • London • New York • Oxford • Philadelphia • St Louis • Sydney • Toronto 2003

MOSBY
An imprint of Elsevier Limited

| | |
|---|---|
| Commissioning editor | **Alex Stibbe** |
| Project Manager | **Frances Affleck** |
| Project Development Manager | **Duncan Fraser** |
| Designer | **Andy Chapman** |
| Cover Design | **Kevin Faerber** |
| Illustration Manager | **Mick Ruddy** |

First edition 1999
Second edition 2003
   Reprinted 2004

ISBN 0723432937

**British Library Cataloguing in Publication Data**
A catalogue record for this book is available from the British Library

**Library of Congress Cataloging in Publication Data**
A catalog record for this book is available from the Library of Congress

**Note**
Medical knowledge is constantly changing. As new information becomes available,
changes in treatment, procedures, equipment and the use of drugs become
necessary. The author, editors and the publishers have taken care to ensure that the
information given in this text is accurate and up to date. However, readers are
strongly advised to confirm that the information, especially with regard to drug
usage, complies with the latest legislation and standards of practice.

Typeset by SNP Best-set Typesetter Ltd., Hong Kong
Printed in Spain

The publisher's policy is to use paper manufactured from sustainable forests

The
Publisher's
policy is to use
**paper manufactured
from sustainable forests**

# Preface

Students often find respiratory medicine difficult when they are first introduced to it. The basic science can be hard going and it isn't always obvious how it relates to real patients with respiratory symptoms. Fortunately, when you have got past the gas laws and acquired a stethoscope, things improve. Once on the ward, you can probably live without a detailed knowledge of Poiseuille's law, but a sound grasp of the basics of the respiratory system will give you confidence when interpreting chest X-rays and examining patients.

In this new edition of *Crash Course: Respiratory System* we have tried to make the science more accessible, linking it wherever possible to clinical situations. We have added to the sections on clinical history taking and examination. Although still discussed, some of the more complex equations have been separated from the main body of the text so if you would rather give them a miss, you can.

I hope this approach makes the basic science more memorable, so that you pass those exams, but at the same time emphasises the point of it all—diagnosing and treating respiratory disease. Good luck!

**Pippa McGowan**

In the second edition of *Crash Course: Respiratory System* we hope to have continued the aim of the first edition by combining pre-clinical and clinical information in an easy-to-use, and importantly, easy-to-remember format. The chapters are more integrated to reflect changes in the curricula seen in many medical schools. We have emphasised the more important, common diseases that are seen in clinical practice and updated the treatment sections to reflect current British Thoracic Society and international guidelines.

Respiratory medicine plays a key part in the working life of all clinicians, whether a general practitioner, physician or surgeon, so understanding the basics is essential. We hope that this book will not only enable you to pass the important exams but will also provide a solid grounding for your future career.

**Dr Ian Adcock**
**Faculty Advisor**

In the six years since the first editions were published, there have been many changes in medicine, and in the way it is taught. These second editions have been largely rewritten to take these changes into account, and keep *Crash Course* up to date for the twenty-first century. New material has been added to include recent research and all pharmacological and disease management information has been updated in line with current best practice. We've listened to feedback from hundreds of students who have been using *Crash Course* and have improved the structure and layout of the books accordingly: pathology material has been closely integrated with the relevant basic medical science; there are more MCQs and the clarity of text and figures is better than ever.

The principles on which we developed the series remain the same, however. Medicine is a huge subject, and the last thing a student needs when exams are looming is to waste time assembling information from different sources, and wading through pages of irrelevant detail. As before, *Crash Course* brings you all the information you need, in compact, manageable volumes that integrate basic medical science with clinical practice. We still tread the fine line between producing clear, concise text and providing enough detail for those aiming at distinction. The series is still written by medical students with recent exam experience, and checked for accuracy by senior faculty members from across the UK.

I wish you the best of luck in your future careers!

**Dr Dan Horton-Szar**
**Series Editor (Basic Medical Sciences)**

# Acknowledgements

I would like to thank Dan Horton-Szar, Alex Stibbe and Duncan Fraser for their hard work in preparing this edition. Thanks also to Richard Denslow, Rosalind Lake and Paola De Carolis for their help during the inevitable last minute panic.

**Figure acknowledgements**

Figs 1.1 and 1.2 adapted with permission from A Stevens and J Lowe. Human Histology, 2nd edition. Mosby, 1997

Figs 5.32, 5.33, 5.34 and 5.35 with kind permission from C J Lote. Principles of Renal Physiology, 4th edition. Kluwer Academic Publishers, 2000

Fig 7.21 adapted with permission from A Stevens and J Lowe. Pathology. Mosby, 1995

Figs 9.21, 9.23 and 9.28 adapted with permission from O Epstein, G D Perkin, D P de Bono and J Cookson. Clinical Examination, 2nd edition. Mosby, 1997

Figs 10.16, 10.17, 10.19, 10.26, 10.27 and 10.28 reproduced from D Sutton and J W R Young. Concise Textbook of Clinical Imaging, 2nd edition. Mosby, 1995

Figs 10.21, 10.22 and 10.23 reproduced from C D Forbes and W F Jackson. Color Atlas and Text of Clinical Medicine, 2nd edition. Mosby, 1997

# Dedication

To Richard.

# Contents

# BASIC MEDICAL SCIENCE
# OF THE RESPIRATORY SYSTEM

# 1. Overview of the Respiratory System

## Overall structure and function

### Respiration
Respiration refers to the processes involved in oxygen transport from the atmosphere to the body tissues and the release and transportation of carbon dioxide produced in the tissues to the atmosphere.

This book will not discuss tissue respiration, in which oxygen is used by the cell to liberate energy; this is also known as internal respiration and is covered in *Crash Course: Metabolism and Nutrition*. The focus of this book is external respiration, or the exchange of gases between the environment and the blood.

Microorganisms rely on diffusion to and from their environment for the supply of oxygen and removal of carbon dioxide. Humans, however, are unable to rely on diffusion because:
- Their surface area : volume ratio is too small
- The diffusion distance from the surface of the body to the cells is too large and the process would be far too slow to be compatible with life.

Remember that diffusion time increases with the square of the distance and as a result, the human body has had to develop a specialized respiratory system to overcome these problems. This system has two components:
- A gas-exchange system that provides a large surface area for the uptake of oxygen from, and the release of carbon dioxide to, the environment. This function is performed by the lungs
- A transport system that delivers oxygen to the tissues from the lungs and carbon dioxide to the lungs from the tissues. This function is carried out by the cardiovascular system.

### Structure
The respiratory system can be neatly divided into upper respiratory tract (nasal and oral cavities, pharynx, larynx and trachea) and lower respiratory tract (main bronchi and lungs) (Fig. 1.1).

### Upper respiratory tract
The upper respiratory tract has a large surface area, a rich blood supply, and its epithelium (respiratory epithelium) is covered by a mucous secretion. Within the nose, hairs are present, which act as a filter. The function of the upper respiratory tract is to warm, moisten, and filter the air so that it is in a suitable condition for gaseous exchange in the distal part of the lower respiratory tract.

### Lower respiratory tract
The lower respiratory tract consists of the lower part of the trachea, the two primary bronchi and the lungs. These structures are contained within the thoracic cavity.

### Lungs
The lungs are the organs of gas exchange and act as both a conduit for air flow (the airway) and a surface for movement of oxygen into the blood and carbon dioxide out of the blood (the alveolar capillary membrane).

The lungs consist of airways, blood vessels, nerves and lymphatics, supported by parenchymal tissue. Inside the lungs, the two main bronchi divide into smaller and smaller airways until the end respiratory unit (acinus) is reached (Fig. 1.2).

### Acinus
The acinus is that part of the airway that is involved in gaseous exchange (i.e. the passage of oxygen from the lungs to the blood and carbon dioxide from the blood to the lungs). The structure of the acinus is considered in detail in Chapter 3.

### Pleurae
The lung, chest wall and mediastinum are covered by two continuous layers of epithelium known as the pleurae. The inner pleura covering the lung is the visceral pleura and the outer pleura covering the chest wall and mediastinum is the parietal pleura. These two pleurae are closely opposed and are separated by only a thin layer of liquid. The liquid acts as a lubricant and allows the two surfaces to slip over each other during breathing.

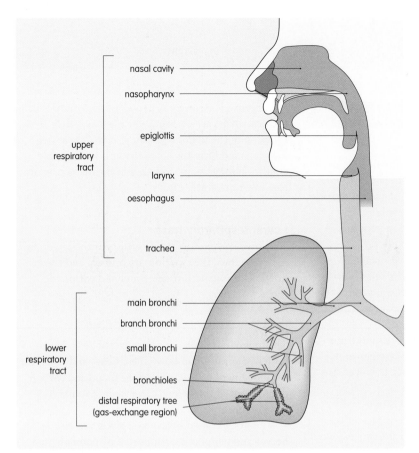

**Fig. 1.1** A schematic diagram of the respiratory tract.

Labels in figure:

upper respiratory tract
- nasal cavity
- nasopharynx
- epiglottis
- larynx
- oesophagus
- trachea

lower respiratory tract
- main bronchi
- branch bronchi
- small bronchi
- bronchioles
- distal respiratory tree (gas-exchange region)

## Basic concepts in respiration

The supply of oxygen to body tissues is essential for life; after only a brief period without oxygen, cells undergo irreversible change and eventually death. The respiratory system plays an essential role in preventing tissue hypoxia by optimizing the oxygen content of arterial blood through efficient gas exchange. The three key steps involved in gas exchange are:
- Ventilation
- Perfusion
- Diffusion.

Together these processes ensure that oxygen is available for transport to the body tissues and that carbon dioxide is eliminated (Fig. 1.3). If any of the three steps are compromised, for example through lung disease, then the oxygen content of the blood will fall below normal (hypoxaemia) and levels of carbon dioxide may rise (hypercapnia) (Fig. 1.4). In clinical practice, we do not directly test for tissue hypoxia but look for:
- Symptoms and signs of impaired gas exchange (e.g. breathlessness or central cyanosis)
- Abnormal results from arterial blood gas tests (see Chapter 10).

Severe hypoxaemia, with or without hypercapnia, is known as respiratory failure (see Chapter 8).

### Ventilation
Ventilation is the movement of air in and out of the respiratory system. It is determined by both:
- The respiratory rate (i.e. number of breaths per minute, normally 12–20)
- The volume of each breath, also known as the tidal volume.

A change in ventilation, in response to the metabolic needs of the body, can therefore be brought about by either:

**Fig. 1.2** The acinus, or respiratory unit. This part of the airway is involved in gas exchange.

- Altering the number of breaths per minute
- Adjusting the amount of air that enters the lungs with each breath.

In practice, the most common response to hypoxaemia is rapid, shallow breathing which increases the elimination of carbon dioxide and often leads to hypocapnia.

A raised respiratory rate, or tachypnoea, is not the same as hyperventilation. The term hyperventilation refers to a situation where ventilation is too great for the body's metabolic needs (see Chapter 5, p. 93).

## The mechanisms of ventilation

The movement of air into and out of the lungs takes place because of pressure differences caused by changes in lung volumes. Air flows from a high-pressure area to a low-pressure area. We cannot change the local atmospheric pressure around us to a level higher than that inside our lungs; the only obvious alternative is to lower the pressure within the lungs. We achieve this pressure reduction by expanding the size of the chest.

The main muscle of inspiration is the diaphragm, upon which the two lungs sit. The diaphragm is dome-shaped; contraction flattens the dome, increasing intrathoracic volume. This is aided by the external intercostal muscles, which raise the rib cage; this results in a lowered pressure within the thoracic cavity and hence the lungs, supply the driving force for air flow into the lungs. Inspiration is responsible for most of the work of breathing; diseases of the lungs or chest wall may increase the work load so that accessory muscles are also required to maintain adequate ventilation.

Expiration is largely a result of elastic recoil of the lung tissue. However, in forced expiration (e.g. during coughing), the abdominal muscles increase intra-abdominal pressure, forcing the contents of the

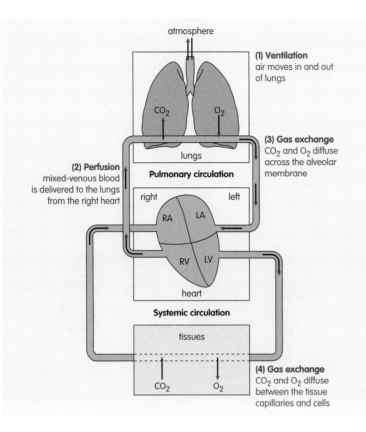

atmosphere

**(1) Ventilation**
air moves in and out
of lungs

$CO_2$     $O_2$

**(3) Gas exchange**
$CO_2$ and $O_2$ diffuse
across the alveolar
membrane

lungs

**Pulmonary circulation**

**(2) Perfusion**
mixed-venous blood
is delivered to the lungs
from the right heart

right                    left

RA     LA

RV     LV

heart

**Systemic circulation**

tissues

**(4) Gas exchange**
$CO_2$ and $O_2$ diffuse
between the tissue
capillaries and cells

$CO_2$          $O_2$

**Fig 1.3** Key steps involved in respiration. (Adapted with permission from *Physiology of Respiration* by M.P. Hlastala and A.J. Berger. Oxford University Press, 2001)

| Common respiratory terms | |
|---|---|
| **Hypocapnia** | Decreased carbon dioxide tension in arterial blood ($P_aCO_2$ < 4.8 kPa or 45 mmHg) |
| **Hypercapnia** | Increased carbon dioxide tension in arterial blood ($P_aCO_2$ > 6 kPa or 45 mmHg) |
| **Hypoxaemia** | Deficient oxygenation of the arterial blood |
| **Hypoxia** | Deficient oxygenation of the tissues |
| **Hyperventilation** | Ventilation that is in excess of metabolic requirements (results in hypocapnia) |
| **Hypoventilation** | Ventilation that is too low for metabolic requirements (results in hypercapnia) |

**Fig. 1.4** Definitions of common respiratory terms.

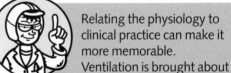

Relating the physiology to clinical practice can make it more memorable.
Ventilation is brought about by altering lung volumes and this can be affected by disease. That is why measurement of lung volumes, and knowing their normal values, is so important in assessing lung function (see Chapter 10).

abdomen against the diaphragm. In addition, the internal intercostal muscles lower the rib cage. These actions greatly increase intrathoracic pressure and enhance expiration.

### Impaired ventilation

There are two main types of disorder which impair ventilation. These are:

- Obstructive disorders in which the airways become narrowed, increasing the resistance to airflow
- Restrictive disorders in which expansion of the lungs is compromised and the volume of gas in the lungs is limited.

Obstructive and restrictive disorders have characteristic patterns of lung function, measured by pulmonary function tests (see Chapter 3).

Ventilatory failure occurs if the work of breathing becomes excessive and muscles fail. In this situation, or to prevent it from occurring, mechanical ventilation is required. Respiratory support is discussed in Chapter 6.

## Perfusion

The walls of the alveoli contain a dense network of capillaries bringing mixed-venous blood from the right heart. The barrier separating blood in the capillaries and air in the alveoli is extremely thin. Perfusion of blood through these pulmonary capillaries allows diffusion, and therefore gas exchange, to take place.

### Ventilation:perfusion inequality

To achieve efficient gaseous exchange, it is essential that the flow of gas (ventilation: V) and the flow of blood (perfusion: Q) are closely matched. The V:Q ratio in a normal, healthy lung is approximately 1. Two extreme scenarios illustrate mismatching of ventilation and perfusion (Fig. 1.5). These are:

- Normal alveolar ventilation but no perfusion (e.g. due a blood clot obstructing flow)
- Normal perfusion but no air reaching the lung unit (e.g. due to a mucus plug occluding an airway).

Ventilation:perfusion inequality is the most common cause of hypoxaemia and underlies many respiratory diseases.

Make sure you grasp the concept of ventilation: perfusion matching—it makes the pathology of many lung diseases easier to understand!

## Diffusion

At the gas exchange surface, diffusion occurs across the alveolar capillary membrane.

Molecules of $CO_2$ and $O_2$ diffuse along their partial pressure gradient.

key

| A | lung unit perfused but not ventilated due to obstruction by mucus plug |
| B | ventilation and perfusion matched |
| C | lung unit ventilated but not perfused due to embolus obstructing branch of pulmonary artery |

**Fig. 1.5** Diagram showing ventilation:perfusion mismatching. (Adapted from *Pulmonary Physiology and Pathophysiology* by J.B. West. Lippincott, Williams & Wilkins, 2001, p. 50.)

| $PO_2$ | Oxygen tension in blood (either arterial or venous) |
| $P_aO_2$ | Arterial oxygen tension |
| $P_vO_2$ | Oxygen tension in mixed-venous blood |
| $P_AO_2$ | Alveolar oxygen tension |

Carbon dioxide tensions follow the same format ($PCO_2$ etc)

**Fig. 1.6** Abbreviations used in denoting partial pressures.

## Partial pressures

Air in the atmosphere, before it is inhaled and moistened, contains 21% oxygen. This means that:

- 21% of the total molecules in air are oxygen molecules
- Oxygen is responsible for 21% of the total air pressure; this is its *partial pressure*, measured in mmHg or kPa and abbreviated as $PO_2$ (Fig. 1.6).

Partial pressure also determines the gas content of liquids, but it is not the only factor. Gas enters the liquid as a solution, and the amount that enters depends on its solubility. The more soluble a gas the more molecules that will enter solution for a given partial pressure. The partial pressure of a gas in a liquid is sometimes referred to as its *tension* (i.e. arterial oxygen tension is the same as $P_aO_2$).

As blood perfusing the pulmonary capillaries is mixed-venous blood:

- Oxygen will diffuse from the higher $PO_2$ environment of the alveoli into the capillaries
- Carbon dioxide will diffuse from the blood towards the alveoli, where $PCO_2$ is lower.

Blood and gas equilibrate as the partial pressures become the same in each and gas exchange then stops.

### Oxygen transport

Once oxygen has diffused into the capillaries it must be transported to the body tissues. The solubility of oxygen in the blood is low and only a small percentage of the body's requirement can be carried in dissolved form. Therefore most of the oxygen is combined with haemoglobin in red blood cells. Haemoglobin has four binding sites and the amount of oxygen carried by haemoglobin in the blood depends on how many of these sites are occupied. If they are all occupied by oxygen the molecule is said to be saturated. The oxygen saturation ($S_aO_2$) tells us the relative percentage of the maximum possible sites that can be bound. Note that anaemia will not reduce $S_aO_2$; lower haemoglobin means there are fewer available sites but the relative percentage of possible sites that are saturated stays the same.

The relationship between the partial pressure of oxygen and % saturation of haemoglobin is represented by the oxygen dissociation curve (see Chapter 5).

### Diffusion defects

If the blood–gas barrier becomes thickened through disease then the diffusion of $O_2$ and $CO_2$ will be impaired. Any impairment is particularly noticeable during exercise, when pulmonary flow increases and blood spends an even shorter time in the capillaries, exposed to alveolar oxygen. Impaired diffusion is, however, a much less common cause of hypoxaemia than ventilation/perfusion mismatching.

## Control of respiration

Respiration must respond to the metabolic demands of the body. This is achieved by a control system within the brainstem (the respiratory centres—see Chapter 6, p. 101) which receives information from various sources in the body where sensors monitor:

It is easy to get confused about $P_aO_2$, $S_aO_2$ and oxygen content. $P_aO_2$ tells us the pressure of the oxygen molecules dissolved in plasma, not those bound to haemoglobin. It is not a measure of how much oxygen is in the arterial blood. $S_aO_2$ tells us how many of the possible haemoglobin binding sites are occupied by oxygen. To calculate the amount of oxygen you would also need to know haemoglobin levels and how much oxygen is dissolved. Oxygen content ($C_aO_2$) is the only value that actually tells us how much oxygen is in the blood and, unlike $P_aO_2$ or $S_aO_2$, it is given in units which denote quantity (ml $O_2$/dl).

- Partial pressures of oxygen and carbon dioxide in the blood
- pH of the extracellular fluid within the brain
- Mechanical changes in the chest wall.

On the basis of information they receive, the respiratory centres modify ventilation to ensure that oxygen supply and carbon dioxide removal from the tissues matches their metabolic requirements. The actual mechanical change to ventilation is carried out by the respiratory muscles: these are known as the effectors of the control system.

Respiration can also be modified by higher centres (e.g. during speech, anxiety, emotion).

## Other functions of the respiratory system

Respiration is also concerned with a number of other functions, including metabolism, excretion, hormonal activity and, most importantly:

- Regulation of the pH of body fluids
- Regulation of body temperature.

### Acid–base regulation

Carbon dioxide forms carbonic acid in the blood, which dissociates to form hydrogen ions, lowering pH. By controlling the partial pressure of carbon dioxide, the respiratory system plays an important role in regulating the body's acid–base status (see Chapter 5); lung disease can therefore lead to acid–base disturbance. In acute disease it is important to test for blood pH and bicarbonate levels and these are included in the standard arterial blood gas results.

## Body temperature regulation

Body temperature is achieved mainly by insensible heat loss. Thus, by altering ventilation, body temperature may be regulated.

## Metabolism

The lungs have a huge vascular supply and thus a large number of endothelial cells. Hormones such as noradrenaline (norepinephrine), prostaglandins and 5-hydroxytryptamine are taken up by these cells and destroyed. Some exogenous compounds are also taken up by the lungs and destroyed (e.g. amphetamine and imipramine).

## Excretion

Carbon dioxide and some drugs (notably those administered through the lungs; e.g. general anaesthetics) are excreted by the lungs.

## Hormonal activity

Hormones (e.g. steroids) act on the lungs. Insulin enhances glucose utilization and protein synthesis. Angiotensin II is formed in the lungs from angiotensin I (by angiotensin-converting enzyme). Damage to the lung tissue causes the release of prostacyclin PG $I_2$, which prevents platelet aggregation.

- Why have humans developed a respiratory system?
- Describe how breathing is brought about.
- What is the difference between the partial pressure of a gas and its concentration?
- How can defects in ventilation, perfusion and diffusion cause hypoxaemia?
- What effect will anaemia have on $P_aO_2$, $S_aO_2$ and on the total oxygen content of the blood?
- Which structures are involved in gas exchange and how does it occur?
- What is the difference between restrictive and obstructive disorders?
- What happens if lung disease increases the work of breathing to excessive levels?
- Describe how respiration is controlled.
- List the main functions of the respiratory system.

# 2. The Upper Respiratory Tract

## Organization of the upper respiratory tract

### Structure of the upper respiratory tract
#### Nose
The nose consists of an external part (the external nose) and an internal part (the nasal cavities, including the nasal septum). These structures are adapted to the main functions of the nose which are olfaction (smelling) and breathing. This book will be concerned only with the internal nose and its function in breathing.

#### Nasal cavities and paranasal sinuses
The lateral wall of the nasal cavity consists of bony ridges called conchae or turbinates (Figs 2.1 and 2.2). These provide a large surface area covered in highly vascularized mucous membrane which warms and humidifies inspired air.

The important role of the nasal cavities in warming and humidifying air is illustrated by patients who have had tracheostomies or endotracheal intubation for long periods. Without nose breathing, the mucosa of the trachea can become dry and crusted.

The anatomy of the paranasal sinuses is important clinically. If the mucosa of the meatuses becomes inflamed (e.g. through a common cold or allergic rhinitis) then the ostia may be blocked. This prevents mucus from draining from the sinuses, leading to increased pressure and infection: sinusitis. It is common clinically for sinusitis to occur in the maxillary, frontal and anterior ethmoidal sinuses; this is because they all drain into a single, small area in the middle meatus. Inflammation here will obstruct all three sinuses. See p. 18 for more on sinusitis.

Under each turbinate there is a groove or meatus. The paranasal air sinuses (frontal, sphenoid, ethmoid and maxillary) drain into these meatuses via small ostia, or openings. The drainage sites of each of the sinuses is shown in Fig. 2.2.

### Blood and nerve supply and lymphatic drainage
The terminal branches of the internal and external carotid arteries provide the rich blood supply for the internal nose. The sphenopalatine artery (from the maxillary artery) and the anterior ethmoidal artery (from the ophthalmic) are the two most important branches. Sensation to the area is provided mainly by the maxillary branch of the trigeminal nerve. Lymphatic vessels drain into the submandibular node, then drain into deep cervical nodes.

### Pharynx
The pharynx extends from the base of the skull to the inferior border of the cricoid cartilage where it is continuous anteriorly with the trachea and posteriorly with the oesophagus. It is described as

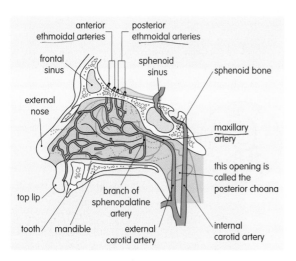

**Fig. 2.1** Lateral view of the nasal cavity showing the rich blood supply.

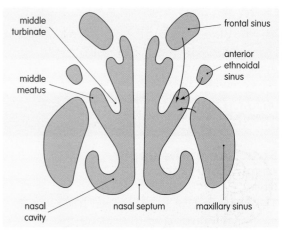

**Fig. 2.2** Frontal view of the nasal cavity drainage sites of the paranasal sinuses.

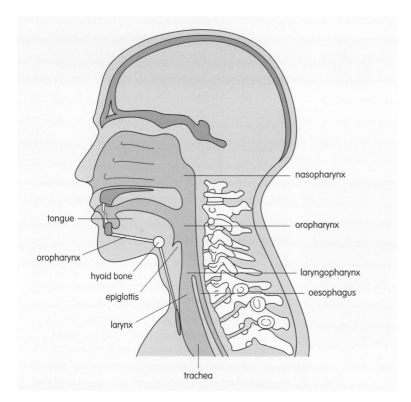

**Fig. 2.3** Schematic diagram showing midline structures of the head and neck.

being divided into three parts: the nasopharynx, oropharynx and the laryngopharynx, which open anteriorly into the nose, the mouth and the larynx, respectively (Fig. 2.3).

The nasopharynx is situated above the soft palate and opens anteriorly into the nasal cavities at the choanae (posterior nares). During swallowing, the nasopharynx is cut off from the oropharynx by the soft palate. The nasopharynx contains the opening of the eustachian canal (pharyngotympanic or auditory tube) and the adenoids, which lie beneath the epithelium of its posterior wall.

Detailed discussion of the oropharynx and laryngopharynx is beyond the scope of this book.

### Musculature, blood and nerve supply and lymphatic drainage

Three muscles surround the fascial tube of the pharynx: the superior, middle and inferior constrictor muscles (Fig. 2.4).

> Muscle tone of the pharynx, particularly at the level of the soft palate, is important in maintaining airway patency. During sleep, the upper airway dilating muscles relax and in some individuals the airway may be partially or completely occluded. This leads to recurrent episodes of sleep apnoea (p. 20).

The arterial blood supply of the pharynx is from the external carotid through the superior thyroid, ascending pharyngeal, facial and lingual arteries. Venous drainage is by a plexus of veins on the outer surface of the pharynx to the internal jugular vein.

Both sensory and motor nerve supplies are from the pharyngeal plexus (cranial nerves IX and X); the maxillary nerve (cranial nerve V) supplies the nasopharynx with sensory fibres.

Lymphatic vessels drain directly into the deep cervical lymph nodes.

### Larynx

At its inferior end, the larynx is continuous with the trachea. At its superior end, it is attached to the U-shaped hyoid bone and lies below the epiglottis of the tongue. The larynx is made up of a cartilaginous skeleton linked by a number of membranes. This cartilaginous skeleton consists of the epiglottis, thyroid, arytenoid and cricoid cartilages. Fig. 2.5 shows an external view and a median section through the larynx.

The larynx has three main functions:
- As an open valve, to allow air to pass when breathing
- Protection of the trachea and bronchi during swallowing. The vocal cords close, the epiglottis folds back covering the opening to the larynx, and

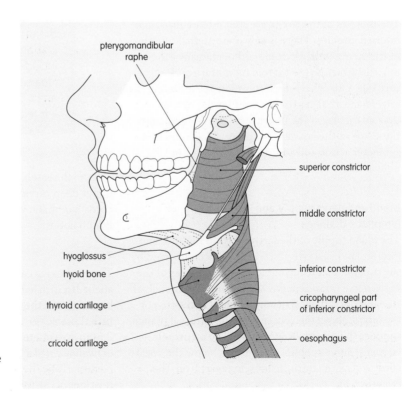

**Fig. 2.4** The pharynx, showing the superior, middle and inferior constrictors.

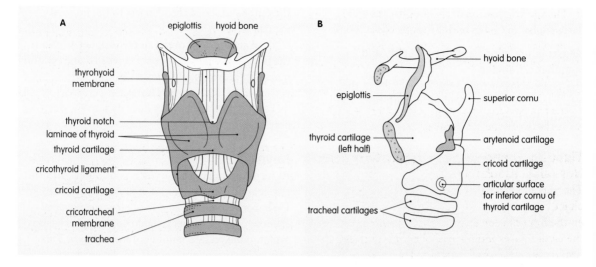

**Fig. 2.5** The larynx. (A) External view—anterior aspect. (B) Median section through the larynx, hyoid bone and trachea.

the larynx is pulled upwards and forwards beneath the tongue
- Speech production (phonation).

### Musculature

The muscles of the larynx are split into external and internal muscles. There is only one external muscle of the larynx (cricothyroid), although many other muscles attach to the thyroid membrane and cartilage. Cricothyroid has its origin at the arch of the cricoid and attaches to the lower border of the thyroid cartilage. The internal muscles may change the shape of the larynx: they protect the lungs by a sphincter action and adjust the vocal cords in phonation.

### Blood and nerve supply and lymphatic drainage

The blood supply of the larynx is from superior and inferior laryngeal arteries, which are accompanied by the superior and recurrent laryngeal branches of the vagus nerve (cranial nerve X). The internal branch of the superior laryngeal nerve supplies the mucosa of the larynx above the vocal cords, the external branch supplies the cricothyroid muscle. The recurrent laryngeal nerve supplies the mucosa below the vocal cords and all the intrinsic muscles apart from the cricothyroid.

The left recurrent laryngeal nerve has a long course through the thorax from the aortic arch, where it leaves the vagus, to the larynx. It is therefore vulnerable to compression by neoplasms, including those of the lung. Hoarseness, loss of voice power and a 'bovine' cough are all signs of left recurrent nerve paralysis.

Lymph vessels above the vocal cords drain into the upper deep cervical lymph nodes; below the vocal cords lymphatic vessels drain into the lower cervical lymph nodes.

### Trachea

The trachea is a cartilaginous and membranous tube of about 10 cm in length. It extends from the larynx to its bifurcation at the carina (at the level of the fourth or fifth thoracic vertebra). The trachea is approximately 2.5 cm in diameter and is supported by C-shaped rings of hyaline cartilage. The rings are completed posteriorly by the trachealis muscle. Important relations of the trachea within the neck are:

- The thyroid gland, which straddles the trachea, its two lobes sitting laterally, and its isthmus anteriorly with the inferior thyroid veins
- The common carotid arteries, which lie lateral to the trachea
- The oesophagus, which lies directly behind the trachea, and the recurrent laryngeal nerve, which lies between these two structures.

## Tissues of the upper respiratory tract

### Nose and nasopharynx

The upper one-third of the nasal cavity is the olfactory area and is covered in yellowish olfactory epithelium. The lower two-thirds of the nasal cavity, the nasal sinuses and the nasopharynx comprise the respiratory area, which is adapted to its main functions of filtering, warming and humidifying inspired air. These areas are lined with pseudostratified ciliated columnar epithelium (Fig. 2.6), also known as respiratory epithelium. With the exception of a few areas, this pattern of epithelium lines the whole of the respiratory tract down to the terminal bronchioles. Throughout these cells are numerous mucus-secreting goblet cells with microvilli on their luminal surface. Coordinated beating of the cilia propels mucus and entrapped particles to the pharynx where it is swallowed.

 The cilia play an important role in preventing microorganisms from causing infection. Abnormal ciliary motility, as seen in Kartagener's syndrome (p. 19), leads to sinusitis and bronchiectasis.

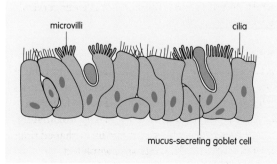

**Fig. 2.6** Respiratory epithelium.

microvilli

cilia

mucus-secreting goblet cell

### Adenoids

The nasopharyngeal tonsil is a collection of mucosa-associated lymphoid tissue (MALT) that lies behind epithelium of the roof and the posterior surface of the nasopharynx. Together with the palatine tonsils and the lymphoid tissue on the dorsum of the tongue these form Waldeyer's ring.

### Oropharynx and laryngopharynx

The oropharynyx and laryngopharynx have two functions as parts of both the respiratory and alimentary tracts. They are lined with non-keratinized stratified squamous (NKSS) epithelium several layers thick and are kept moist by numerous salivary glands.

### Larynx and trachea

The epithelium of the larynx is made up of two types: NKSS epithelium and respiratory epithelium. NKKS epithelium covers the vocal folds, vestibular fold and larynx above this level. Below the level of the vestibular fold (with the exception of the vocal folds, which are lined with keratinized stratified squamous epithelium), the larynx and trachea are covered with respiratory epithelium.

## Development of the upper respiratory tract

### Branchial arches and pharyngeal pouches

During week 4 of development, the branchial arches are formed; these are gill-like pairs of folds at the cranial (head) end of the embryo. Eventually, six pairs of branchial arches are formed, which are numbered craniocaudally (head to tail) from first to sixth arches. Not all arches are present at once; the first two branchial arches degenerate before the sixth arch is formed. The branchial arches form the major part of the branchial apparatus, which consists of:

- Branchial arches
- Pharyngeal pouches: evaginations of endodermal tissue, situated inside the primitive pharynx
- Branchial grooves: located between the branchial arches
- Branchial membrane: bilaminar layer of ectodermal and endodermal tissue between the branchial arches.

The branchial arches form the skeletal and muscular components of the head and neck. Mesenchymal cells group together within the arches to form clusters called branchial arch cartilages, which form skeletal structures. Mesenchymal cells also form myoblasts (primitive muscle cells), which migrate to form the musculature of the head and neck.

Figure 2.7 shows the formation of structures from the branchial arches and pharyngeal pouches.

The nerve supply of the branchial arches is derived from the cranial nerves. The first and second branchial arches receive sensory fibres from cranial nerve V and motor fibres from cranial nerve VII. The nerve supply to the third branchial arch is from cranial nerve IX, which also supplies the stylopharyngeus. The fourth and sixth branchial arches are supplied by two branches of the vagus nerve (cranial nerve X): the superior laryngeal and recurrent laryngeal nerves.

## Primitive mouth, nasal and oral cavities

The primitive mouth is formed by a depression in the ectoderm at the cranial end of the embryo called the stomodeum, initially separated from the primitive pharynx by a bilaminar membrane called the oropharyngeal membrane. This membrane ruptures at about day 24–26, by which time the ectoderm of the cranial end of the embryo has

| A | Branchial arch derivatives | | | |
|---|---|---|---|---|
| Arch No. | Bones and cartilage | Muscles | Nerves | Ligaments |
| 1 | incus and malleus | tensor tympani<br>tensor veli palatini<br>muscles of mastication<br>mylohyoid<br>anterior belly of digastric | cranial nerve V<br>(trigeminal nerve) | anterior ligament of malleus<br>sphenomandibular ligament |
| 2 | stapes<br>styloid process<br>lesser coruna of the hyoid bone<br>superior part of hyoid | stapedius<br>stylohyoid<br>posterior belly of digastric<br>muscles of facial expression | cranial nerve VII<br>(facial nerve) | stylohyoid ligament |
| 3 | inferior part of body of hyoid<br>greater coruna of hyoid | stylopharyngeus | cranial nerve IX<br>(glossopharyngeal nerve) | |
| 4/6 | thyroid cartilage<br>cricoid cartilage<br>arytenoid cartilage<br>corniculate and cuneiform cartilage | cricothyroid<br>levator veli palatini<br>pharyngeal constrictors<br>intrinsic laryngeal muscles<br>striated oesophageal muscle | cranial nerve X<br>recurrent laryngeal nerve<br>superior laryngeal nerve<br>branches of the vagus nerve | |

| B | Pharyngeal pouch derivatives |
|---|---|
| Pouch No. | Development |
| 1 | tubotympanic recess ⟶ auditory tube and tympanic cavity |
| 2 | mostly obliterate ⟶ intratonsillar cleft<br>endoderm ⟶ epithelium of tonsil and crypts |
| 3 | endoderm (dorsal) ⟶ inferior parathyroids<br>endoderm (ventral) ⟶ thymus |
| 4 | endoderm (dorsal) ⟶ superior parathyroid<br>endoderm (ventral) ⟶ ultimobranchial bodies, which fuse with the thyroid gland to form the parafollicular cells |

**Fig. 2.7** Derivatives of (A) branchial arches and (B) pharyngeal pouches.

**Fig. 2.8** Formation of the trachea and larynx: (A) lateral view; (B) cross-section on X–X. Note how defects in formation of the septum can lead to a fistula between trachea and oesophagus.

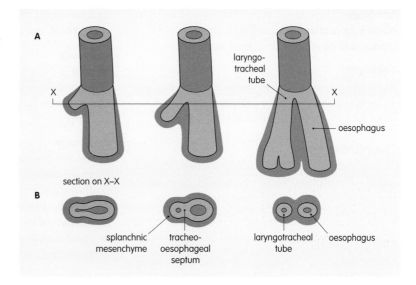

already invaginated, forming the nasal and oral cavities.

### Respiratory tract: larynx and trachea

The respiratory tract starts as a groove in the median plane of the primitive pharynx, the laryngotracheal groove. This groove deepens to form the laryngotracheal diverticulum and continues caudally (towards the tail) into the splanchnic mesenchyme, its distal end forming the lung bud. The cartilage and smooth muscle of the larynx are formed from the mesenchyme surrounding the diverticulum (Fig. 2.8). The foregut is separated from the diverticulum by the tracheo-oesophageal septum; when the diverticulum lengthens this is called the laryngotracheal tube. Defects in development may result in a tracheo-oesophageal fistula.

The connective tissue, cartilages and smooth muscle of trachea develop from the splanchnic mesenchyme, the glandular tissue developing from the endoderm.

## Disorders of the nose

### Inflammatory conditions
#### Infectious rhinitis (acute coryza or common cold)

The term 'rhinitis' indicates that the mucosal membrane lining the nose is inflamed. Inflammation in the common cold is caused by a number of viral infections:

- Rhinovirus
- Coronavirus
- Adenovirus
- Parainfluenza virus
- Respiratory syncitial virus.

The common cold is a highly contagious self-limiting condition, with the highest incidence in children. Symptoms are nasal obstruction, rhinorrhoea (runny nose) and sneezing. Complications include sinusitis, otitis media and lower respiratory tract infections such as bronchitis.

Many different disorders affecting the upper respiratory tract are described here; some are much commoner than others. The commonest disorders of the upper respiratory tract are those that involve inflammation of the lining of the nose (rhinitis), particularly when associated with infection (e.g. the common cold). Another important condition associated with the upper respiratory tract is sleep apnoea (p. 20). In contrast, many of the nasal neoplasms are very rare.

## Pathology
Acute inflammation with oedema, glandular hypersecretion and loss of surface epithelium.

## Treatment
Treat symptomatically with decongestants and analgesics. Unless bacterial complications ensue, antibiotics are useless because of viral aetiology.

# Chronic rhinitis
Chronic rhinitis may follow an acute inflammatory episode. Predisposing factors include inadequate drainage of sinuses, nasal obstruction caused by polyps, and enlargement of the adenoids.

# Allergic rhinitis
Allergic rhinitis is a common condition, affecting up to 30% of the Western population (Fig. 2.9). It is classified as either seasonal rhinitis (hayfever) or perennial rhinitis.

## Seasonal rhinitis
Has a maximum prevalence in patients aged 10–20 years. It occurs during summer months. Approximately 20% of patients with allergic rhinitis also suffer from asthma.

## Perennial rhinitis
The incidence of perennial rhinitis decreases with age. It is most common in patients aged 10–30 years.

There is no seasonal variation in symptoms which are mainly caused by Der p1 allergen in faecal particles of the house dust mite. Proteins from the urine and saliva of domestic pets, especially cats, also cause problems.

In some cases the pathology of perennial rhinitis is non-allergic and is due to abnormalities of the autonomic nervous system; this is termed vasomotor, or intrinsic, rhinitis. Nasal polyps may also present with perennial rhinitis secondary to nasal obstruction.

## Aetiology
Rhinitis is caused by hypersensitivity to allergens; commonest allergens are highly soluble proteins or glycoproteins (e.g. from pollens, moulds, cat dander and dust mite).

## Pathology
Symptoms are caused by a type I IgE mediated hypersensitivity reaction. IgE fixes onto mast cells in nasal mucous membranes. Upon re-exposure to allergen, cross-linking of the IgE receptor occurs on the surface of the mast cells leading to mast cell degranulation and release of histamine and leukotrienes.

## Investigations
Diagnosis of rhinitis is clinical. Skin prick tests, nasal smears and provocation tests can be used. Blood tests are:
- PRIST (plasma radioimmunosorbent test)—measures total plasma IgE levels
- RAST (radioallergosorbent test)—measures specific serum IgE antibody.

## Treatment
Treatment is by allergen avoidance and drug treatment with antihistamines, anti-inflammatory drugs (e.g. nasal corticosteroids) and sodium cromoglycate.

# Acute sinusitis
Sinusitis is an inflammatory process involving the lining of paranasal sinuses. The maxillary sinus is most commonly clinically infected (see p. 12). The majority of infections are rhinogenic in origin and are classified as either acute or chronic.

## Aetiology
The causes of acute sinusitis are:
- Secondary bacterial infection (by *Streptococcus pneumoniae* or *Haemophilus influenzae*), often after upper respiratory tract viral infection
- Dental extraction or infection
- Swimming and diving
- Fractures involving sinuses.

## Clinical features
Symptoms occur over several days with yellow–green nasal discharge, malaise, sinus tenderness and disturbed sense of smell. There may be fullness and pain over the cheeks, maxillary toothache

| Clinical features of rhinitis | |
|---|---|
| **Seasonal rhinitis** | **Perennial rhinitis** |
| Sneezing | Sneezing |
| Watery nasal discharge | Watery nasal discharge |
| Nasal irritation | Nasal blockage |
| Watery eyes | |

**Fig. 2.9** Clinical features of rhinitis.

or a frontal headache. Pain is classically worse on leaning forward. Postnasal discharge may lead to cough.

### Pathology

Hyperaemia and oedema of the mucosa occurs. Blockage of sinus ostia and mucus production increases. Cilia stop beating; therefore, stasis of secretions leads to secondary infection.

### Investigations

The investigations are:
- Blood—white cell count and erythrocyte sedimentation rate (may be raised but are often normal)
- Culture of pus from nose
- Radiology of paranasal sinuses—CT scan.

### Treatment

Medical treatment is by analgesia, broad-acting antibiotic for 7 days, and a decongestant. Discourage smoking and alcohol consumption. If no response to two regimens of antibiotics, refer to ear, nose and throat (ENT) specialist.

## Chronic sinusitis

Chronic sinusitis is an inflammation of the sinuses which has been present for more than three months. It usually occurs after recurrent acute sinusitis and is common in patients who are heavy smokers and work in dusty environments (Fig. 2.10).

### Clinical features

Clinical features are similar to those of acute sinusitis but are typically less severe.

### Pathology

Prolonged infection leads to irreversible changes in the sinus cavity, including:
- An increase in vascular permeability
- Oedema and hypertrophy of the mucosa
- Goblet-cell hyperplasia
- Chronic cellular infiltrate
- Ulceration of the epithelium, resulting in granulated tissue formation.

### Investigations

The investigations are through sinus radiographs, high definition coronal section CT and diagnostic endoscopy.

### Treatment

This condition is difficult to treat. Treatments are:
- Medical—broad-acting antibiotics and decongestant
- Surgical—antral lavage, inferior meatal intranasal antrostomy and functional endoscopic sinus surgery.

Rarely, recurrent sinusitis may be caused by Kartagener's syndrome, a congenital mucociliary disorder due to the absence of the ciliary protein dynein. It is characterized by sinusitis, bronchiectasis, otitis media, dextrocardia and infertility.

## Necrotizing lesions
### Mucromycotic infections

Mucomycosis (or zygomycosis) is a virulent fungal infection caused by *Rhizopus oryzae*. The organism rarely causes disease in immunocompetent hosts, but

| Predisposing factors of sinusitis | | | |
|---|---|---|---|
| Acute factors | | Chronic factors (same as for acute, plus the following) | |
| Local | General | Local | General |
| Pre-existing rhinitis | Debilitation | | |
| Nasal polyps | Immunocompromised | Anatomical variants | Atmospheric irritants |
| Nasal foreign bodies | Mucociliary disorders | Dental disease | |
| URTI | | Recurrent sinus infection | |
| Nasal tumours | | | |

**Fig. 2.10** Predisposing factors of sinusitis.

acidotic diabetics, patients with extensive burns, leukaemia or lymphoma are at risk of infection after inhalation of spores. The spores invade blood vessels causing thrombi and ischaemic necrosis. The primary sites of infection are nasal turbinates; patients present with sinusitis, inflammation of the orbit with proptosis, and meningoencephalitis.

Treatment is by systemic amphotericin B. Prognosis is poor.

### Wegener's granulomatosis

Wegener's granulomatosis is a rare, necrotizing vasculitis of unknown aetiology affecting small arteries and veins. It classically involves the upper and lower respiratory tract and the kidneys (glomerulonephritis). Mucosal thickening and ulceration occur, producing the clinical features of rhinorrhoea, cough, haemoptysis and dyspnoea.

If untreated, mortality after 2 years is 93%, but the disease responds well to high-dose prednisolone and cyclophosphamide.

### Lethal midline granuloma (lymphoma)

Malignant midline granuloma of the nose is a T-cell lymphoma that presents as an ulcerated lesion and which progressively destroys midfacial structures. The lesion consists of proliferating lymphocytes and macrophages. Treatment is by radiotherapy combined with surgical excision.

## Neoplasms

Neoplasms of the nose and paranasal sinuses (Fig. 2.11) are rare, with malignant tumours accounting for only 1% of all malignancies. Known nasal carcinogens include hardwood dust, nickel dust, snuff and radiation. Clinical features depend on the location and spread of the neoplasia; patients may present with unilateral nasal obstruction and epistaxis or symptoms may be predominantly dental, orbital, rertroantral or facial. Inverted papilloma is one of the more important benign tumours as it is associated with squamous carcinoma.

### Inverted papilloma (transitional cell papilloma)

Inverted papilloma is a benign epithelial tumour affecting men and women in the ratio of 5:1. The disease accounts for 5% of all nasal tumours. Aetiology is unclear.

#### Pathology

A papilliferous exophytic mass arises from the lateral walls of the nose. The epithelium invaginates into underlying tissue, and microcyst formation occurs resembling nasal polyps. Approximately 10% of these tumours are associated with squamous carcinoma.

## Disorders of the pharynx

### Sleep apnoea

Sleep apnoea syndrome is characterized by recurrent upper airway obstruction during sleep. Predisposing factors include the male sex, middle-age and obesity. A cycle is generated during sleep in which:

- The upper airway dilating muscles lose tone
- The airway is occluded
- The patient wakes
- The airway reopens.

As a consequence of this cycle, sleep is unrefreshing and daytime sleepiness is common, particularly during monotonous situations such as motorway driving. Each arousal also causes a transient rise in blood pressure, which may lead to sustained hypertension, pulmonary hypertension and cor pulmonale, ischaemic heart disease and stroke.

| Neoplasms of the nose and paranasal sinuses | |
| --- | --- |
| **Benign** | **Malignant** |
| Papilloma (squamous cell, transitional cell) | plastocytoma (lymphoma) |
| Osteoma | olfactory neuroblastoma |
| | adenocarcinoma |
| | squamous cell carcinoma |

**Fig. 2.11** Neoplasms of the nose and paranasal sinuses.

Sleep apnoea can markedly reduce a patient's quality of life. It is also a public health problem—patients with sleep apnoea are at an increased risk of road accidents as they have difficulty concentrating when driving and may even fall asleep at the wheel.

### Investigations and treatment

Patients are referred to a sleep or respiratory specialist for overnight studies. Fifteen apnoeas/hypoapnoeas (of 10 seconds or longer) per hour of sleep is diagnostic.

Some patients can be managed conservatively and are advised to lose weight and avoid alcohol and sedatives as these relax the upper airway dilating muscles. However, for most patients nightly continuous positive airway pressure (CPAP) is recommended.

## Neoplasms
### Nasopharyngeal carcinoma

Nasopharyngeal carcinoma is commonly a poorly differentiated squamous cell carcinoma. Men are more likely to suffer from the disease, which usually presents in patients aged 50–70 years. The disease is common in South East Asia, and is associated with the Epstein–Barr virus and salted preserved fish. Nasopharyngeal carcinoma presents with epistaxis, nasal obstruction or a neck lump. Seventy per cent of patients have metastatic lymph node involvement at presentation. Overall 5-year survival rate is 35%. Treatment is by radiotherapy.

### Nasopharyngeal angiofibroma

Nasopharyngeal angiofibroma is a benign neoplasm occurring in childhood affecting boys more than girls. It arises unilaterally and frequently coincides with a pubertal growth spurt. The disease presents with epistaxis and nasal obstruction.

### Pathology

An enlarging vascular tumour is present, which contains a fibrous component. The disease can cause bone erosion and destruction by pressure atrophy. The sphenopalatine foramen is always involved.

### Investigations and treatment

Investigate by MR imaging or CT scanning. Surgical treatment is possible, but vascularity may be a problem. Radiotherapy is used only in unresectable cases.

## Disorders of the larynx

## Inflammatory conditions
### Acute laryngitis

Acute laryngitis is a common condition, usually caused by viral infection, although secondary infection with streptococci or staphylococci can occur. Patients typically present with a hoarse voice and feel unwell. Rarely, dysphagia and pain on phonation occur.

Acute laryngitis is usually a self-limiting condition. If symptoms persist, refer to an ENT specialist.

### Chronic laryngitis

Chronic laryngitis is inflammation of the larynx and trachea associated with excessive smoking, continued vocal abuse and excessive alcohol.

The mucous glands are swollen and the epithelium hypertrophied. Heavy smoking leads to squamous metaplasia of the larynx. Biopsy is mandatory to rule out malignancy. Management is directed at avoidance of aetiological factors.

### Laryngotracheobronchitis (croup) and acute epiglottitis

The features of laryngotracheobronchitis (croup) and acute epiglottitis are described in Fig. 2.12.

### Pathology

In laryngotracheobronchitis, there is necrosis of epithelium and formation of an extensive fibrous membrane on the trachea and main bronchi. Oedema of the subglottic area occurs, with subsequent danger of laryngeal obstruction.

In acute epiglottitis, there is an acute inflammatory oedema and infiltration by neutrophil polymorphs. No mucosal ulceration occurs. Acute epiglottitis may also occur in adults, although it is much more common in children (see Fig. 2.12).

### Treatment

To treat laryngotracheobronchitis, keep the patient calm and hydrated. Nurse in a warm room in an upright position. Drug treatment, if required, includes steroids, oxygen and nebulized adrenaline.

Acute epiglottitis is a medical emergency. Call for anaesthetist, ENT surgeon and, if appropriate, the paediatric team. Never attempt to visualize the epiglottis. Keep calm and reassure the patient. Never leave the patient alone.

### Reactive nodules

Reactive nodules are common, small, inflammatory polyps usually measuring less than 10mm in diameter. They are also known as singer's nodules. They present in patients aged 40–50 years and are

| Laryngotracheobronchitis (croup) and acute epiglottitis | | |
|---|---|---|
| | Croup | Epiglottitis |
| Aetiology | Viral | Bacterial |
| Organism | Parainfluenza, respiratory syncytial virus | Group B haemophilus influenza |
| Age range | 6 months to 3 years | 3–7 years |
| Onset | Gradual over days | Sudden over hours |
| Cough | Severe barking | Minimal |
| Temperature | Pyrexia <38.5°C | Pyrexia >38.5°C |
| Stridor | Harsh | Soft |
| Drooling | No | Yes |
| Voice | Hoarse | Reluctant to speak |
| Able to drink | Yes | No |
| Active | Yes | No, completely still |
| Mortality | Low | High |

**Fig. 2.12** Features of laryngotracheobronchitis (croup) and acute epiglottitis.

more common in men. Reactive nodules are caused by excessive untrained use of vocal cords. Patients present with hoarseness of the voice.

## Pathology
Keratosis develops at the junction of the anterior and middle thirds of the vocal cord on each side. Oedematous myxoid connective tissue is covered by squamous epithelium. The reactive nodules may become painful because of ulceration.

Some of these conditions may seem more relevant to an ENT specialist. However, a working knowledge is also important to the respiratory physician when considering differential diagnoses; for example, laryngeal disease may present as airway obstruction and hoarseness and chronic sinusitis may present as a persistent cough.

# Neoplasms
## Squamous papilloma
Squamous papilloma is the commonest benign tumour of larynx; it usually occurs in children aged 0–5 years, but can also affect adults.

### Aetiology
The disease is caused by infection of the epithelial cells with human papillomavirus (HPV) types 6 and 11, and can be acquired at birth from maternal genital warts.

### Clinical features
Clinical features include hoarseness of the voice and an abnormal cry (Fig. 2.13).

### Pathology
Tumours may be sessile or pedunculated. They can occur anywhere on the vocal cords. Lesions are commoner at points of airway constriction (Figs 2.14A and B).

### Investigations and treatment
Investigations include endoscopy, followed by histological confirmation.

Surgical treatment is by removal with a carbon dioxide laser. Medical treatment is with alpha interferon.

**Fig. 2.13** Features of squamous papilloma.

| Features of squamous papilloma | | |
|---|---|---|
| | **Adult** | **Child** |
| **Incidence** | Rare | Common |
| **Number of lesions** | Single mass | Multiple masses |
| **Outcome** | Surgical removal | Regress spontaneously at puberty |

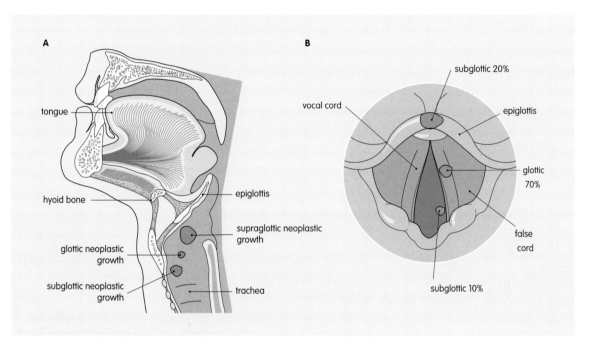

**Fig. 2.14** Position of laryngeal carcinoma (A) and as seen on mirror examination (B).

## Squamous cell carcinoma

Squamous cell carcinoma is the commonest malignant tumour of the larynx affecting men and women in the ratio of 5:1. The disease accounts for 1% of all male malignancies. Incidence increases with age, with peak incidence occurring in those aged 60–70 years. Patients present with hoarseness, although dyspnoea and stridor are late signs.

Predisposing factors include alcohol and tobacco smoke (the condition is very rare in non-smokers).

### Pathology

Carcinoma of vocal cord appears first, and subsequently ulcerates. Carcinoma of larynx infiltrates and destroys surrounding tissue. Infection may follow ulceration.

### Investigations and treatment

Investigations include chest radiography, full blood count, serum analysis (liver function tests for metastatic disease), direct laryngoscopy under general anaesthesia, and full paraendoscopy and bronchoscopy. Treatment is by radiotherapy and surgery.

### Prognosis

Prognosis is poor if the tumour involves the upper part of the larynx or subglottic region.

- Describe the anatomy of the upper respiratory tract, giving significant clinical details where appropriate.
- Where does the maxillary sinus open into the nasal cavity and what is the clinical significance of this position?
- Draw respiratory epithelium, indicating the functions of each cell type.
- List the derivatives of the branchial arches and pharyngeal pouches.
- Describe the pathology and management of allergic rhinitis.
- What are the different ways in which sinusitis can present?
- How does sleep apnoea affect the patient and why is it a public health issue?
- How do nasopharyngeal neoplasms commonly present?
- Describe the difference between croup and acute epiglottitis.
- List the causes of hoarseness of the voice.

# 3. The Lower Respiratory Tract

## Organization of the lower respiratory tract

### Structure of the lower respiratory tract

The lower respiratory tract consists of:
- The lower part of the trachea
- The two main bronchi
- Lobar bronchi, segmental bronchi and smaller bronchi
- Bronchioles and terminal bronchioles
- The end respiratory unit.

These structures make up the tracheobronchial tree (Fig. 3.1). The structures distal to the two main bronchi are contained within a tissue known as the lung parenchyma.

### Thorax

The cone-shaped thoracic cavity is bounded superiorly by the first rib and inferiorly by the diaphragm. The thorax is narrow at the top (thoracic inlet) and wide at its base (thoracic outlet).

The thoracic wall is supported and protected by the bony thoracic cage consisting of:
- Thoracic vertebrae
- Manubrium
- Sternum
- Twelve pairs of ribs with associated costal cartilages (Fig. 3.2A).

Each rib makes an acute angle with the spine and:
- Articulates with the body and transverse process of its equivalent thoracic vertebra
- Articulates with the body of the vertebra above.

The upper seven ribs (true ribs) articulate anteriorly through their costal cartilages with the sternum. The eighth, ninth, and tenth ribs (false ribs) articulate with the costal cartilages of the next rib above. The eleventh and twelfth ribs (floating ribs) are smaller and their tips are covered with a cap of cartilage.

The space between each rib is known as the intercostal space. Lying obliquely between adjacent ribs are the internal and external intercostal muscles.

The intercostal muscles support the thoracic cage; their other functions include:
- External intercostal muscles—raise the rib cage and increase intrathoracic volume
- Internal intercostal muscles—lower the rib cage and reduce intrathoracic volume.

The mechanics of ventilation breathing will be covered in detail in Chapter 4. Deep to the intercostal muscles and under cover of the costal groove lies a neurovascular bundle of vein, artery and nerve (see Fig. 3.2B). This anatomy is important during some procedures (e.g. when inserting a chest drain into a pneumothorax, the drain is inserted through the intercostal space just above the rib to avoid hitting the subcostal vessels).

The thorax contains:
- Lungs, heart and major vessels
- Oesophagus, lower part of the trachea and main bronchi.

### Mediastinum

The mediastinum is situated in the midline and lies between the two lungs. It contains the:
- Heart and great vessels
- Trachea and oesophagus
- Phrenic and vagus nerves
- Lymph nodes.

### Pleurae and pleural cavities

The pleurae consist of a continuous serous membrane, which covers the external surface of the lung and is then reflected to cover the inner surface of the thoracic cavity (Fig. 3.3).

The differences between the visceral and parietal pleurae are:
- The visceral pleura lines the surface of the lungs
- The parietal pleura lines the thoracic wall and the diaphragm.

The pleurae form a double layer, creating a potential space known as the pleural cavity. The visceral and parietal pleurae are so closely apposed that only a thin film of fluid is contained within the pleural cavity. This allows the pleurae to slip over each other

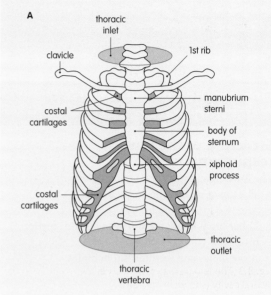

**Fig. 3.1** Tracheobronchial tree. Schematic showing the divisions of the airway down to the end respiratory unit (acinus).

during breathing, thus reducing friction. Normally, no cavity is actually present, although in pathological states this potential space may expand.

Where the pleura is reflected off the diaphragm onto the thoracic wall, a small space is created which is not filled by the lung tissue; this space is known as the costodiaphragmatic recess. At root of the lung (the hilum), the pleurae become continuous and form a double layer known as the pulmonary ligament.

The parietal pleura has a blood supply from intercostal arteries and branches of the internal thoracic artery. Venous and lymph drainage follow a return course similar to the arterial supply. Nerve supply is from the phrenic nerve; thus, if the pleura becomes inflamed this may cause ipsilateral (on the same side of the body) shoulder-tip pain.

The visceral pleura has a blood supply from bronchial arteries. Venous drainage is through the bronchial veins to the azygous and hemiazygous veins. Lymph vessels drain through the superficial plexus over the surface of the lung to bronchopulmonary nodes at the hilum. The visceral pleura has an autonomic nerve supply and therefore does not give rise to the sensation of pain.

**Fig. 3.2** The thoracic cage (A) and details of the subcostal neurovascular bundle (B).

Inflammation of the pleurae can cause an increase in fluid between the parietal and visceral pleurae. This inflammation may give rise to a pleural rub on auscultation, which is said to mimic the sound of a foot crunching through fresh snow. Excess liquid or air may be present within the pleural cavity caused by:

- Pneumothorax
- Haemothorax
- Pleurisy and pneumonia
- Malignancy.

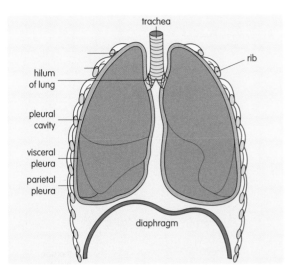

Fig. 3.3 The two pleurae form a potential space called the pleural cavity (shown in dark blue).

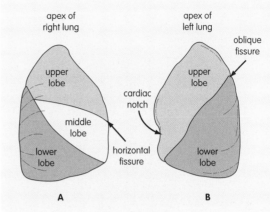

Fig. 3.4 Lateral aspect of the lungs. The outer surfaces show impression of the ribs. (A) Left lung; (B) right lung.

## Lungs

The two lungs are situated within the thoracic cavity and lie on either side of the mediastinum. During life, they appear pink and spongy, although carbon deposits give patchy discoloration. The lungs contain:

- Airways: bronchi, bronchioles, respiratory bronchioles, alveolar ducts, alveolar sacs and alveoli
- Vessels: pulmonary artery and vein and bronchial artery and vein
- Lymphatics and lymph nodes
- Nerves
- Supportive connective tissue (lung parechyma), which has elastic qualities.

Figures 3.4 and 3.5 show the lateral and medial surfaces of the lung.

Lists are more difficult to remember than diagrams. Try to memorize Fig. 3.4 and construct a list of medial relations from it.

## Hilum of the lung

The hilum or root of the lung (Fig. 3.6) consists of:

- Bronchi
- Vessels: pulmonary artery and vein
- Nerves
- Lymph nodes and lymphatic vessels
- Pulmonary ligament.

### Bronchopulmonary segments

The trachea divides to form the left and right primary bronchi, which in turn divide to form lobar bronchi, supplying air to the lobes of each lung. The lobar bronchi divide again to give segmental bronchi, which supply air to regions of lung known as bronchopulmonary segments. The bronchopulmonary segment is both anatomically and functionally distinct. This is important because it means that a segment of diseased lung can be removed surgically (e.g. in tuberculosis).

### Surface anatomy

The surface anatomy of the lungs is shown in Fig. 3.7.

## Airways and the blood–air interface
### Airways (respiratory tree)

Inside the thorax, the trachea divides into the left and right primary bronchi. The right main bronchus is shorter and more vertical than the left; for this reason, inhaled foreign bodies are more likely to pass into the right lung.

The primary bronchi within each lung divide into secondary or lobar bronchi. The lobar bronchi divide again into tertiary or segmental bronchi. The airways continue to divide, always splitting into two daughter airways of progressively smaller calibre until eventually forming bronchioles.

Figure 3.1 outlines the structure of the respiratory tree. Each branch of the tracheobronchial tree can be

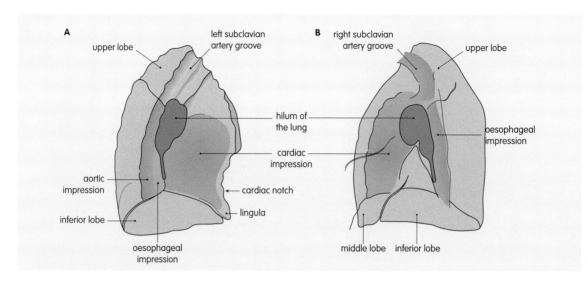

**Fig. 3.5** Relations of the lung. (A) Left lung; (B) right lung.

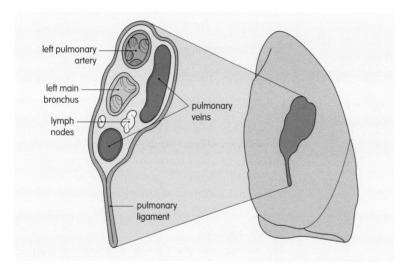

**Fig. 3.6** Contents of the hilum.

classified by its number of divisions (called the generation number); the trachea is generation number 0. The trachea and bronchi contain cartilage in their walls for support and to prevent collapse of the airway. At about generation 10 or 11, the airways contain no cartilage in their walls and are known as bronchioles. Airways distal to the bronchi that contain no cartilage rely on lung parenchymal tissue for their support and are kept open by subatmospheric intrapleural pressure (radial traction).

Bronchioles continue dividing for up to 20 or more generations before reaching the terminal bronchiole.

Terminal bronchioles are those bronchioles which supply the end respiratory unit (the acinus).

The tracheobronchial tree can be classified into two zones:
- The conducting zone (airways proximal to the respiratory bronchioles), involved in air movement by bulk flow to the end respiratory units
- The respiratory zone (airways distal to the terminal bronchiole), involved in gaseous exchange.

As the conducting zone does not take part in gaseous exchange, it can be seen as an area of

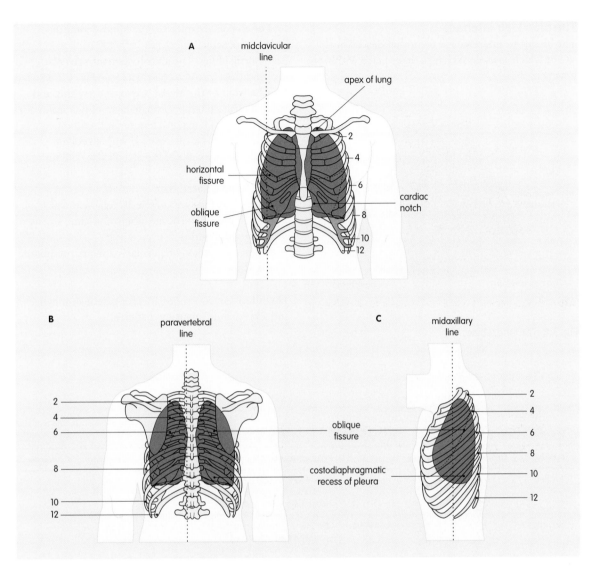

**Fig. 3.7** Surface anatomy of the lungs and pleura (shaded area). (A) Anterior aspect; (B) posterior aspect; (C) lateral aspect.

'wasted' ventilation and is described as anatomical dead space.

## Acinus

The acinus is that part of the airway that is involved in gaseous exchange (i.e. the passage of oxygen from the lungs to the blood and carbon dioxide from the blood to the lungs). The acinus consists of:

- Respiratory bronchioles, leading to the alveolar ducts
- Alveolar ducts, opening into two or three alveolar sacs, which in turn open into several alveoli (see Fig. 1.2 on page 5)

- Alveoli also open directly into alveolar ducts and a few open directly into the respiratory bronchiole.

## Lung lobules

Lung lobules (Fig. 3.8) are areas of lung containing groups of between three and five acini surrounded by parenchymal tissue. Each lobule is separated from a neighbouring lobule by an interlobular septum.

### Structure of the airways

The structure of the airways changes as the tracheobronchial tree descends; these differences are outlined in Fig. 3.9.

## The blood–air interface

The blood–air interface is a term that describes the site at which gaseous exchange takes place within the lung (Fig. 3.10).

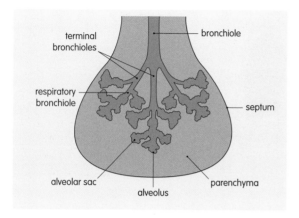

Fig. 3.8  The lung lobule.

The alveoli are microscopic blind-ending air pouches, of which there are 150–400 million in each normal lung. The alveoli open into alveolar sacs and then into alveolar ducts (see Fig. 1.2 on page 5). The walls of the alveoli are extremely thin and the alveoli are lined by a single layer of pneumocytes (types I and II) lying on a basement membrane. The alveolar surface is covered with alveolar lining fluid. The walls of the alveoli also contain capillaries.

It should be noted that:

- Average surface area of the alveolar–capillary membrane = 50–100m² (about the same size as two tennis courts)
- Average thickness of alveolar–capillary membrane = 0.4μm.

This allows an enormous area for gaseous exchange and a very short diffusion distance.

| | | | Differences in structure of the airways | | | |
|---|---|---|---|---|---|---|
| Airway | Generation No. | Lining | Wall structure | Diameter | Function | Contractile |
| trachea | 0 | respiratory epithelium | membranous tube supported by C-shaped rings of cartilage loose submucosa and glands | 25 mm | Con | No |
| bronchus | 1–11 | respiratory epithelium | fibromuscular tubes containing smooth muscle reinforced by β-receptors; incomplete rings of cartilage | 1–10 mm | Con | Yes |
| bronchiole | 12–16 | simple ciliated cuboidal epithelium and Clara cells | membranous and smooth muscle in the wall; no submucosal glands and no cartilage | 1.0 mm | Con | Yes |
| respiratory bronchiole | 18+ | simple ciliated cuboidal epithelium and Clara cells | merging of cuboidal epithelium with flattened epithelial lining of alveolar ducts; membranous wall | 0.5 mm | Con/Gas | Yes |
| alveolar duct | 20–23 | flat nonciliated epithelium; no glands | outer lining of spiral smooth muscle; walls of ducts contain many openings laterally into alveolar sacs | 0.5 mm | Gas | Yes |
| alveolus | 24 | pneumocytes types I and II | types I and II pneumocytes lie on an alveolar basement membrane; capillaries lie on the outer surface of the wall and form the blood–air interface | 75–300 mm | Gas | No |

Fig. 3.9  Differences in structure of the airways. Function: Con = conduction of air; Gas = gas exchange.

A common short-answer question in exams is: 'Name the differences in structure between the the bronchi and the bronchioles'. It is a good idea to memorize the information in Fig. 3.9.

bronchioles and distal airways means that these airways must be kept open by radial traction (see Chapter 4). The walls of the airways are composed of:

- Respiratory epithelium (ciliated columnar type)
- Basement membrane
- Lamina propria
- Elastic fibres
- Smooth muscle
- Cartilage.

## Tissues of the lower respiratory tract

The basic structural components of the walls of the airways are shown in Fig. 3.11. The proportions of these components vary in different regions of the tracheobronchial tree. The absence of cartilage in the

## Trachea

The respiratory epithelium of the trachea is tall and sits on a particularly thick basement membrane separating it from the lamina propria. The lamina propria of the trachea is loose and highly vascular,

**Fig. 3.10** Blood–air interface.

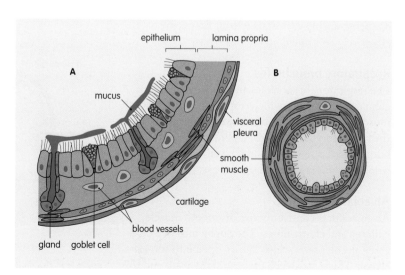

**Fig. 3.11** Structure of the airways: (A) bronchial structure; (B) bronchiolar structure. Note there are no submucosal glands or cartilage in the bronchiole. (Redrawn with permission from *Respiratory Physiology* 2e, by J. G. Widdecombe and A. Davies. Arnold, 1991.)

with a fibromuscular band of elastic tissue. Under the lamina propria lies a loose submucosa containing numerous glands that secrete mucinous and serous fluid. The C-shaped cartilage found within the trachea is hyaline in type and merges with the submucosa.

## Bronchi

Respiratory epithelium of the bronchi is shorter than the epithelium of the trachea and contains fewer goblet cells. The lamina propria is denser with more elastic fibres and it is separated from the submucosa by a discontinuous layer of smooth muscle. The lamina propria also contains mast cells.

The cartilage of the bronchi forms discontinuous flat plates and there are no C-shaped rings.

## Tertiary bronchi

The epithelium in the tertiary bronchi is similar to that in the bronchi. The lamina propria of the tertiary bronchi is thin and elastic, being completely encompassed by smooth muscle. Submucosal glands are sparse and the submucosa merges with surrounding adventitia. Mucosa-associated lymphoid tissue (MALT) is present (see p. 33).

## Bronchioles

The epithelium of a bronchiole is ciliated cuboidal and contains clara cells, which are nonciliated and secrete proteinaceous fluid. Bronchioles contain no cartilage and no glands in the submucosa. The smooth muscle layer is prominent. Adjusting the tone of the smooth muscle layer alters airway diameter, enabling resistance to air flow to be effectively controlled.

## Respiratory bronchioles

The respiratory bronchioles are lined by ciliated cuboidal epithelium, which is surrounded by smooth muscle. Clara cells are present within the walls of the respiratory bronchioles. Goblet cells are absent but there are a few alveoli in the walls; thus, the respiratory bronchiole is a site for gaseous exchange.

## Alveolar ducts

Alveolar ducts consist of rings of smooth muscle, collagen and elastic fibres. They open into two or three alveolar sacs, which in turn open into several alveoli. There are alveoli present in the walls and this is a site for gaseous exchange.

## Alveoli

An alveolus is a blind-ending terminal sac of respiratory tract (Fig. 3.12). Most gaseous exchange occurs in the alveoli. Because alveoli are so numerous, they provide the majority of lung volume and surface area. The majority of alveoli open into the alveolar sacs. Communication between adjacent alveoli is possible through perforations in the alveolar wall called pores of Kohn. The alveoli are lined with type I and type II pneumocytes, which sit on a basement membrane. Type I pneumocytes are structural, whereas type II pneumocytes produce surfactant (see Chapter 4).

Layers through which gas exchange occurs are:
- Alveolar lining fluid.
- Pneumocytes.
- Alveolar basement membrane.
- Capillary endothelium.

### Type I pneumocytes

To aid gaseous diffusion, type I pneumocytes are very thin; they contain flattened nuclei and few mitochondria. Type I pneumocytes make up 40% of the alveolar cell population and 90% of the surface lining of the alveolar wall. Cells are joined by tight junctions.

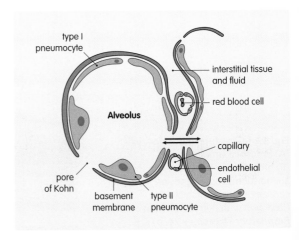

**Fig. 3.12** The alveolus. Note communication between alveoli through pores of Kohn.

### Type II pneumocytes

Type II pneumocytes are rounded cells containing rounded nuclei; their cytoplasm is rich in mitochondria and endoplasmic reticulum, and microvilli exist on their exposed surface. Type II pneumocytes make up 60% of the alveolar cell population and 5–10% of the surface lining of the alveolar wall. They produce surfactant.

### Alveolar macrophages

Alveolar macrophages are derived from circulating blood monocytes. They lie on an alveolar surface lining or on alveolar septal tissue. The alveolar macrophages phagocytose foreign material and bacteria; they are transported up the respiratory tract by mucociliary clearance. They are discussed further under the lung defences below (p. 40).

### Mucosa-associated lymphoid tissue (MALT)

The immune system has a major role in the defence of the respiratory tract against pathogens (see below). To aid this key role, lymphoid cells concentrate in the mucosal surfaces of the body to provide immunological protection. This specialized local system of lymphoid tissue is known as mucosa-associated lymphoid tissue (MALT).

MALT is non-capsulated lymphoid tissue located in the walls of the gastrointestinal, respiratory and urogenital tracts, providing immunological protection. These tissues are also a main site of lymphocyte activation and activated lymphocytes will specifically return to respiratory mucosa.

Examples of MALT were mentioned among the tissues of the upper respiratory tract (e.g. the adenoids and the tonsils). MALT in the lung is termed BALT (bronchus-associated lymphoid tissue). BALT is located beneath the mucosa of the bronchi and is covered by M cells, specialized epithelial cells that sample and transport antigen to the lymphoid tissue.

The lymphoid tissue of the respiratory tract is similar to that in the gut; aggregates are a diffuse distribution of mostly B lymphocytes within the lamina propria, covered by similar antigen-targeting and antigen-transporting cells (M cells). The lymphatic vessels associated with MALT are all efferent lymphatics, which drain to regional (hilar) lymph nodes. Large aggregations function in a similar manner to lymph nodes, containing T-cell and B-cell zones.

## Development of the lower respiratory tract

### Development of the bronchi

The laryngotracheal diverticulum develops into the lung bud, which divides into two bronchial buds by the end of week 4 (Fig. 3.13). As the bronchial bud enlarges, it forms two primary bronchi: the right and left primary bronchi (occurring in week 5). The right main bronchus is slightly larger and more vertical than the left. By the end of week 5, the secondary bronchi start to form.

By week 8, the segmental bronchi develop and together with the splanchnic mesenchyme form the bronchopulmonary segment. The splanchnic mesenchyme forms:

• Visceral pleura (mesoderm)
• Pulmonary capillaries and vasculature

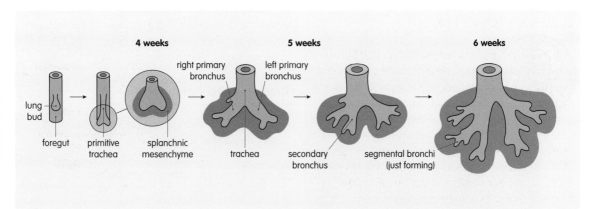

**Fig. 3.13** Development of primary bronchi and the formation of the secondary and segmental bronchi.

- Bronchial smooth muscle
- Pulmonary connective tissue.

## Development of the lungs

Lung development is divided into four stages: pseudoglandular, canalicular, terminal sac and alveolar periods.

### Stage 1—pseudoglandular period

During the pseudoglandular period, the major parts of the lung are formed; however, because there are no areas for gaseous exchange, respiration is not possible, and babies born at this stage do not survive.

### Stage 2—canalicular period

During the canalicular period, there are increases in the diameter of airways, bronchi and terminal bronchioles. The lung vasculature develops, and primitive end respiratory units are formed: respiratory bronchiole, alveolar duct and terminal sac (primitive alveolus). Some gaseous exchange is possible, and there is a very small chance of survival if born after week 22 (although intensive care is required).

### Stage 3—terminal sac period

During the terminal sac period, numerous terminal sacs develop; there is thinning of epithelial lining of terminal sacs. The squamous epithelium (type I pneumocytes) develops at about week 24, whereas secretory cells (type II pneumocytes) develop at around weeks 24–28. Type II pneumocytes produce surfactant, reducing surface tension within the liquid film within an alveolus and thus preventing alveolar collapse. After week 32, sufficient surfactant has been produced to allow the neonate to inflate its own lungs and allow the alveoli to continue to develop.

The formation of surfactant is an essential part of lung development. The first breath requires high pressures to inflate the lungs; less force is needed to generate subsequent breaths due to the action of surfactant in reducing surface tension. It is primarily lack of surfactant that causes ventilatory failure in premature babies.

### Stage 4—alveolar period

During the alveolar period, clusters of primitive alveoli are formed. Breathing occurs *in utero* by aspiration of amniotic fluid. The lungs are half full of liquid at birth; fluid is emptied through the mouth and also absorbed into the blood and lymph. The alveoli mature after birth: for the first 3 years after birth, alveoli increase only in number, not size; between the ages of 3 and 8 years, alveoli increase in both size and number.

## The pulmonary circulation

## Blood vessels

The lungs have a dual blood supply from the pulmonary and bronchial circulations. The bronchial circulation is part of the systemic circulation.

### Pulmonary circulation
#### Function

The primary function of the pulmonary circulation is to allow the exchange of oxygen and carbon dioxide between the blood in the pulmonary capillaries and air in the alveoli. Oxygen is taken up into the blood while carbon dioxide is released from the blood into alveolar air.

#### Anatomy

Mixed venous blood is pumped from the right ventricle through the pulmonary arteries and thence through the pulmonary capillary network, which is in contact with the respiratory surface (Fig. 3.14). Gaseous exchange occurs (carbon dioxide given up by the blood, oxygen taken up by the blood) and the oxygenated blood returns through the pulmonary venules and veins to the left atrium. The pulmonary capillary network offers a huge gas exchange area of approximately 50–100 $m^2$.

### Bronchial circulation

The bronchial circulation is part of the systemic circulation; bronchial arteries are branches of the descending aorta.

#### Function

The function of the bronchial circulation is to supply oxygen, water and nutrients to:
- Lung parenchyma
- Airways—smooth muscle, mucosa and glands

**Fig. 3.14** Pulmonary circulation. The pulmonary capillaries lie within the lungs, situated in the alveolar walls. They are in contact with alveolar gas and this is the site where gaseous exchange takes place.

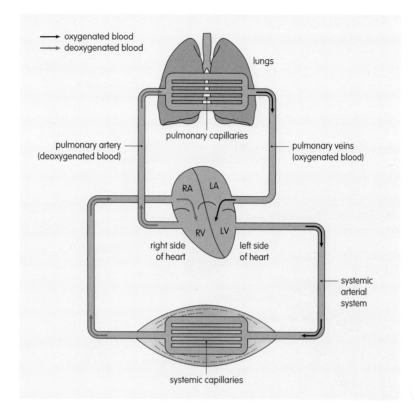

- Pulmonary arteries and veins
- Pleurae.

An additional function of the bronchial circulation is in the conditioning (warming) of inspired air. The airways distal to the terminal bronchiole are supplied only by alveolar wall capillaries. For this reason, a pulmonary embolus may result in infarction of the tissues supplied by the alveolar wall capillaries shown as a wedge-shaped opacity on the lung periphery of a chest X-ray.

## Development of the pulmonary circulation

The primitive heart is divided into four chambers during weeks 4 and 5. This involves:
- Formation of endocardial cushions.
- Division of the primitive atrium.

During week 6, the six primitive aortic arches are transformed into the adult arterial layout. However, the ductus arteriosus is still patent. For further information on development of the heart see *Crash Course: Cardiovascular System*.

## Fetal circulation

The main difference between adult and fetal circulation (Fig. 3.15) is that oxygenation of the fetal blood is by the maternal placental circulation. Consequently, the pulmonary circulation is largely bypassed through:
- The foramen ovale—which connects the right atrium to the left atrium
- The ductus arteriosus—which connects the pulmonary artery to the aorta.

Deoxygenated fetal blood flows through the two umbilical arteries (branches of the common iliacs) to the placenta (Fig. 3.15). Oxygen and nutrients are taken up from the maternal blood by the fetal circulation. Waste products of metabolism and carbon dioxide are passed from fetal blood to the maternal circulation. Oxygenated blood returns back to the fetal heart through the umbilical vein, ductus venosus and inferior vena cava. The oxygenated blood from the umbilical vein mixes with deoxygenated blood from the portal circulation and lower limbs and is returned to the right side of the

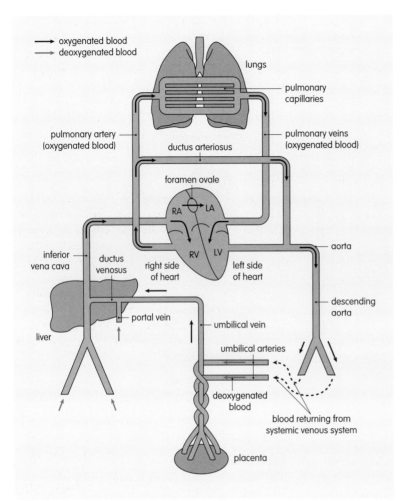

**Fig. 3.15** Fetal circulation. A large proportion of blood entering the right atrium passes through the foramen ovale into the left atrium. A large proportion of blood entering the pulmonary artery passes along the ductus arteriosus directly to the aorta.

heart. The majority of the fetal blood bypasses the pulmonary circulation, passing through the foramen ovale into the left atrium (see large arrow in Fig. 3.15).

In fetal life, the pressure in the pulmonary circulation is greater than systemic circulation and less than one-third of the right ventricular output passes through the lungs; the remainder flows from the pulmonary artery through the ductus arteriosus into the aorta.

## Changes of circulation after birth

At birth, blood flow through the umbilical vessels stops. When blood flow through the umbilical vein ceases, the ductus venosus, a thick-walled vessel with a muscular sphincter, closes. As the neonate takes its

first breath, the lungs fill with air and pulmonary vascular resistance falls to 10% of its value before lung expansion. Left atrial pressure is raised above that in the inferior vena cava by three methods:

- Decreased pulmonary vascular resistance leading to a large increase in blood flow through the lungs to the left atrium
- Decreased blood flow to the right atrium caused by occlusion of the umbilical vein
- Increased resistance to the left ventricular output produced by occlusion of the umbilical arteries.

The reversal of pressure gradient between the atria closes the valve over the foramen ovale. Fusion of the septal leaflets occurs over a period of several days.

The fall in pulmonary arterial pressure reverses the flow through the ducus arteriosus, but within a few moments of birth the ductus arteriosus begins to constrict, producing a turbulent flow heard as a murmur in the newborn child. The constriction is progressive and usually complete within 1–2 days after birth.

The exact mechanism for closure of the ductus arteriosus is not entirely clear, although it is thought to involve bradykinin, prostaglandins (because indomethacin can delay closure) and adenosine.

The following factors have been suggested as causes of closure of the ductus arteriosus:
- Cutting of the umbilical cord
- Exposure to cold air
- Increase in arterial partial pressure of oxygen
- Pressure difference between pulmonary and systemic circulations.

At birth, the walls of the left and right ventricles are the same thickness. After birth, the thickness of the right ventricular wall diminishes whereas that of the left ventricle increases.

The following fetal vessels lose their function and become ligaments at birth:
- Ductus arteriosus—becomes the ligamentum arteriosum.
- Ductus venosus—becomes the ligamentum venosum.
- Umbilical arteries—become the medial umbilical ligaments.
- Umbilical veins—become the ligamentum teres.

## Patent ductus arteriosus

Patent ductus arteriosus (PDA) is a common congenital heart defect, especially in girls. It is associated with maternal rubella (togavirus infection) in early pregnancy. As discussed above, the ductus arteriosus normally closes within 24 hours of birth. If closure fails to occur, blood flows from the aorta through the patent ductus and into the pulmonary artery (a left-to-right shunt). This increases pulmonary artery pressure (hydrodynamic pulmonary hypertension). The defect is classified as either small ductus or large ductus. The murmur heard has a machine-like quality and extends throughout the cardiac cycle. The treatment of choice is surgical ligation of the ductus. If the defect is large, the infant may require medical treatment to alleviate heart failure.

### Atrial septal defect

Atrial septal defect (ASD) is a defect in the atrial septum around the area of the fossa ovalis, caused by a defect in the ostium secundum. Blood flows from the left atrium to the right atrium and then into the right ventricle (a left-to-right shunt), increasing the pulmonary blood flow, causing hydrodynamic pulmonary hypertension. Symptoms do not usually occur until about 30–40 years of age, when patients present with heart failure; at presentation, a soft heart murmur is usually heard, and a fixed splitting of the second heart sound.

## Defence mechanisms of the lungs

### Overview

The lungs have a very large surface area for gaseous exchange and present a small barrier to diffusion between air and the blood flowing through the lungs. In fact, they possess the largest surface area of the body in contact with the environment and, therefore, are extremely susceptible to damage by foreign material and provide an excellent gateway for infection. The lungs are exposed to many foreign materials:
- Dust particles
- Pollen
- Fungal spores
- Bacteria
- Viruses
- Airborne pollutants.

Therefore, it is necessary for defence mechanisms to prevent infection and reduce the risk of damage by inhalation of foreign material (Fig. 3.16). There are three main mechanisms of defence:
- Physical
- Humoral – *endocrine factors, as opposed*
- Cellular. *to neural / somatic*

**Fig. 3.16** Summary of defences of the respiratory system.

Physical defences are particularly important in the upper respiratory tract, whilst at the level of the alveoli other defences, such as alveolar macrophages predominate.

## Physical defences
### Preventing entry to distal lower respiratory tract
Entry is restricted by the following three mechanisms:

- Filtering at the nasopharynx—hairs within the nose act as a coarse filter for inhaled particles; sticky mucus lying on the surface of the respiratory epithelium traps particles, which are then transported by the wafting of cilia to the nasopharynx; the particles are then swallowed into the gastrointestinal tract
- Swallowing—during swallowing, the epiglottis folds back, the laryngeal muscles constrict the opening to the larynx, and the larynx itself is lifted; this prevents aspiration of food particles
- Irritant C fibres—stimulation of receptors within the bronchi by inhalation of chemicals, particles, or infective material produces a reflex contraction of bronchial smooth muscle; this reduces the diameter of airways and increases mucus secretion, thus limiting the penetration of the offending material.

### Airway clearance
#### Cough reflex
Inhaled material and material brought up the bronchopulmonary tree to the trachea and larynx by mucociliary clearance can trigger a cough reflex (see Chapter 8). This is achieved by a reflex deep inspiration, increasing intrathoracic pressure while the larynx is closed. The larynx is suddenly opened, producing a high-velocity jet of air, which ejects unwanted material at high speed through the mouth.

#### Mucociliary clearance
Mucociliary clearance deals with a lot of the large particles trapped in the bronchi and bronchioles and debris brought up by alveolar macrophages. Respiratory epithelium is covered by a layer of mucus

secreted by goblet cells and submucosal glands. Approximately 10–100mL of mucus is secreted by the lung daily. The mucus film is divided into two layers:

- Periciliary fluid layer about 6μm deep, immediately adjacent to the surface of the epithelium. The mucus here is hydrated by epithelial cells. This reduces its viscosity and allows movement of the cilia
- Superficial gel layer about 5–10μm deep. This is a relatively viscous layer forming a sticky blanket, which traps particles.

The cilia beat synchronously at 1000–1500 strokes per minute. Coordinated movement causes the superficial gel layer, together with trapped particles, to be continually transported towards the mouth at 1–3cm/min. The mucus and particles reach the trachea and larynx where they are swallowed or expectorated (coughed up).

Mucociliary clearance is inhibited by:
- Tobacco smoke
- Cold air
- Many drugs (e.g. general anaesthetics)
- Sulphur oxides
- Nitrogen oxides.

It is possible to measure the efficiency of the cilia with a simple clinical test. The saccharin screening test establishes the amount of time it takes for saccharin placed in the anterior nares to taste sweet.

The importance of mucociliary clearance is illustrated by cystic fibrosis, in which a defect in chloride channels throughout the body leads to hyperviscous secretions. In the lung, inadequate hydration causes excessive stickiness of the mucus lining the airways, preventing the action of the cilia in effecting mucociliary clearance. Failure to remove bacteria leads to repeated severe respiratory infections, which progressively damage the lungs. Impaired mucociliary clearance is the major cause of morbidity and mortality in cystic fibrosis.

Smaller inhaled particles will travel further down the respiratory tract. The method that is used to deal with inhaled particles depends upon which area of the respiratory tract the particle finally reaches (e.g. large particles may be filtered out by the nasopharynx).

## Humoral defences

Lung secretions contain a wide range of proteins which defend the lungs by various different mechanisms.

Humoral and cellular aspects of the immune system are considered only briefly here; for more information see *Crash Course: Immunology and Haematology*.

### Antimicrobial peptides

A number of proteins in lung fluid have antibacterial properties. These are generally low molecular weight proteins such as:
- Defensins
- Lysozyme
- Lactoferrin.

### Surfactant

The alveoli are bathed in surfactant and this reduces surface tension and prevents the lungs from collapsing (see p. 58). Surfactant also contains proteins which play an important role in defending the host. Surfactant protein A (Sp-A) is the most abundant of these proteins; it has been shown to enhance phagocytosis of microorganisms by alveolar macrophages.

### Immunoglobulins

Effector B lymphocytes (plasma cells) in the submucosa produce immunoglobulins. All classes of antibody are produced, but IgA production predominates. The immunoglobulins are contained within the mucous secretions in the respiratory tract and are directed against specific antigens.

### Complement

Complement proteins are found in lung secretions in particularly high concentrations during inflammation and they play an important role in propagating the inflammatory response. Complement components can be secreted by alveolar macrophages (see below) and act as chemotactants for the migration of cells such as neutrophils to the site of injury.

## Antiproteases

Lung secretions contain a number of enzymes (antiproteases) that break down the destructive proteases released from dead bacteria, macrophages and neutrophils. One of the most important of these antiproteases is $\alpha_1$-antitrypsin.

Cigarette smoke increases the number of pulmonary macrophages; these release a chemical that attracts leucocytes to the lung. The leucocytes in turn release proteases, including elastase, that attack elastic tissue in the lungs. This process is usually inhibited by $\alpha_1$-antitrypsin, but this itself is inhibited by oxygen radicals released by leucocytes. The result is a protease–antiprotease imbalance that leads to the destruction of lung tissue and the development of emphysema.

A deficiency in $\alpha_1$-antitrypsin (inherited as an autosomal dominant condition) leads to a reduction in the breakdown of proteolytic enzymes, such as elastase, released from neutrophils during acute inflammation. This results in increased destruction of the alveolar wall and lung parenchymal tissue. Thus, any insult to the lungs (e.g. smoking) will lead to increased destruction of tissue and emphysema. It should be noted, however, that only 2% of individuals who have emphysema have $\alpha_1$-antitrypsin deficiency; the vast majority of cases of emphysema are related to smoking alone.

Inherited defects in any of these humoral mechanisms can lead to lung disease. Patients with deficiencies in IgA or complement (C3) are prone to recurrent respiratory tract infections.

## Cellular defences
### Alveolar macrophages

Alveolar macrophages are differentiated monocytes, and are both phagocytic and mobile. They normally reside in the lining of the alveoli where they ingest

bacteria and debris, before transporting it to the bronchioles where it can be removed from the lungs by mucociliary clearance. Alveolar macrophages can also initiate and amplify the inflammatory response by secreting proteins that recruit other cells. These proteins include:

- Complement components
- Cytokines (e.g. IL-1, IL-6) and chemokines
- Growth factors.

## Neutrophils

Neutrophils are the predominant cell recruited in the acute inflammatory response. Neutrophils emigrate from the intravascular space to the alveolar lumen where intracellular killing of bacteria takes place by two mechanisms:

- Oxidative—via reactive oxygen species
- Non-oxidative—via proteases.

In some cases, defence mechanisms can cause injury to lung tissue. Uncontrolled degranulation of neutrophils releases large amounts of elastase, damaging the lung parenchyma in diseases such as emphysema.

## Metabolic functions of the lungs

### Overview

The lungs, in addition to their role as gas exchange organs, have some important metabolic functions, notably:

- Conversion of angiotensin I to angiotensin II
- Deactivation of vasoactive substances
- Arachidonic acid metabolism
- Phospholipid synthesis
- Protein synthesis.

### Angiotensin converting enzyme

Renin released from the juxtaglomerular cells of the kidney enters the blood stream where it acts on a plasma protein, angiotensinogen, to produce angiotensin I (Fig. 3.17). Angiotensin I is further converted by angiotensin-converting enzyme (ACE) to angiotensin II, which stimulates aldosterone

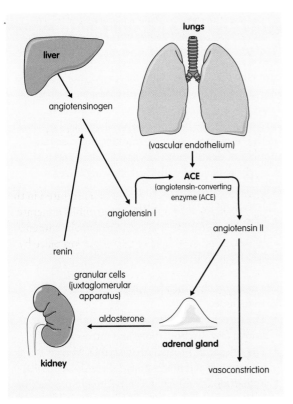

**Fig. 3.17** The renin–angiotensin system. Conversion of angiotensin I to angiotensin II by angiotensin-converting enzyme (ACE) occurs mainly in the pulmonary vascular endothelium.

**Fig. 3.18** Bradykinin degradation.

**Fig. 3.19** Arachidonic acid metabolism. The production of endoperoxides and leukotrienes.

secretion and acts as a potent vasoconstrictor. ACE is produced by the vascular endothelial cells of the lungs.

## Deactivation of vasoactive substances

Many different vasoactive substances are deactivated as they pass through the lungs. An example of this is the degradation of bradykinin (a potent vasodilator) to inactive peptides by ACE (Fig. 3.18).

The administration of an ACE inhibitor (such as captopril) inhibits both the production of angiotensin II and the breakdown of bradykinin.

## Arachidonic acid metabolism

The lungs are capable of both production and removal of arachidonic acid metabolites. The following metabolites are removed by the lung:

- Prostaglandin $E_2$
- Prostaglandin $F_{2\alpha}$
- Leukotrienes.

## Arachidonic acid synthesis

Arachidonic acid is released from membrane phospholipids by the action of phospholipase $A_2$ (Fig. 3.19). Arachidonic acid is converted into endoperoxides (e.g. prostaglandins) by the action of cyclo-oxygenase or into leukotrienes by the action of lipoxygenase.

Leukotrienes ($LTB_4$, $LTC_4$, $LTD_4$) are implicated as a cause of bronchoconstriction in asthma (Chapters 6 and 7). Thromboxane $A_2$ increases platelet aggregation and vasoconstriction, whereas prostacyclin has opposite effects. The prostaglandins produced have vasodilatory and vasoconstrictory effects.

## Phospholipid synthesis

Type II pneumocytes produce surfactant which contains an important phospholipid (dipalmitoyl phosphatidylcholine, DPC). As noted above, surfactant has the property of reducing surface tension in proportion to its surface concentration and plays an important role in defence.

Phospholipids are produced from fatty acids in association with smooth endoplasmic reticular membrane. Synthesis occurs at the interface between cytosol and the endoplasmic reticular membrane. The synthesized phospholipids are transported to vesicles by 'membrane budding' (endoplasmic reticular membrane fuses with the vesicle).

The surfactant mixture is extruded into the alveolus and lowers the surface tension. The synthesis is rapid and allows quick turnover of surfactant.

## Protein synthesis

Structural proteins, collagen, and elastin form the parenchyma of the lung; their synthesis and breakdown are important to the normal functioning of the lung. An increase in their breakdown is associated with increased protease activity (as seen in $\alpha_1$-antitrypsin deficiency) and leads to emphysema.

## The effect of smoking on the lower respiratory tract

Smoking is associated with increased morbidity and mortality in many different diseases, e.g. ischaemic heart disease, peripheral vascular disease and carcinoma of the oesophagus and bladder. Focusing on the respiratory system, smoking increases the number of deaths from laryngeal cancer and is strongly associated with the following lower respiratory tract diseases:

- Lung cancer (see p. 156)
- Chronic obstructive pulmonary disease (COPD) (see p. 133)
- Cor pulmonale.

The main mechanisms by which smoking causes harm include:

- The direct effect of toxic compounds in tobacco smoke (e.g. hydrocarbons and nitrosamines)
- The release of proteolytic enzymes from neutrophils and macrophages (see above, p. 40)
- Reduction in endogenous nitric oxide production
- Increased permeability of blood vessel walls.

Smoking cessation is discussed in Chapter 6.

- Describe the anatomy and function of the pleurae.
- List the medial relations of the lungs and the contents of the hilum.
- Describe the structure of the tracheobronchial tree and define the differences between conducting and respiratory zones.
- Give an account of the blood–air interface.
- List the differences between bronchi and bronchioles.
- Describe the ultrastructure of the airways.
- Describe the differences in function between the pulmonary and bronchial circulations.
- Outline the fetal circulation.
- How does the circulation change at birth?
- Explain why the lungs are susceptible to damage.
- Describe the mechanisms available to the lung to prevent entry of particulate matter.
- Describe the key functions of the alveolar macrophage.
- List the metabolic functions of the lung.
- Describe with the use of a diagram the conversion of angiotensin I.
- Outline with the aid of a diagram arachidonic acid metabolism.

# 4. Ventilation and Gas Exchange

## Overview

Ventilation is the flow of air in and out of the respiratory system (breathing); it is defined physiologically as the amount of air breathed in and out in a given time. The function of ventilation is to maintain blood gases at their optimum level, by delivering air to the alveoli where gas exchange can take place. The movement of air in and out of the lungs occurs due to pressure differences brought about by changes in lung volume. The respiratory muscles bring about these changes, but other factors are also involved, namely the physical properties of the lungs, including their elasticity and the resistance of the airways. Lung diseases that affect these physical properties therefore impair gas exchange by reducing the delivery of fresh gas to the lungs, ultimately leading to a mismatch in ventilation:perfusion.

## Ventilation

### Anatomical dead space

Not all of the air entering the respiratory system actually reaches the alveoli and takes part in gas exchange. Chapter 3 introduced the concept of anatomical dead space, or those areas of the airway not involved in gaseous exchange (i.e. the conducting zone). Included in this space are:

- Nose and mouth
- Pharynx
- Larynx
- Trachea
- Bronchi and bronchioles, down to and including the terminal bronchioles.

Inspired air held within these areas is referred to as dead air. The volume of the anatomical dead space ($V_D$) is usually about 150 mL (or 2 mL/kg of bodyweight). Anatomical dead space varies with the size of the subject and also increases with increased inspiration because greater expansion of the lungs lengthens and widens the conducting airways.

Anatomical dead space can be measured using Fowler's method which is based on the single-breath nitrogen test. This test is described in Chapter 10.

### Physiological dead space

Anatomical dead space is not the only cause of 'wasted' ventilation, even in the healthy lung. The total dead space is known as physiological dead space and includes gas in the alveoli that does not participate in gas exchange.

Physiological dead space = anatomical dead space + alveolar dead space

Alveolar dead space comes about because gas exchange is less than optimal in some parts of the lung. If each acinus (or end respiratory unit) were perfect, the amount of air received by each alveolus would be matched by the flow of blood through the pulmonary capillaries. In reality:

- Some areas receive less ventilation than others
- Some areas receive less blood flow than others.

In a normal, healthy person, anatomical and physiological dead space are almost equal, alveolar dead space being very small (<5 mL). However, when lung disease alters ventilation:perfusion relationships, the volume of alveolar dead space increases. $V/Q$ mismatch.

### Measurement of physiological dead space

Physiological dead space is measured using the Bohr equation (Fig. 4.1).

Respiratory physiology involves a number of equations and you may find this aspect difficult. Memorizing these equations is less important than understanding the underlying concepts and being able to relate them to clinical practice. For this reason, in most cases we have separated the equations from the main body of the text; if you want more detail or need to memorize them for your exams, you will find the equations and brief explanations in the figures.

**Fig. 4.1** The Bohr equation.

The Bohr equation is used in measuring physiological dead space

$$V_D/V_T = (P_A CO_2 - P_E CO_2)/ P_A CO_2$$

$V_D$ = Volume of dead space
$V_T$ = Tidal volume
$P_A CO_2$ = Partial pressure of carbon dioxide in alveolar air
$P_E CO_2$ = Partial pressure of carbon dioxide in mixed expired air

Normally, the partial pressures of carbon dioxide in alveolar gas and arterial blood are the same.

The equation can therefore be shown as:
$$V_D/V_T = (P_a CO_2 - P_E CO_2)/P_a CO_2$$

The method requires a sample of arterial blood and involves the analysis of carbon dioxide in expired air. Knowing that carbon dioxide is not blown off from end respiratory units that are not perfused, and that carbon dioxide in air is almost zero, it is possible to carry out a component balance for carbon dioxide to establish the volume of physiological dead space.

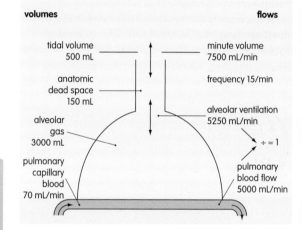

**Fig. 4.2** Ventilation in the simplified lung. (From *Pulmonary Pathophysiology* by G. Criner and G. D'Alonzo. Fence Creek Publishing, 1999, p. 38.)

A component balance works on the basis of conservation of mass (i.e. what goes into a system must equal what comes out). Several tests in respiratory medicine (e.g. helium dilution, nitrogen washout) are based on this principle.

## Minute ventilation

Minute ventilation ($\dot{V}_E$) is the volume of gas moved in and out of the lungs in 1 minute (Fig. 4.2).
    In order to calculate $\dot{V}_E$ you need to know:
- The number of breaths per minute
- The volume of air moved in and out with each breath (the tidal volume: $V_T$).

The normal frequency of breathing varies between 12 and 20 breaths per minute. Normal tidal volume is approximately 500 mL in quiet breathing. If a subject with a tidal volume of 500 mL took 12 breaths a minute, it would seem obvious that the volume exhaled per minute (minute ventilation) would be $500 \times 12 = 6000$ mL/min. Or, more generally:

$$\dot{V}_E = V_T f$$

where $\dot{V}_E$ = minute ventilation, $V_T$ = tidal volume, and $f$ = the respiratory rate (breaths/minute).

## Alveolar ventilation

We have already noted that not all the air inspired reaches the alveoli; some stays within the trachea or other conducting airways.
    Therefore, two values of minute ventilation need to be considered:
- Minute ventilation ($\dot{V}_E$), as described above
- Minute alveolar ventilation ($\dot{V}_A$), which is the amount of air that reaches the alveoli in 1 minute.

From our understanding of anatomical dead space, we can say that for one breath:

$$V_A = V_T - V_D$$

where $V_A$ = the volume reaching the alveolus in one breath, and $V_D$ = the volume of dead space. Hence, in 1 minute:

$$\dot{V}_A = (V_T - V_D)f$$

## Variation in ventilation within the lung

Not all regions of the lungs are ventilated equally. Ventilation per unit volume can be measured by inhalation of a radioactive isotope of xenon ($^{133}$Xe). If radiation counters are placed at different levels of the lungs, the volume of inhaled radioactive xenon in various areas of the lung can be measured.

It has been shown that the lower zones of the lungs are ventilated better than the upper zones. The causes of regional differences in ventilation will be discussed in the next section.

Note that at this stage we are still considering the healthy lung. In clinical practice, disease has a much greater effect on variation of ventilation.

## Lung volumes

The gas held by the lungs can be thought of in terms of subdivisions, or specific lung volumes. Some of these volumes can be measured using spirometry, a technique which is described in Chapter 10. A trace from a spirometer, showing key lung volumes, is reproduced in Fig. 4.3. Note that one of the subdivisions shown here, tidal volume, has already been introduced above under the concept of minute ventilation. Definitions of all the lung volumes and capacities (combinations of two or more volumes) are given in Fig. 4.4 .

## Measuring lung volumes

There are four main methods of measuring lung volumes:

- Spirometry
- Nitrogen washout
- Helium dilution
- Plethysmography.

**Fig. 4.3** Typical spirometer trace. Note that functional residual capacity (FRC) and residual volume (RV) cannot be measured using a spirometer; thus, neither can total lung capacity (TLC). ERV = expiratory reserve volume; IRV = inspiratory reserve volume; TV = tidal volume; IC = inspiratory capacity; VC = vital capacity.

These techniques are considered in detail in Chapter 10.

## Effect of disease on lung volumes

Understanding lung volumes is important because they can be affected by disease. Two particular volumes are important in common diseases such as asthma and COPD and are considered in more detail below. These are residual volume (RV) and functional residual capacity (FRC).

### Residual volume and functional residual capacity

After breathing out, the lungs are not completely emptied of air. A completely deflated lung would require a much greater amount of energy to inflate it than one in which the alveoli have not collapsed (see Fig. 4.17). Even a maximum respiratory effort (forced expiration) fails to expel all the air from the lungs. When the expiratory muscles contract, all the structures in the lungs (not only the alveoli but also the airways) are compressed by the positive intrapleural pressure. During forced expiration, the smaller airways collapse before the alveoli empty completely. Thus, some air remains within the lungs; this is known as the residual volume (Fig. 4.3).

During normal breathing (quiet breathing), the lung volume oscillates between inhalation and exhalation. In quiet breathing, after the tidal volume has been expired:

| Descriptions of lung volumes and capacities | |
|---|---|
| **Air in lungs is divided into 4 volumes** | |
| tidal volume (TV) | volume of air breathed in and out in a single breath: 0.5 L |
| inspiratory reserve volume (IRV) | volume of air breathed in by a maximum inspiration at the end of a normal inspiration: 3.3 L |
| expiratory reserve volume (ERV) | volume of air that can be expelled by a maximum effort at the end of a normal expiration: 1.0 L |
| residual volume (RV) | volume of air remaining in lungs at end of a maximum expiration: 1.2 L |
| **Pulmonary capacities are combinations of 2 or more volumes** | |
| inspiratory capacity (IC) = TV + IRV | volume of air breathed in by a maximum inspiration at the end of a normal expiration: 3.8 L |
| functional residual capacity (FRC) = ERV + RV | volume of air remaining in lungs at the end of a normal expiration. Acts as buffer against extreme changes in alveolar gas levels with each breath: 2.2 L |
| vital capacity (VC) = IRV +TV + ERV | volume of air that can be breathed in by a maximum inspiration following a maximum expiration: 4.8 L |
| total lung capacity (TLC) = VC + RV | only a fraction of TLC is used in normal breathing: 6.0 L |
| **Most of these volumes can be measures with a spirometer (see Fig. 4.3)** | |

**Fig. 4.4** Descriptions of lung volumes and capacities.

- Pressure outside the chest is equal to pressure inside the alveoli (i.e. atmospheric pressure)
- Elastic forces tending to collapse the lung are balanced by the elastic recoil trying to expand the chest (Fig. 4.5)
- This creates a subatmospheric (negative) pressure in the intrapleural space.

The lung volume at this point is known as functional residual capacity. RV and FRC can be measured using nitrogen washout, helium dilution and plethysmography (see Chapter 10).

## Patterns of lung function

Disease affects lung volumes in specific patterns, depending on the pathological processes. Diseases can be classified as obstructive, restrictive or mixed, with each showing characteristic changes in lung volumes. Figs 4.6 and 4.7 summarize the common patterns seen.

### Obstructive disorders

This group of disorders is characterized by obstruction of normal airflow due to airway narrowing and includes:

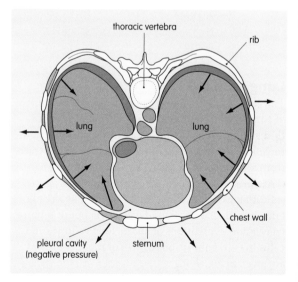

**Fig. 4.5** Pressures within the thoracic cavity. The tendency for the lungs to collapse (elastic recoil) and the opposing forces tendency to expand the chest wall creates a subatmospheric (negative) pressure in the intrapleural space.

**Fig. 4.6** Lung volumes in health, and in obstructive and restrictive disease. See Fig. 4.4 for abbreviations. Note that in obstructive diseases TLC and FRC are increased. VC may be entirely normal or reduced. In restrictive diseases all lung volumes are reduced. (From *Pulmonary Pathophysiology* by G. Criner and G. D'Alonzo. Fence Creek Publishing, 1999, p. 128.)

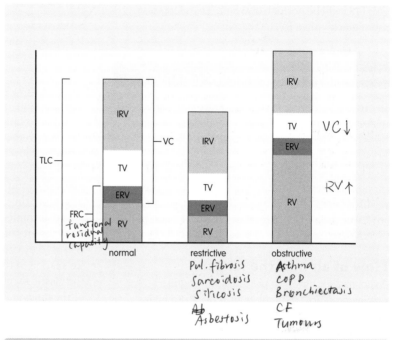

**Fig. 4.7** Patterns of lung function.

| | Patterns of lung function | | |
|---|---|---|---|
| | **Obstructive** | **Restrictive** | **Mixed** |
| $FEV_1$ | ↓ | ↓ | ↓ |
| FVC | N or δ/L | ↓ | ↓ |
| $FEV_1$/FVC ratio | ↓ | N | ↓ |
| TLC | N or ↑ | ↓ | ↓ |
| VC | N or ↓ | ↓ | ↓ |
| RV | ↑ | N or ↓ | N or ↑ |
| RV/TLC ratio | ↑ | N or ↑ | ↑ |

- Asthma
- COPD
- Bronchiectasis
- Cystic fibrosis
- Tumours (inside or outside the airways).

Within this group, the mechanisms causing the airway narrowing differ. They include obstruction by a mucus plug, airway compression and smooth muscle constriction.

In general, obstructive disorders lead to hyperinflation of the lungs as air is trapped behind closed airways. RV is increased, as is the ratio of RV:TLC. In patients with severe obstruction, air trapping is so extensive that vital capacity is decreased.

### Restrictive disorders
A large number of disorders can be classifed as restrictive, including:
- Pulmonary fibrosis
- Sarcoidosis
- Silicosis
- Asbestosis.

Each of these disorders results in stiffer lungs which cannot expand to normal volumes. All the subdivisions of volume are decreased and the ratio of

RV:TLC will be normal, or where VC decreases more quickly than RV, increased.

## Mechanics of breathing

In order to understand ventilation we must also understand the mechanism by which it takes place: breathing. This section reviews the mechanics of breathing including:
- The pressure differences which generate airflow
- The respiratory muscles that effect these pressure differences
- Tissue properties that influence how easily the lungs expand.

### Flow of air into the lungs

To achieve air flow into the lungs, we require a driving pressure (remember air flows from high pressure to low pressure). Pressure at the entrance to the respiratory tract (i.e. at the nose and mouth) is atmospheric ($P_{atm}$). Pressure inside the lungs is alveolar pressure ($P_A$).

Therefore:

- If $P_A = P_{atm}$, no air flow occurs (e.g. at functional residual capacity)
- If $P_A < P_{atm}$, air flows into the lungs
- If $P_A > P_{atm}$, air flows out of the lungs.

Because we cannot change atmospheric pressure, alveolar pressure must be altered to achieve air flow. Thus, if the volume inside the lungs is changed, Boyle's law predicts that pressure inside the lungs will also change. How can this be achieved? (Fig. 4.8).
- The lungs contain no muscle that can actively expand or contract
- Therefore the chest must be expanded, which lowers intrapleural pressure, expanding the lungs
- The majority of chest expansion in quiet breathing is caused by contraction of the diaphragm
- Relaxation of the muscles of the chest wall allows the elastic recoil of the lungs to cause contraction of the lungs and expulsion of gas.

### Intrapleural pressure

In the previous section, we saw that at FRC elastic recoil of the lungs is exactly balanced by the elastic recoil of the chest wall trying to expand the chest.

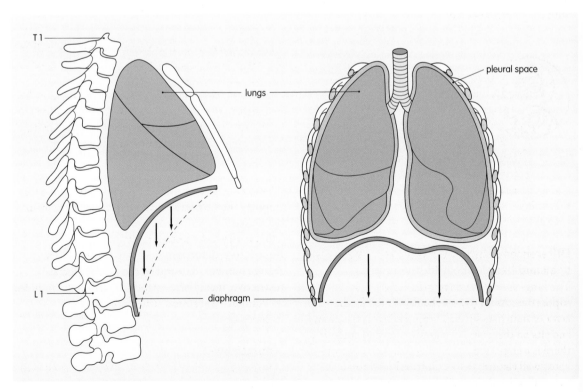

**Fig. 4.8** Expanding the lungs to draw in air. Flattening the diaphragm increases the thoracic volume, lowering the intrapleural pressure and expanding the lungs.

These two opposing forces create a subatmospheric (negative) pressure within the intrapleural space; as the alveoli communicate with the atmosphere, the intrapleural pressure is also less than the pressure inside the lungs (Fig. 4.9). The intrapleural pressure fluctuates during breathing (Fig. 4.10) but is about −0.5kPa at the end of quiet expiration. In summary, there is a gradient between the pressure on the inside and the outside of the lungs, or across the lung walls; this is known as the transmural pressure. It is transmural pressure (caused by the negative pressure in the pleural space) that ensures that the lungs are held partially expanded in the thorax. It effectively links the lungs (which are like suspended balloons) with the chest wall.

On inspiration, intrathoracic volume is increased; this lowers intrapleural pressure making it more negative, causing the lungs to expand and air to enter. On expiration, the muscles of the chest wall relax and the lungs return to their original size by elastic recoil, with the expulsion of air.

It should be noted that during quiet breathing, intrapleural pressure is always negative. In forced expiration, however, the intrapleural pressure becomes positive, forcing a reduction in lung volume with the expulsion of air.

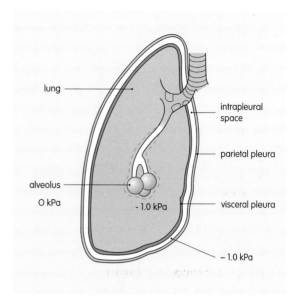

**Fig. 4.9** Transmural pressure and inflation pressure. The transmural pressure is the difference in pressure across the walls of the airways. There is a slight difference in pressure between the intrapleural space and the outside of the airway, but this has been ignored in this example and the inflation pressure can be considered as the pressure difference between the intrapleural pressure and the pressure inside the alveoli (−1.0kPa).

Puncture wounds through the thorax can mean that the intrapleural space is open to the atmosphere— a pneumothorax. The pressures equilibrate and the lungs are no longer held expanded, leading to collapse.

### Differences in intrapleural pressure between apex and base

The lungs are not rigid and therefore not self-supportive. As we pass vertically down the lung, each layer of lung hangs down from the layer of lung above and sits on the layer of lung below. Thus, at the apex, there is a larger weight of lung pulling away from the chest wall causing the intrapleural pressure to be more negative at the apex than at the base. For an upright subject at functional residual capacity (before inspiration) the intrapleural pressure at the

apex is −0.8kPa and at the base about −0.2kPa. The lung base is compressed compared with the apex.

It should be noted that:
- Alveolar volumes at the base and the apex of the lung are of different values before inspiration
- However, intrapleural pressure changes at lung base and apex during breathing are of equal magnitude.

These two factors will be important later when we look at why ventilation varies from lung base to apex.

## Muscles of respiration

We have seen that the chest must be expanded in order to reduce intrapleural pressure and drive air into the lungs. This section describes the muscles of respiration that bring about this change in volume.

### Thoracic wall

The thoracic wall is made up of (from superficial to deep):
- Skin and subcutaneous tissue
- Ribs, thoracic vertebra, sternum and manubrium

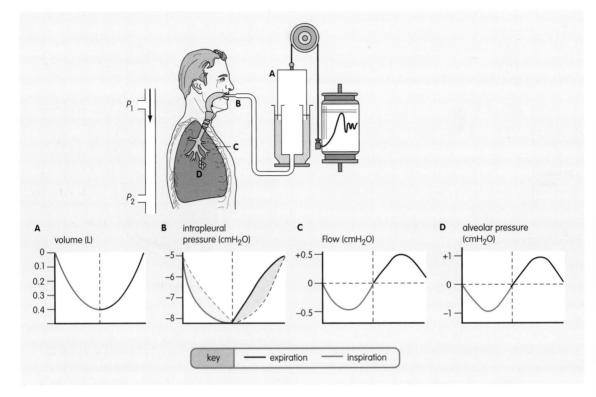

**Fig. 4.10** Negative pressure within the intrapleural space and during breathing. Lung volume (A), change in intrapleural pressure (B), air flow (C) and alveolar pressure (D). All measurements are relative to inspiration and expiration. Note that intrapleural pressure becomes more negative during inspiration as intrathoracic volume increases.

- Intercostal muscles: external, internal and thoracis transversus
- Parietal pleura.

Situated at the thoracic outlet is the diaphragm, which attaches to the costal margin, xyphoid process and lumbar vertebrae.

### Intercostal muscles
The action of the intercostal muscles is to pull the ribs closer together. There are therefore two main actions:
- If the first rib is fixed by scalene muscle, the external intercostal muscles pull the ribs upwards
- If the last rib is fixed by quadratus lumborum, the internal intercostal muscles pull the ribs downwards.

Their action during respiration is discussed in function of the respiratory muscles.

### External intercostal muscles
External intercostal muscles span the space between each rib and originate from the inferior border of the upper rib, attaching to the superior border of the rib below. The muscle attaches along the length of the rib, from the tubercle to the costal chondral junction and its fibres run forward and downward (Fig. 4.11A).

### Internal intercostal muscles
Internal intercostal muscles span the space between each rib and originate from the subcostal groove of the rib above and attach to the superior border of the rib below. The muscle attaches along the length of the rib from the angle of the rib to the sternum and its fibres run downward and backward (Fig. 4.11B).

### Thoracis transversus
Thoracis transversus muscle is incomplete and has the parietal pleura and neurovascular bundle as its relations.

### Diaphragm
The diaphragm is the main muscle of respiration (Fig. 4.12). The central region of the diaphragm is

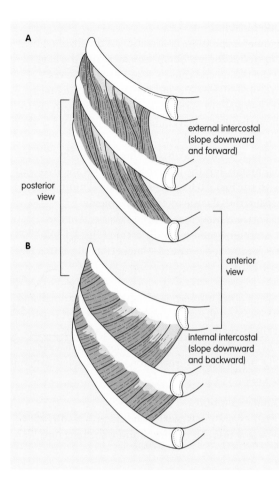

**Fig. 4.11** Intercostal muscles. (A) External intercostal muscles; (B) internal intercostal muscles.

tendinous; the outer margin is muscular, originating from the borders of the thoracic outlet.

The diaphragm has right and left domes. The right dome is higher than the left to accommodate the liver below. There is a central tendon that sits below the two domes, attaching to the xiphisternum anteriorly and the lumbar vertebrae posteriorly.

Several important structures pass through the diaphragm:

- The inferior vena cava passes through the right dome at the level of the eighth thoracic vertebra (T8)
- The oesophagus passes through a sling of muscular fibres from the right crus of the diaphragm at the level of the tenth thoracic vertebra (T10)
- The aorta pierces the diaphragm anterior to the twelfth thoracic vertebra (T12).

The diaphragm attaches to the costal margin anteriorly and laterally. Posteriorly, it attaches to the lumbar vertebrae by the crura (left crus at L1 and L2, right crus at L1, L2 and L3). In addition, the position of the diaphragm changes relative to posture: it is lower when standing than sitting.

The motor and sensory nerve supply of the diaphragm is from the phrenic nerve. Blood supply of the diaphragm is from pericardiophrenic and musculophrenic branches of the internal thoracic artery.

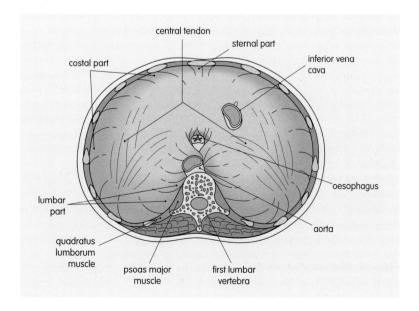

**Fig. 4.12** The diaphragm. Many structures pass through the diaphragm, notably the inferior vena cava, the aorta and the oesophagus.

The phrenic nerve supplies the diaphragm (60% motor, 40% sensory). Remember, 'nerve roots 3, 4 and 5 keep the diaphragm alive'. Thus, if you break your neck at C3, you die.

The diaphragm of a patient with COPD may become flatter as air is trapped in the lungs. Sometimes this change is visible on a chest X-ray. There may also be evidence in the way the patient breathes: a flattened diaphragm pulls the lower rib cage forward during inspiration (Hoover's sign).

## Function of the muscles of respiration

Breathing can classified into inspiration and expiration, quiet or forced.

### Quiet inspiration

In quiet inspiration, contraction of the diaphragm flattens its domes. This action increases the length of the thorax and thus its volume. This lowers intrapleural pressure and draws air into the lungs. At the same time, the abdominal wall must relax to allow the abdominal contents to be displaced as the diaphragm moves down.

The main muscle in quiet breathing is the diaphragm, but the intercostal muscles are involved. With the first rib fixed, the intercostal muscles can expand the rib cage by two movements:

- Forward movement of the lower end of the sternum—pump-handle action (Fig. 4.13A)
- Upward and outward—bucket-handle action (Fig. 4.13B).

During quiet inspiration, these actions are small and the intercostal muscles mainly prevent deformation of the tissue between the ribs, which would otherwise lower the volume of the thoracic cage (Fig. 4.14). The internal intercostal muscles carry out this role.

### Quiet expiration

Quiet expiration is passive and there is no direct muscle action. During inspiration, the lungs are

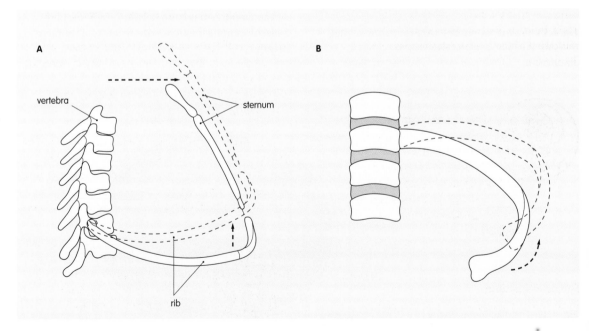

**Fig. 4.13** Posterior (A) and lateral (B) expansion of the chest. (A) Note the expansion of the chest in a forward and upward movement (pump-handle action) and (B) an outward and upward movement (bucket-handle action).

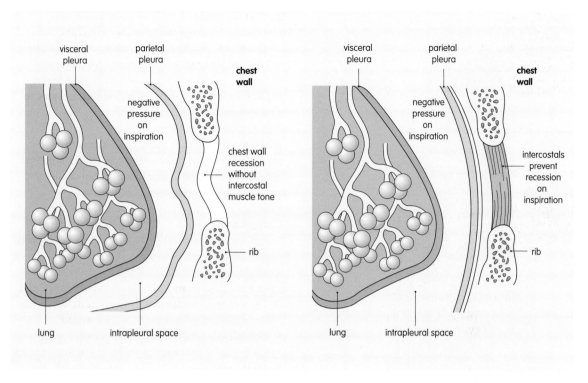

**Fig. 4.14** The intercostal muscles: they prevent deformation of the thoracic wall in quiet breathing, thus maintaining thoracic volume.

expanded against their elastic recoil. This recoil is sufficient to drive air out of the lungs in expiration. Thus, quiet expiration involves the controlled relaxation of the intercostal muscles and the diaphragm.

> The change in intrathoracic volume is mainly caused by the movement of the diaphragm downwards. Contraction of the diaphragm comprises 75% of the energy expenditure during quiet breathing.

### Forced inspiration

In addition to the action of the diaphragm:
- Scalene muscles and sternocleidomastoids raise the ribs anteroposteriorly, producing movement at the manubriosternal joint

- Intercostal muscles are much more active and raise the ribs to a much greater extent than in quiet inspiration
- The twelfth rib, which is attached to quadratus lumborum, allows forcible downward movement of the diaphragm
- Arching the back using erector spinae also increases thoracic volume.

During respiratory distress, the scapulae are fixed by trapezius muscles, rhomboid muscles and levator scapulae; pectoralis minor and serratus anterior raise the ribs; the arms can be fixed (e.g. by holding the back of a chair), allowing the use of pectoralis major.

> Use of the accessory muscles of inspiration and fixing of the torso are signs that you should look for when assessing a patient with dyspnoea.

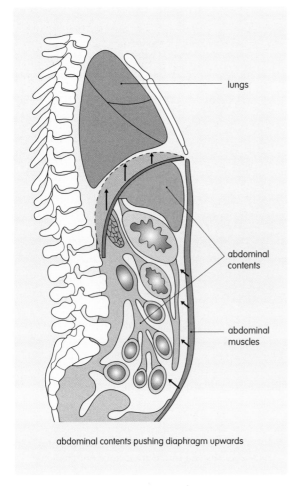

abdominal contents pushing diaphragm upwards

**Fig. 4.15** Forced expiration. Note the abdominal contents pushing the diaphragm upwards.

### Forced expiration

Elastic recoil of the lungs is reinforced by contraction of the muscles of the abdominal wall. These force the abdominal contents against the diaphragm, pushing it up (Fig. 4.15).

In addition, quadratus lumborum pulls the ribs down, thus adding to the force of the abdominal contents against the diaphragm. Intercostal muscles prevent outward deformation of the tissue between the ribs. Latissimus dorsi and serratus posterior inferior also may play some role.

## Elastic properties of the lung

In order for ventilation to take place, the respiratory muscles described above must overcome the

mechanical properties of the lungs and thorax, specifically their tendency to elastic recoil.

The elastic properties of the lung are caused by:

- Elastic fibres and collagen in the tissues in the lung
- Surface tension forces in the lung caused by the alveolar–liquid interface.

When we discuss the elastic properties of the lung, we often focus not on recoil but on stretch; the capacity of the lung to stretch is known as compliance and is discussed below.

### Compliance

Compliance describes the distensibility or ease of stretch of a material when an external force is applied to it. Elasticity ($E$) is the resistance to that stretch:

Therefore, $C = 1/E$

In respiratory physiology, we deal with:

- Compliance of the lung ($C_L$)
- Compliance of the chest wall ($C_w$)
- Total compliance ($C_{TOT}$) of the chest wall and lung together.

### Lung compliance

Lung compliance is the ease with which the lungs expand under pressure. The pressure to inflate comes from the transmural pressure (i.e. the difference between the intrapleural pressure and the intrapulmonary pressure); this is plotted against the change in volume on a pressure–volume curve (Fig. 4.16). Compliance represents the slope of the curve ($\Delta V:\Delta P$).

Lung mechanics are often categorized as static or dynamic. This can sometimes be confusing. As the name implies, static qualities do not change with time; lung statics help us to explore certain qualities of the lungs in isolation. Obviously, in real life, air in the respiratory tree flows (i.e. it changes with time). Therefore lung dynamics give us a fuller picture of what actually happens during respiration.

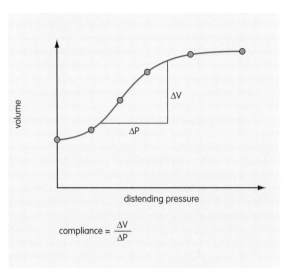

compliance = $\dfrac{\Delta V}{\Delta P}$

**Fig. 4.16** The pressure–volume curve.

Lung compliance can be looked at in two ways:
- Static lung compliance
- Dynamic lung compliance.

Dynamic lung compliance is a measure of the change in volume of the lung during breathing and will thus include the work required to overcome airway resistance. This will be discussed later.

Static lung compliance involves the inflation of the lungs in steps of various inflating pressures and recording the volume at the new inflation pressure. The lungs are expanded from complete collapse to total lung capacity, and measurements are also taken in deflation (see dotted line in Fig. 4.17A). This is carried out *in vitro* because, in life, we cannot completely deflate the lungs. Why is there a difference between inflation and deflation curves? This difference is called hysteresis and will be explained later.

Figure 4.17B also shows the pressure–volume curve for inflation of the lungs from functional residual capacity to total lung capacity. The curve still shows hysteresis, but not to the extent of the pressure–volume curve from complete lung collapse to total lung capacity. The slope of the curve (i.e. compliance) varies with lung volume. It can be seen that compliance is greatest at the lower lung volumes and is smallest at higher lung volumes. For these reasons, lung compliance is sometimes quoted as specific lung compliance (sp.$C_L$).

$$sp.C_L = C_L/V_L$$

You can see from the pressure–volume curve that expanding the lung is like blowing up a balloon. At first high pressure is required for a small increase in volume. Then the slope becomes steeper before flattening out again.

This change in lung compliance helps explain the difference in ventilation of the lung between apex and base.

The lung *alveolar* volume in the base is less (because it is compressed) relative to the apex (see p. 49). Thus, the base of the lung has greater initial compliance than that of the apex. Because both base and apex are subject to intrapleural pressure changes of the same magnitude during inspiration, the base of the lung will therefore expand to a greater extent than the apex. This explains in part the regional difference of ventilation.

### Chest wall compliance
As we have discussed before, the chest wall has elastic properties; at functional residual capacity, these are equal and opposite to those in the lung (i.e. tending to expand the chest). If the sternum were cut (e.g. in surgery) or if air were introduced into the intrapleural space then this would cause the chest wall to spring open.

As we breathe in, elastic forces (tending to expand the chest wall) aid inflation; however, at about two-thirds of total lung capacity, the chest wall has reached its resting position and any expansion beyond this point requires a positive pressure to stretch the chest wall.

Below this resting position, the chest wall is being compressed by the pressure difference between atmospheric pressure and intrapleural pressure. Thus, if we plot inflation pressure against volume of the chest wall, the inflation pressure is negative below two-thirds of total lung capacity (the dashed line in Fig. 4.18). However, compliance (the slope of the pressure–volume curve for the chest wall) remains positive, because we are looking at the change in volume caused by a change in inflation pressure. Above the resting position the inflation pressure required to expand the chest is positive.

**Fig. 4.17** Pressure–volume curves for inflation of the lungs (A) *in vitro*. (B) in life, from residual volume to total lung capacity. Note the curve still shows hysteresis but to a lesser extent.

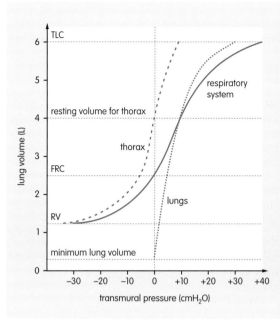

**Fig. 4.18** Pressure–volume curve of the entire respiratory system. Only at functional residual capacity does the passively inflated lung–thorax system (respiratory system) have no pressure difference between the alveoli and the body surface.

Compliance of the lung is also plotted (dotted line in Fig. 4.18). Total compliance is plotted on the same graph and is derived from:

$$1/C_{TOT} = 1/C_L + 1/C_W$$

### Effect of disease on compliance

Structural change in the thorax (e.g. kyphoscoliosis) may alter compliance of the chest wall; however, in practice, disease more often has an effect on compliance of the lung. Emphysema and pulmonary fibrosis (Fig. 4.19) represent two extremes of lung compliance in disease. In emphysema the compliance of the lung is increased, that is it becomes more easily distended. This is due to

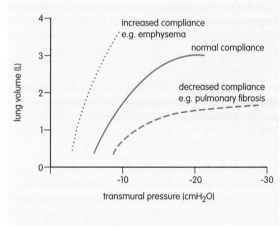

**Fig. 4.19** Pressure–volume curves in disease.

the destruction of the normal lung architecture, including the elastic fibres and collagen. Impaired elastic recoil means that the lungs do not deflate as easily, contributing to air trapping.

In diseases that cause fibrosis, scar tissue replaces normal interstitial tissue. As a result, the lungs become stiffer and compliance decreases.

## Surface tension and surfactant

As noted above, the elasticity, and therefore compliance of the lungs, is dependent on two factors. The first is the elastic fibres in lung tissue. The second is the surface tension of the alveolar lining. This lining is a thin film of liquid, the main component of which is surfactant.

### Surface tension

Surface tension is a physical property of liquids and arises because fluid molecules have a stronger attraction to each other than to air molecules (Fig. 4.20). Molecules on the surface of a liquid in contact with air are therefore pulled close together and act like a skin.

When molecules of a liquid lie on a curved surface (e.g. in a bubble), surface tension acts to pull that surface inwards. If the bubble is to be prevented from collapsing there must be an equal and opposite force tending to expand it. This is provided by a positive pressure within the bubble.

The alveoli are lined with liquid and are in contact with air. They can therefore can be considered similar to tiny bubbles. Laplace's Law (Fig. 4.21) tells us that the smaller a bubble, the greater the internal pressure needed to keep it inflated (Fig. 4.22). If a bubble of about the same size as an alveolus was made of interstitial fluid and filled with air it would require an internal pressure in the order of 3 kPa to prevent it from collapsing. The lungs would have a very low compliance and the forces involved in breathing would be extremely large. This would seem to argue against the lungs having a liquid lining.

This problem was investigated by von Neergaard, who measured the compliance of excised lungs, first using air to inflate them and then using saline (Fig. 4.23). He noticed that:

- Lungs were much easier to inflate (i.e. more compliant) with saline than air
- When he used air, the pressure required was greater during inflation than during deflation.

This phenomenon is called hysteresis.

Since there was no surface tension when saline was used, the alveoli did seem to have a liquid lining; surface tension was contributing to the elastic recoil of the lungs making them harder to inflate. However, the pressure needed to inflate the lungs was actually

**Fig. 4.20** Surface tension. (Adapted with permission from *Physiology* 3e, by R.M. Berne and M.N. Levy. Mosby Year Book, 1993.)

---

Laplace's law: states that 'The pressure within a bubble is equal to twice the surface tension divided by the radius'

$$P = \frac{2T}{r}$$

$P$ = pressure within bubble
$T$ = surface tension
$r$ = radius

The smaller a bubble (i.e. the more curved the surface) the larger the radial component.
The larger the radial component the greater the tendency to collapse.
Smaller bubbles must have a greater internal pressure to keep them inflated.

**Fig. 4.21** Laplace's law.

much lower than if the fluid were water or interstitial fluid. Something in the fluid lining the lungs reduces surface tension, making the lungs more compliant and therefore easier to expand.

This leads us to three questions:

- How is this low surface tension achieved?
- Laplace's law says that small bubbles have higher internal pressure than larger ones. If two bubbles of different sizes were connected, air would flow from the small bubble to the large, causing the small bubble to collapse (Fig. 4.24). Why does this not happen to alveoli?
- How does the phenomenon of hysteresis of the pressure–volume curve occur?

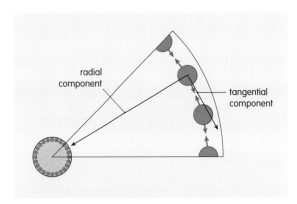

**Fig. 4.22** Surface tension of a bubble. Radial forces tend to collapse the bubble and there must be a positive pressure inside the bubble to prevent it from collapsing. The smaller the bubble, the greater the internal pressure.

The answers to all these questions are linked to surfactant.

### Surfactant

Surfactant is secreted by type II pneumocytes and contains a phospholipid (dipalmitoyl phosphatidyl choline). Surfactant has three functions:

- Prevention of alveolar collapse (gives alveolar stability)
- Increase in lung compliance by reducing surface tension of alveolar lining fluid
- Prevention of transudation of fluid into alveoli.

### Prevention of alveolar collapse

Because of two factors, alveoli of different sizes do not collapse:

- Surface tension of the alveolar lining fluid varies with surface area. This is because surfactant reduces surface tension in proportion to its surface concentration. Surfactant is insoluble in water and floats on the surface of the alveolar lining fluid. In larger alveoli the surfactant is more spread out (dilute) and the surface tension is higher (Fig. 4.25)
- There is interaction between adjacent groups of alveoli. Therefore, collapsing alveoli pull on adjacent alveoli preventing further collapse. This is termed alveolar interdependence.

### Prevention of transudation of fluid into alveoli

Surfactant reduces the surface tension in the alveolar lining fluid, which reduces the tendency for the alveolus to collapse. If the alveoli were lined with interstitial fluid, their collapse would cause a more

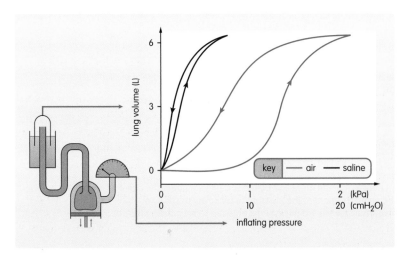

**Fig. 4.23** Note the marked difference between the pressure–volume curves of air-filled and saline-filled lungs. It is much easier to inflate the lung without air. (Adapted with permission from *Physiology* 3e, by R.M. Berne and M.N. Levy. Mosby Year Book, 1993.)

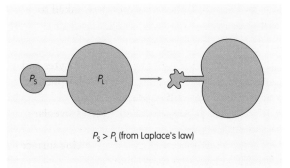

$P_S > P_L$ (from Laplace's law)

**Fig. 4.24** The pressure in the smaller bubble ($P_s$) from Laplace's law. The smaller bubble collapses, emptying into the larger, lower pressure bubble.

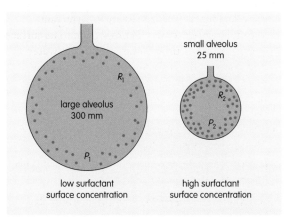

**Fig. 4.25** The surface tension ($T_1$) within the larger alveolus (with radius $R_1$) is greater than the surface tension ($T_2$) within the smaller alveolus (with radius $R_2$). This is because the surfactant is more spread out in the larger alveolus. Thus, the T:R ratio remains constant and the same pressure is required to inflate alveoli of all sizes ($P_1 = P_2$).

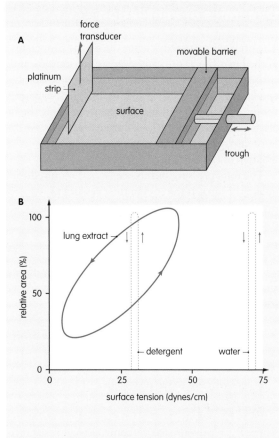

**Fig. 4.26** (A) Surface balance. The area of the surface is altered and the surface tension is measured from the force exerted on a platinum strip dipped into the surface. (B) Plots of surface tension and area obtained with a surface balance. Note that lung washings show a change in surface tension with area and that the minimum tension is very small. (Adapted with permission from *Respiratory Physiology* 5e, by J. West. Lippincott Williams & Wilkins, 1994.)

negative pressure in the interstitial space. This would lead into an increase in hydrostatic pressure difference between the pulmonary capillary and the interstitial space, leading to transudation of fluid.

## Hysteresis

Hysteresis of the pressure–volume curve is explained by a property of surfactant. The surface tension of surfactant shows different values when being expanded (e.g. during inspiration) or compressed (e.g. during expiration) (Fig. 4.26). Because lung compliance is dependent upon surface tension, this explains why hysteresis of the pressure–volume curve occurs.

## Respiratory distress syndrome

Respiratory distress syndrome (RDS) occurs in premature babies of less than 32 weeks' gestation; it is caused by a deficiency of surfactant production by type II pneumocytes. Difficulty in breathing occurs; breathing is rapid and laboured, often with an expiratory grunt. There is diffuse damage to alveoli with hyaline membrane formation. Treatment is with high-concentration oxygen therapy, which reverses the hypoxaemia.

## Dynamics of ventilation

The previous section discusses the elastic properties of the lungs (i.e. those caused by surface tension and tissue elasticity). These were looked at under static conditions; however, if we inflate the lungs, dynamic conditions exist. So, in addition to overcoming the elastic properties of the lung during breathing, we must also overcome the dynamic resistance to inflation of the lungs.

The total pressure difference ($P_{TOT}$) required to inflate the lungs is the sum of the pressure to overcome lung compliance and the pressure to overcome dynamic resistance:

$$P_{TOT} = P_{COM} + P_{DYN}$$

where $P_{COM}$ = pressure to overcome lung compliance and $P_{DYN}$ = pressure to overcome the dynamic resistance.

Dynamic resistance itself comprises:
- Resistance presented by the airways to flow of air into the lungs—airway resistance
- Resistance to tissues as they slide over each other—viscous tissue resistance.

$$P_{DYN} = P_{AR} + P_{VTR}$$

where $P_{AR}$ = pressure to overcome airways resistance and $P_{VTR}$ = pressure to overcome viscous tissue resistance.

Viscous tissue resistance comprises approximately 20% of the total dynamic resistance i.e. the vast majority of the total resistance is provided by the airways.

### Dynamic lung compliance

Now that we have introduced dynamic conditions, in which airway resistance is a factor, we need to review our measurements of lung compliance. If a pressure–volume curve is plotted under dynamic conditions, the pressure–volume loop is widened when compared with the curve under static conditions (Fig. 4.27). Dynamic lung compliance is the slope of this curve at any one point. Dynamic lung compliance is less than static lung compliance.

### Airway resistance

Airway resistance is an important concept because it is increased in common diseases such as asthma and COPD. It is defined as the resistance to flow of gas within the airways of the lung.

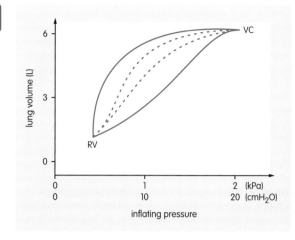

**Fig. 4.27** Difference in pressure–volume relationships in lungs inflated and deflated (measurements made under static conditions with no air flowing: dotted lines; dynamic conditions with air flowing continuously into or out of the lung: solid lines).

**Fig. 4.28** Laminar flow in which the coloured filament remained central. The flow occurs in streamlines, or laminae. The greatest velocity of flow is centrally and the velocity profile is parabolic. (Adapted with permission from *Physiology* 3e, by R.M. Berne and M.N. Levy. Mosby Year Book, 1993.)

Before we discuss airway resistance, it is important to outline pattern of flow.

### Pattern of flow

The pattern of fluid flowing through a tube (e.g. an airway or blood vessel) varies with the velocity and physical properties of the fluid. This was established by a French engineer, Reynolds, who injected a coloured dye into the centre of a clear pipe of water flowing at various velocities. He discovered two phenomena, which he described as laminar flow (which appeared at low flow rates; Fig. 4.28) and turbulent flow (which appeared at high flow rates; Fig. 4.29).

Figure 4.30 describes some of the differences between laminar and turbulent flow. Both types of flow are seen in the respiratory system.

### Turbulent flow

Turbulent flow is much more likely to occur with:

- High velocities (e.g. within the airways during exercise)
- Larger diameter airways
- Low-viscosity, high-density fluids.

Branching or irregular surfaces can also initiate turbulence.

### Laminar flow

Laminar flow is described by Poiseuille's law (Fig. 4.31). In basic terms, Poiseuille's law means that the wider the tube, the lower the resistance to airflow. Importantly, the change in width is not directly proportional to the change in resistance: for a given reduction in the radius there is a four-fold increase in resistance. Narrower or longer pipes or a higher fluid viscosity have a higher resistance to flow and so flow rate is reduced.

> Remembering Poiseuille's law isn't drastically important, but understanding it is! So, remember that in laminar flow: A small change in radius significantly affects either flow rate or pressure drop required to achieve the same flow. An example of this is bronchoconstriction in asthma.
> - Flow varies directly with pressure drop.
> - Flow varies inversely with viscosity (e.g. during scuba diving).

### Sites of airway resistance

Considering the whole respiratory system, approximately one-half of the resistance to airflow occurs in the upper respiratory tract when breathing through the nose. This is significantly reduced when mouth breathing. Thus, approximately one-half of

vortices

**Fig. 4.29** Turbulent flow in which the coloured filament broke up into eddies. (Adapted with permission from *Physiology* 3e, by R.M. Berne and M.N. Levy. Mosby Year Book, 1993.)

| Differences between laminar and turbulent flow | |
| --- | --- |
| **Laminar** | **Turbulent** |
| fluid moves parallel to walls only | flow has some movement at right angles |
| no mixing between fluid other than by diffusion | well-mixed flow eddies and diffusion |
| non erosive flow regime | flow regime can be erosive |
| flow is quiet | may account for murmurs heard clinically |
| poor flow for arterial thrombi but venous stasis may lead to thrombi | arterial thrombi more likely to form |
| resistance to flow is independent of surface roughness | resistance to flow is dependent on surface roughness |
| flow is proportional to the radius to the power 4 | flow is proportional to diameter to the power 5 |

**Fig. 4.30** Differences between laminar and turbulent flow.

**Fig. 4.31** Poiseuille's law.

Poiseuille's law: states that for a fluid under laminar flow conditions, the flow rate is directly related to the pressure drop between the two ends of a tube and the fourth power of the radius but inversely related to viscosity and length of pipe:

$$F = \frac{P\pi r^4}{8\,\eta\,L}$$

$(F)$ = flow rate
$(P)$ = pressure drop
$(r)$ = radius
$(\eta)$ = viscosity
$(L)$ = length of pipe

Remember, Poiseuille's law applies to laminar, not turbulent, flow.

the resistance lies within the lower respiratory tract.

Assuming laminar air flow, Poiseuille's law would predict that the major resistance to air flow would occur in the airways with a smaller radius. This is not the case because although the individual diameter of each airway is small, the total cross-sectional area for flow increases (large number of small airways) as we go down the tracheobronchial tree.

In exercise, the airway resistance may increase significantly due to high air flows inducing turbulence. It is normal under these conditions to switch to mouth breathing to reduce airway resistance.

It is important to note that resistance of the smaller airways is difficult to measure. Thus, these small airways may be damaged by disease and it may be some time before this damage is detectable, thus representing a 'silent' zone.

### Factors determining airway resistance

Factors affecting airway resistance are:
- Lung volume
- Bronchial smooth muscle tone
- Altered airway calibre
- Change in density and viscosity of inspired gas.

### Lung volume

Airways are supported by radial traction of lung parenchyma and thus their diameter and resistance to flow are affected by lung volume (Fig. 4.32):
- Low lung volumes tend to collapse and compress the airways, reducing their diameter and thus increasing resistance to flow
- High lung volumes tend to increase radial traction, increasing the length and diameter of airways

- The increase in diameter reduces airway resistance. The increase in length has a much smaller effect of increasing resistance, which is explained by Poiseuille's law.

Things to remember:
- The major site of airway resistance is medium-sized bronchi.
- 80% of the resistance of the lower respiratory tract is presented by the trachea and bronchi.
- Less than 20% of airway resistance is caused by airways less than 2 mm in diameter.

### Bronchial smooth muscle tone

Motor innervation of the smooth muscle of the airways is via the vagus nerve. The muscle has resting tone determined by the autonomic nervous system. This tone can be affected by a number of factors (Fig. 4.33).

Factors acting to decrease the airway diameter include:
- Irritant and cough receptors, C fibre reflex—reflex and bronchoconstriction act to close the airway
- Pulmonary stretch receptors
- Mediator release—inflammatory mediators (histamine, leukotrienes etc.) cause bronchoconstriction.

Factors acting to increase the airway diameter include:

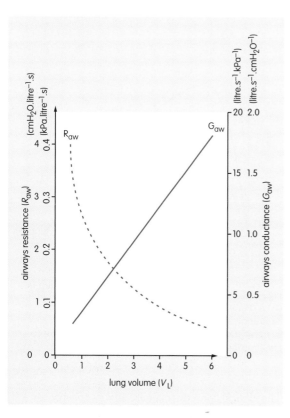

**Fig. 4.32** The relationship between lung volume ($V_L$) and airway resistance ($R_{aw}$) and conductance ($G_{aw}$). Note that at low lung volumes, $R_{aw}$ is high and $G_{aw}$ is low. (Adapted with permission from *Respiratory Physiology* 2e, by J. Widdicombe and A. Davies. Edward Arnold, 1991.)

- Carbon dioxide
- Catecholamine release
- Other nerves—non-adrenergic, non-cholinergic (NANC) nerves cause bronchodilation.

Reduced airway calibre can be caused either by disease or by an inhaled foreign body. A change in density and viscosity of gas occurs in scuba diving (Chapter 6).

Increased smooth muscle tone is very important in asthma. Inflammatory mediators act to narrow the airways and increase resistance to airflow.

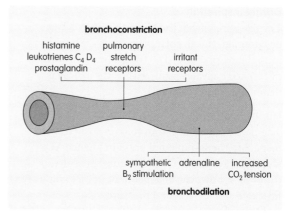

**Fig. 4.33** Factors affecting bronchial motor tone. (Adapted with permission from *Physiology* 3e, by R.M. Berne and M.N. Levy. Mosby Year Book, 1993.)

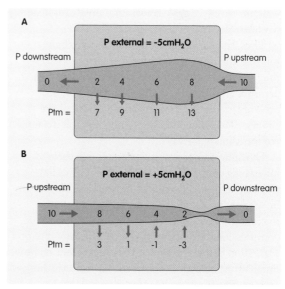

**Fig. 4.34** Transmural pressure, (A) during inspiration; (B) during expiration. Ptm = transmural pressure.

## Effect of transmural pressure on airway resistance

Remember that the airways are not rigid tubes; they are affected by the pressures around them. The pressure difference between the gas in the airway and the pressure outside the airway is known as the transmural pressure difference. The pressure outside the airway reflects the intrapleural pressure (Fig. 4.34).

### During inspiration

The pressure within the pleural cavity is always negative and the alveolar pressure is greater than intrapleural pressure. The transmural pressure difference is always positive thus the airway is distended (radial traction).

### During expiration

The pressure within the alveolus is positive with respect to the intrapleural pressure; hence, the alveolus stays open. The transmural pressure difference, however, is dependent upon expiratory flow rate and intrapleural pressure.

During forced expiration, the positive intrapleural pressure is transmitted through the lungs to the external wall of the airways. In addition, there is a dynamic pressure drop from alveolus to the airway caused by airway resistance. This is greater at high expiratory flow rates. Thus, the pressure in the lumen of the airway may be lower than the external wall pressure (negative transmural pressure), leading to collapse of the airways.

Thus, the harder the subject tries to exhale forcibly, the more the airways are compressed, so the rate of expiration does not rise as the increased pressure gradient (from alveoli to atmospheric pressure) is offset by the reduced calibre of the airways. This phenomenon is known as the dynamic compression of airways.

Dynamic compression of airways is greater at lower lung volumes because the effect of radial traction holding the airways open is less. Thus it can be seen that for a specific lung volume there is a maximum expiratory flow rate caused by dynamic compression of the airways (Fig. 4.35). Any rate of expiration below this flow rate is dependent on how much effort is made to expel the air from the lungs and the flow is said to be effort dependent. At maximum expiratory flow rate, any additional effort does not alter the expiratory flow rate (because of dynamic compression of airways) and the flow is said to be effort independent.

### Dynamic compression in disease

In patients with COPD, dynamic compression limits expiratory flow even in tidal breathing. The main reasons for this are:

- Loss of radial traction (due to destruction of the lung architecture) means the airways are more readily compressed
- Increased lung compliance, leading to lower alveolar pressure and less force driving air out of the lungs.

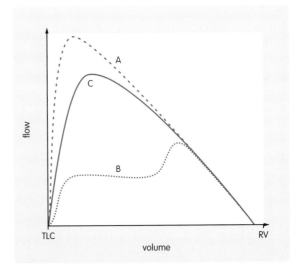

**Fig. 4.35** Flow–volume curves made with a spirometer. (A) Maximum inspiration and forced expiration. (B) Slow expiration initially then forced. (C) Expiratory flow almost to maximum effort. Note that the three descending curves are almost superimposed.

The clinical consequences are airway collapse on expiration and air trapping in the alveoli. Patients sometimes demonstrate pursed lip breathing as they attempt to increase pressure on expiration and reduce the amount of air trapped.

### Measuring airway resistance

Airway resistance can be measured by plethysmography. In practice, estimates of airway resistance are made every day using simpler methods which rely on the relationship between resistance and airflow. Peak expiratory flow rate (PEFR) measures the maximum airflow achieved in a rapid, forced expiration. Spirometry measures the volume exhaled in a specified time (e.g. the forced expired volume in 1 second or $FEV_1$). These investigations are described in Chapter 10.

## The work of breathing

The work of breathing is the work done by the respiratory muscles to overcome the forces described above, i.e. resistance to airflow and the elastic recoil of the lungs.

The work done ($W$) to change a volume ($\Delta V$) of gas at constant pressure ($P$) is shown by the relationship below:

$$W = P \cdot \Delta V$$

Work done is measured in joules; a volume change of 10L at a pressure of $1\,cmH_2O = 1J$ of energy.

Respiration normally represents just a small fraction of the total cost of metabolism (approximately 2%). However, the work required to inflate the lungs, along with this percentage, will rise if:

- Lungs are inflated to a larger volume (e.g. COPD and chronic severe asthma)
- Lung compliance decreases (e.g. fibrotic lungs)
- Airway resistance increases (e.g. COPD and asthma)
- Turbulence is induced in the airways (e.g. in high flow rates experienced during strenuous exercise).

In contrast, the work of breathing is reduced by bronchodilators which act to decrease airway resistance.

The increased work requirement can be dramatic in patients with severe COPD; a great deal of energy is required just in order to breathe. This can also be understood in terms of the efficiency of ventilation (i.e. the amount of work done divided by energy expenditure). Efficiency of normal quiet breathing is low (about 10%) even in health. In COPD, efficiency decreases, and the work done increases, so much that all the oxygen supplied from increasing ventilation is consumed by the respiratory muscles.

The work of breathing can be illustrated by volume–pressure curves (Fig. 4.36). Figure 4.37 shows the effect of disease on these curves. Figure 4.38 shows the effect of the pattern of breathing on work; there is an optimal balance between volume and rate of breathing at which the work of breathing is minimal.

Try to relate these concepts to respiratory failure. A patient with lung disease may be able to respond to impaired gas exchange by raising the ventilatory rate, leading to rapid, shallow breaths. This increases the work of breathing. If lung disease is severe, the work of breathing may become unsustainable. Respiratory muscles tire, ventilatory failure ensues and the patient must be mechanically ventilated, to reduce the work of breathing.

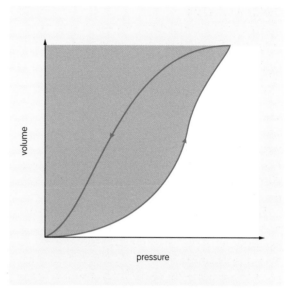

**Fig. 4.36** Graph of normal lung volume against trans-lung pressure. The shaded area is the inspiratory work of breathing. (Adapted with permission from *Respiratory Physiology* 2e, by J. Widdicombe and A. Davies. Arnold, 1991.)

## Gaseous exchange in the lungs

This section discusses how gas is transferred from the alveoli to the bloodstream and from the bloodstream to the alveoli. A brief outline of how the laws of diffusion apply to the diffusion of gas from the airways to the circulation is given below. Time for diffusion and diffusion–perfusion limitations are also discussed.

### Diffusion

Gas exchange between alveolar air and blood in the pulmonary capillaries takes place by diffusion.

Diffusion is the process in which molecules move due to their random motion (Brownian motion). The process of diffusion is seen to be a net movement of particles:

- Diffusion occurs from an area of high concentration to an area of low concentration. Thus, the driving force for diffusion is concentration difference ($\Delta C$)
- Diffusion will occur until the concentration in the two areas is equalized (i.e. net movement has ceased). Random movement of particles continues to occur and this is known as dynamic equilibrium.

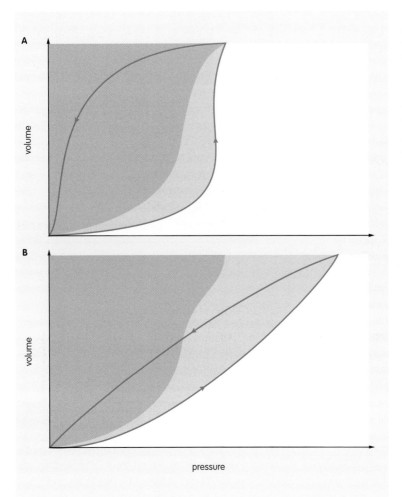

**A**

volume

**B**

volume

pressure

**Fig. 4.37** Changes to breathing work during diseased states. Paler shading denotes disease state; dark shading shows the normal work prefills from Fig. 4.36. (A) Increased airway resistance (e.g. in asthma); (B) decreased compliance (e.g. in fibrotic lung disease). (Adapted with permission from *Respiratory Physiology* 2e, by J. Widdicombe and A. Davies. Arnold, 1991.)

Diffusion in the lungs occurs across a membrane and is therefore governed by Fick's law (Fig. 4.39). Fick's law tells us that the rate of diffusion of a gas increases:

- As the surface area of the membrane increases
- The thinner the membrane
- The greater the partial pressure gradient across the membrane
- The more soluble the gas.

It is clear that the blood–gas interface with its large surface area of 50–100m$^2$ and average thickness of 0.4μm permits the high rate of diffusion required by the body.

We can also see that the rate of diffusion across the alveoli is directly dependent upon the difference in partial pressures between a gas in the alveoli ($P_A$) and in arterial blood ($P_a$).

Henry's law states that at equilibrium, the amount of gas dissolved in a given volume of liquid at a given temperature is proportional to the partial pressure ($P$) of the gas in the gas phase and its solubility in the liquid ($S$).

$C = S \cdot P$

The following will increase the rate of oxygen diffusion into the blood:
- Increased surface area of the alveolus.
- Decreased thickness of the alveolar wall.
- Increased alveolar partial pressure of oxygen (oxygen therapy).

## Partial pressures of respiratory gases

The partial pressure of a gas can be calculated by Dalton's law. Dalton's law states that 'The pressure exerted by a mixture of nonreacting gases is equal to the sum of the partial pressures of the separate components.' In other words, each gas in a mixture of gases exerts the same pressure as it would if it were present alone in the volume occupied by the mixture (Fig. 4.40).

From Dalton's law we see that:
- The total pressure of a gas is the sum of all the partial pressures of its constituents
- The partial pressure of a gas can be calculated from its fractional concentration.

If we consider the total barometric pressure of air ($P_{atm}$, about 760 mmHg at sea level), this is composed of the sum of all the partial pressures of its constituent gases:

$$P_{atm} = PO_2 + PN_2 + PCO_2 + PH_2O$$

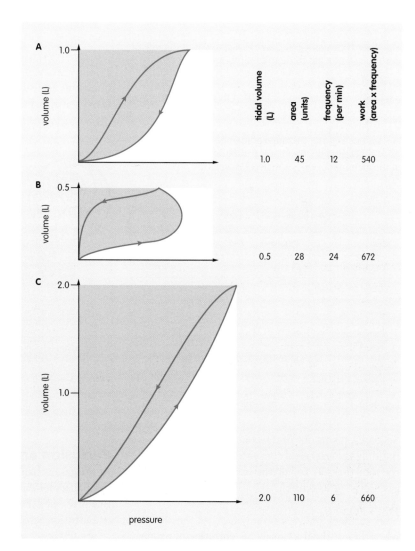

**Fig. 4.38** The work done in breathing is altered by the pattern of breathing. (A) Optimal pattern; (B) increased frequency and decreased volume; (C) decreased frequency and increased volume. Note that the work of breathing is highest when frequency decreases and volume increases. (Adapted with permission from *Respiratory Physiology* 2e, by J. Widdicombe and A. Davies. Arnold, 1991.)

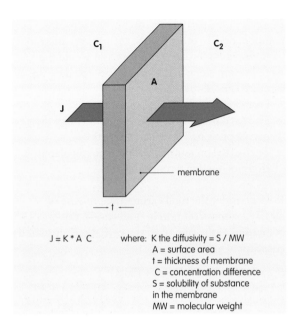

$J = K * A \ C$  where: K the diffusivity = S / MW
A = surface area
t = thickness of membrane
C = concentration difference
S = solubility of substance
in the membrane
MW = molecular weight

**Fig. 4.39** Diffusion—Fick's law. Fick stated that the rate of diffusion ($J$) of a gas through a membrane was:

$$J = K \times A \times \Delta C / t$$

where

$$K = S/\text{wt}_{mol}$$

$A$ = surface area; $t$ = thickness of membrane; $\Delta C$ = concentration difference; $S$ = solubility of substance in the membrane; $\text{wt}_{mol}$ = molecular weight.

| Partial pressures of respiratory gases | | | |
|---|---|---|---|
| Gas | $PO_2$ (kPa) | $PCO_2$ (kPa) | $PH_2O$ (kPa) |
| atmosphere | 21 | 0 | variable |
| trachea (inspiration) | 20 | 0 | 6.3* |
| alveolar gas | 13.5 | 5.3 | 6.3 |
| exhaled breath | 16 | 3.5 | variable |

*note inspired air is fully saturated with water vapour before it enters the lungs

**Fig. 4.40** Partial pressures of respiratory gases.

Secondly, taking one of the constituent gases, we can multiply the fractional concentration of that gas by the total pressure to find the partial pressure that the gas exerts, or its tension:

$$PO_2 = FO_2 \times P_{atm}$$

where $FO_2$ is the fractional concentration of oxygen.

Dry air has a fractional concentration of oxygen of 21%; inserting this value into the equation above gives us an oxygen tension at sea level of 159mmHg.

We specified sea level because the partial pressure of a gas in a system will alter with total pressure. If atmospheric pressure is reduced (e.g. when climbing Mount Everest), so is the partial pressure of oxygen.

### Water vapour pressure

Dry gas pressures are, however, of little relevance in respiratory medicine. On inspiration, air is warmed and humidified. Therefore water vapour also exerts a pressure, which reduces the pressure available to the partial pressures of the gases.

The water vapour pressure of a gas depends on:
- Saturation of the gas (quoted as % saturation)
- Temperature of the gas (increases as temperature rises).

It is important to know that for fully (100%) saturated air, the water vapour pressure at 37°C is 47mmHg. Using this value we can calculate the partial pressure of oxygen in inspired (or 'tracheal') air.

$$PO_2 = 0.21 \times (760 - 47) = 150\text{mmHg}$$

The following will decrease the rate of oxygen diffusion into the blood:
- Reduction in the overall alveolar surface area (e.g. emphysema).
- Increased distance for diffusion (e.g. emphysema).
- Increased thickness of the alveolar wall (e.g. fibrosing alveolitis).
- Reduction in the alveolar partial pressure of oxygen (e.g. altitude).

Partial pressures are also expressed in kPa. 1kPa is 7.5mmHg.

### Perfusion and diffusion limitation

At the gas exchange surface, gas transfer occurs through a membrane into a flowing liquid. There are two processes (Fig. 4.41) occurring:
- Diffusion across the alveolar capillary membrane

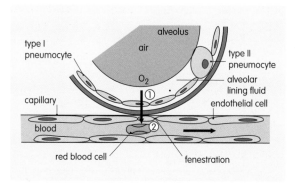

**Fig. 4.41** Gas transfer across alveolar capillary membrane. (1) Diffusion across membrane; (2) perfusion of blood through pulmonary capillaries.

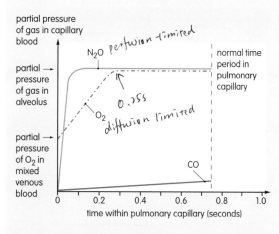

**Fig. 4.42** Graph of partial pressure of respiratory gases against time within the pulmonary capillary bed. Transfer of $N_2O$ is perfusion limited, transfer of CO is diffusion limited. Transfer of $O_2$ is usually perfusion limited but may change with diseased states.

- Perfusion of blood through pulmonary capillaries.

Uptake of a gas into the blood is dependent on its solubility and the chemical combination (e.g. with haemoglobin: Hb). If the chemical combination is strong, the gas is taken up by the blood with little rise in arterial partial pressure.

The solubility of nitrous oxide ($N_2O$) in the blood is low, and it does not undergo chemical combination with any component of the blood. Thus, rate of transfer of gas into the liquid phase is slow and partial pressure of the gas in the blood rises rapidly (Fig. 4.42). This reduces the partial pressure difference between alveolar gas and the blood and hence the driving force for diffusion. Nitrous oxide is, therefore, an example of a gas that is said to be perfusion limited. Thus, the amount of nitrous oxide taken up by the blood is dependent almost solely upon the rate of blood flow through the pulmonary capillaries.

In the case of carbon monoxide (CO), the gas is taken up rapidly and bound tightly by haemoglobin; the arterial partial pressure rises slowly (Fig. 4.42). Thus, there is always a driving force (partial pressure difference) for diffusion (even at low perfusion rates), and the overall rate of transfer will be dependent on the rate of diffusion. This type of transfer is said to be diffusion limited. Thus the amount of carbon monoxide taken up by the blood is dependent on the rate of diffusion of carbon monoxide from the alveoli to the blood.

The transfer of oxygen is normally perfusion limited because the arterial partial pressure of oxygen ($P_aO_2$) reaches equilibrium with the alveolar gas ($P_AO_2$) by about one-third of the way along the pulmonary capillary (Fig. 4.42); there is, therefore, no driving force for diffusion after this point. However, if the diffusion is slow because of emphysematous changes to the lung, then $P_aO_2$ may not reach equilibrium with the alveolar gas before the blood reaches the end of the capillary. Under these conditions, the transfer of oxygen is diffusion limited.

## Oxygen uptake in the capillary network

The time taken for the partial pressure of oxygen to reach its plateau is approximately 0.25 seconds. The pulmonary capillary volume under resting conditions is about 75 mL, which is approximately the same size as the stroke volume of the right ventricle. Pulmonary capillary blood is therefore replaced with every heart beat, approximately every 0.75 seconds. This far exceeds the time for transfer of oxygen into the bloodstream.

During exercise, however, the cardiac output increases and the flow rate though the pulmonary capillaries also increases. Because the lungs have the ability to recruit new capillaries and distend already open capillaries (see Chapter 5), the effect of increased blood flow rate on the time allowed for diffusion is not as great as one might expect. In strenuous exercise, the pulmonary capillary network volume may increase by up to 200 mL. This helps

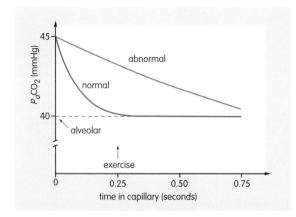

**Fig. 4.44** Change in $P_aCO_2$. Calculated when alveolar capillary membrane is normal or abnormal. (Adapted with permission from *Respiratory Physiology* 5e, by J. West. Lippincott Williams & Wilkins, 1994.)

**Fig. 4.43** Pulmonary capillary partial pressure of oxygen vs. time in the pulmonary capillary network. (A) Alveolar $PO_2$ normal; (B) low alveolar $PO_2$. Curves are for normal blood gas interface and abnormal in diseased state. Note that the difference between the normal and abnormal lungs increases at low alveolar $PO_2$. (Adapted with permission from *Respiratory Physiology* 5e, by J. West. Lippincott Williams & Wilkins, 1994.)

maintain the time allowed for diffusion, although it cannot keep it to the same value as at rest (Fig. 4.43).

## Carbon dioxide transfer

Fick's is not the only law that describes the diffusion of gases in the lung. Graham's law tells us that gases with greater molecular weights diffuse more slowly than those that are lighter.

However, we are also concerned with the diffusion rates of gas in blood. Diffusion in liquids is directly dependent upon the solubility of the gas, but inversely proportional to the square root of its molecular weight. Carbon dioxide diffuses 20 times more rapidly than oxygen, but has a similar molecular weight. Thus, the difference in rates of diffusion is caused by the much higher solubility of carbon dioxide.

Under normal conditions, the transfer of carbon dioxide is not diffusion limited (Fig. 4.44).

## Measuring diffusion

As we have already seen (p. 68), gas transfer ($J$) can be calculated using Fick's law:

$$J = K \cdot A \cdot (P_A - P_a)/t.$$

It is not possible to measure the area and thickness of a complex structure like the blood–gas barrier, so the equation is rewritten:

$$J = D_L(P_A - P_a)$$

Where $D_L$ is the diffusing capacity of the lung, defined as the ease of diffusion of gas into the blood (the rate of uptake of a gas divided by the partial pressure difference between alveoli and blood).

$$D_L = J/(P_A - P_a)$$

Carbon monoxide is the gas most commonly used to study diffusing capacity. Because carbon monoxide is taken up into the liquid phase very quickly, the rate of perfusion of pulmonary capillaries does not significantly affect the partial pressure difference between alveolar gas and the bloodstream. In addition, carbon monoxide binds irreversibly to haemoglobin and is not taken up by the tissues.

In contrast, oxygen is not a good candidate for calculating diffusing capacity because it binds reversibly to haemoglobin; thus, mixed venous partial pressure may not be the same as that of blood entering the pulmonary capillary bed. In addition, because oxygen is taken up less quickly than CO, perfusion has more of an effect.

We therefore use the diffusing capacity of carbon monoxide ($D_{L(CO)}$) as a general measure of the diffusion properties of the lung.

The terms diffusing capacity ($D_{L(CO)}$) and transfer factor ($T_{L(CO)}$) are interchangeable.

The partial pressure of carbon monoxide in the blood ($P_{a(CO)}$) is negligible, so the equation can be rewritten:

$$D_{L(CO)} = J_{(CO)}/P_{A(CO)}$$

One of the methods used to measure diffusion across the blood–gas interface is the single-breath method. A single breath of a mixture of carbon monoxide and air is taken. The breath is then held for approximately 10 seconds. The difference between inspiratory and expiratory concentrations of carbon dioxide is measured and therefore the amount of carbon monoxide taken up by the blood in 10 secs is known. If the lung volume is also measured by the helium dilution method, it is possible to determine the transfer coefficient ($K_{CO}$) or diffusion rate per unit of lung volume. This is a more useful measure of diffusion where lung volume has been lost, for example after surgery or in pleural effusion. Because there can be many causes of a reduction in diffusing capacity, it is not a specific test for lung disease. It is, however, a sensitive test; it is able to demonstrate minor impediments to gas diffusion.

Factors that decrease the rate of diffusion include:
- Thickening of the alveolar capillary membrane (e.g. in fibrosing alveolitis)
- Oedema of the alveolar capillary walls
- Increased lining fluid within the alveoli
- Increased distance for gaseous diffusion (e.g. in emphysema)
- Reduced area of alveolar capillary membrane (e.g. in emphysema)
- Reduced flow of fresh air to the alveoli from terminal bronchioles
- Hypoventilation.

- Define minute ventilation and alveolar ventilation.
- Define anatomical dead space, quoting its normal value. Describe two methods of measuring anatomical dead space.
- Define all lung volumes and capacities, giving normal values. State the significance of each volume and capacity.
- Name four methods for measuring lung volume.
- Outline the regional variations in ventilation of the lung and how this might be measured.
- Explain why intrapleural pressure is negative. Describe its variation during breathing.
- Describe how breathing is brought about, naming the muscles involved and their actions.
- Define lung compliance and explain what is meant by static and dynamic lung compliance, including a description of the pressure–volume curve.
- Describe the role of surfactant.
- Define airway resistance and viscous tissue resistance.
- List the factors determining airway resistance.
- Describe how airway resistance is altered in asthma.
- Explain what is meant by dynamic compression of the airways.
- Summarize the mechanisms that impair ventilation in COPD.
- Which factors affect the rate of diffusion across the blood–air interface? What is the driving force for diffusion?
- Give the normal values of the partial pressures of carbon dioxide and oxygen within the respiratory system.
- Explain the terms 'partial pressure of a gas' and 'vapour pressure'.
- Name three conditions that lower the transfer of oxygen to the blood. How do these conditions affect diffusion?
- Using examples, define perfusion limitation and diffusion limitation.
- Define diffusing capacity. How can diffusing capacity be measured?

# 5. Perfusion and Gas Transport

## Overview

The pulmonary circulation is a highly specialized system which is adapted to accommodate the entire cardiac output both at rest and during exercise. It is able to do this because it is:

- A low-pressure, low-resistance system
- Able to recruit more vessels with only a slight increase in arterial pulmonary pressure.

However, good perfusion is not enough to ensure that the blood is adequately oxygenated. The most important determinant in arterial blood gas composition is the way in which ventilation and perfusion are matched to each alveolus. Mismatching of ventilation:perfusion is the central mechanism in many common lung diseases.

The ability of the lungs to change minute ventilation, and therefore alter the rate of excretion of $CO_2$, gives the respiratory system a key role in maintaining the body's acid–base status. This chapter therefore also reviews the fundamentals of acid–base balance and discusses the common acid–base disturbances.

## Pulmonary blood flow

### Outline of pulmonary circulation

An outline of the pulmonary blood flow was given in Fig. 3.14. Venous blood returning from the body enters the right atrium and passively fills the right ventricle during diastole. During systole, the right ventricle contracts, ejecting its contents into the pulmonary artery (note the pulmonary artery contains deoxygenated blood).

Blood flows along the pulmonary arteries and arterioles, which closely follow the course of the airways. Blood enters the pulmonary capillaries (situated within the walls of the alveoli) and gaseous exchange takes place. Blood then returns to enter the left atrium through postcapillary venules and pulmonary veins (which contain oxygenated blood).

## Mechanics of the circulation

The flow of blood through the pulmonary vasculature is slightly less than the systemic output of the left ventricle. This is because a proportion of the coronary circulation from the aorta drains directly into the left ventricle. In addition, the bronchial circulation from the aorta drains into pulmonary veins, thus bypassing the lungs. However, we can consider the flow through the pulmonary artery to be equal to cardiac output.

Pressures within the pulmonary circulation are much lower than those equivalent regions within the systemic circulation (Fig. 5.1). Because the volume of blood flowing through both circulations is approximately the same, the pulmonary circulation must offer lower resistance.

Pulmonary capillaries and arterioles cause the main resistance to flow in the pulmonary circulation. This low resistance is achieved in two ways:

- A large number of resistance vessels exist, which are usually dilated; thus, the total area for flow is very large
- Small muscular arteries contain much less smooth muscle than equivalent arteries in the systemic circulation; they are more easily distended.

Many other factors affect pulmonary blood flow and pulmonary vascular resistance. These are discussed below.

### Hydrostatic pressure

Hydrostatic pressure has three effects.

- It distends blood vessels: as hydrostatic pressure rises, distension of the vessel increases
- It is capable of opening previously closed capillaries (recruitment)
- It causes flow to occur; in other words, a pressure difference ($\Delta P$) between the arterial and venous ends of a vessel provides the driving force for flow (see Fig. 5.2).

| Normal pressures in the pulmonary circulation | | |
|---|---|---|
| Site | Pressure (mmHg) | Pressure (cmH₂O) |
| Pulmonary artery<br>Systolic/diastolic pressure | 24/9 | 33/11 |
| Mean pressure | 14 | 19 |
| Arteriole (mean pressure) | 12 | 16 |
| Capillary (mean pressure) | 10.5 | 14 |
| Venule (mean pressure) | 9.0 | 12 |
| Left atrium (mean pressure) | 8.0 | 11 |

**Fig. 5.1** Pressures within the pulmonary circulation. The pulmonary arterial and left atrial pressures are measured during cardiac catheterization, the former directly, the latter by wedging the arterial catheter into a branch of the pulmonary artery. The capillary pressure is computed by a standard equation. (Adapted with permission from *Physiology* 3e, by R.M. Berne and M.N. Levy. Mosby Year Book, 1993.)

**Fig. 5.2** Hydrostatic pressure in terms of driving force. $P_2 - P_1$ i.e. $\Delta P$ provides the driving force of the flow.

Pulmonary $\Delta P$ is small compared with the systemic circulation, so $R$ must be small to achieve the same flow rate.

Flow = driving force/resistance
= $\Delta P/R$

Poiseuille's law tells us that the calibre of a vessel significantly affects resistance to flow and hence the flow rate through a vessel when a particular pressure difference is applied. The pulmonary circulation is therefore a low-pressure, low-resistance system.

In situations where increased pulmonary flow is required (e.g. during exercise), the cardiac output is increased, which raises pulmonary vascular pressure. This causes recruitment of previously closed capillaries and distension of already open capillaries (Fig. 5.3). In turn, this reduces the pulmonary vascular resistance to flow; it is for this reason that resistance to flow through the pulmonary vasculature decreases with increasing pulmonary vascular pressure.

Remember, any resistance to flow causes a drop in pressure; therefore, the hydrostatic pressure in postcapillary venules will be less than that within the capillaries.

### Pressure outside pulmonary blood vessels

Pressure outside a vessel can tend either to compress or collapse the vessel if the pressure is positive, or to aid the distension of the vessel if the pressure is negative.

The tendency for a vessel to distend or collapse is also dependent on the pressure inside the lumen. Thus, it is the pressure difference across the wall (or the transmural pressure) which determines whether a vessel compresses or distends (Fig. 5.4).

Pulmonary vessels can be considered in two groups (Fig. 5.5): alveolar and extra-alveolar vessels.

### Alveolar vessels

Remember that there is a dense network of capillaries in the alveolar wall; these are the alveolar vessels. External pressure is alveolar pressure (normally atmospheric pressure). As the lungs

**Fig. 5.3** In order to minimize pulmonary vascular resistance when pulmonary arterial pressure increases, new vessels are recruited and vessels that are already open are distended.

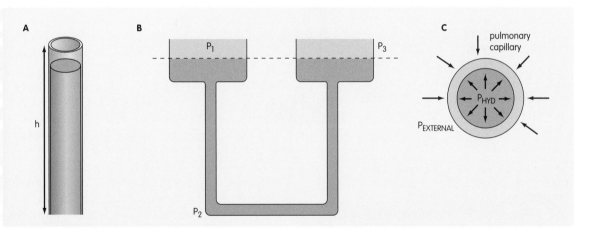

**Fig. 5.4** Hydrostatic pressure. (a) Hydrostatic pressure = $\rho \cdot g \cdot h$ [$\rho$ = density of liquid; $g$ = gravity; $h$ = height]. (b) $P_2 > P_1$ because of the height of the column of liquid. $P_3 = P_1$ because they are at the same height. (c) Hydrostatic pressure tends to distend pulmonary vessels, whereas the external pressure tends to collapse them.

expand, these vessels are compressed. The diameter of these vessels (capillaries) is dependent on the transmural pressure (i.e. the difference between hydrostatic pressure within the capillary lumen and pressure within the alveolus). If the alveolar pressure is greater than capillary hydrostatic pressure, the capillary will tend to collapse.

Vessels in the top of the lung may collapse as the alveoli expand. This is much more likely during diastole when the venous (capillary) pressure falls below alveolar pressure (Fig. 5.4).

### Extra-alveolar vessels

Extra-alveolar vessels are arteries and veins contained within the lung tissue. As the lungs expand, these vessels are distended by radial traction. The external pressure is similar to intrapleural pressure (subatmospheric—negative).

Because extra-alveolar vessels have an external pressure that is almost always negative, transmural pressure tends to distend these vessels.

During inspiration, intrapleural pressure and thus the pressure outside the extra-alveolar vessels becomes even more negative, causing these vessels to distend even further, reducing vascular resistance and increasing pulmonary blood flow. At large lung volumes, the effect of radial traction is greater and the extra-alveolar vessels are distended more.

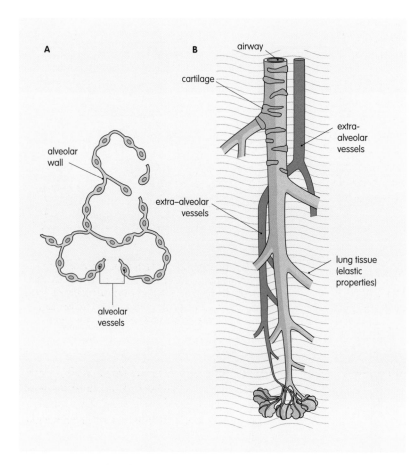

**Fig. 5.5** Diagram of (A) alveolar vessels, which are subject to external pressures of alveolar gas, and (B) extra-alveolar vessels contained within lung tissue, subject to intrapleural pressure.

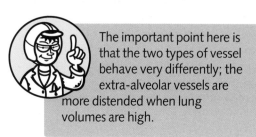

The important point here is that the two types of vessel behave very differently; the extra-alveolar vessels are more distended when lung volumes are high.

## Lung volume

Extra-alveolar vessels are distended by increased radial traction associated with increased lung volumes. The capillary, however, is affected in several ways.

Hydrostatic pressure within the capillaries during deep inspiration is lowered. This is caused by a negative intrapleural pressure around the heart. This changes the transmural pressure and the capillaries tend to be compressed, increasing pulmonary vascular resistance (Fig. 5.6).

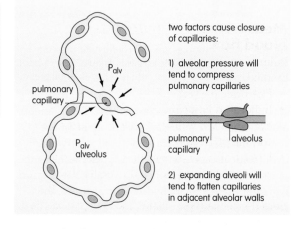

two factors cause closure of capillaries:

1) alveolar pressure will tend to compress pulmonary capillaries

2) expanding alveoli will tend to flatten capillaries in adjacent alveolar walls

**Fig. 5.6** Alveolar pressure and capillary compression. The transmural pressure is the difference between hydrostatic pressure inside the capillary and alveolar pressure outside the capillary. $P_{alv}$ = pressure in the alveolus.

At large lung volumes, the alveolar wall is stretched and becomes thinner, compressing the capillaries and increasing vascular resistance.

## Smooth muscle within the vascular wall

Smooth muscle in the walls of extra-alveolar vessels tends to reduce their diameter. Thus, the forces caused by radial traction and hydrostatic pressure within the lumen are trying to distend these vessels, whereas the tone of the vascular smooth muscle opposes this action. Drugs that lead to contraction of smooth muscle therefore increase pulmonary vascular resistance.

The factors affecting the capillary blood flow are:
• Hydrostatic pressure.
• Alveolar air pressure.
• Lung volume.

The factors affecting extra-alveolar vessels are:
• Hydrostatic pressure.
• Intrapleural pressure.
• Lung volume.
• Smooth muscle tone.

## Measurement of pulmonary blood flow

Pulmonary blood flow can be measured by three methods:
• Fick principle (Fig. 5.7)
• Indicator dilution method: a known amount of dye is injected into venous blood and its arterial concentration is measured
• Uptake of inhaled soluble gas (e.g. $N_2O$): the gas is inhaled and arterial blood values measured.

Both the first and second methods give average blood flow, whereas the third method measures instantaneous flow. The third method relies upon $N_2O$ transfer across the gas exchange surface being perfusion limited.

Fick theorized that because of the laws of conservation of mass, the difference in oxygen concentration between mixed venous blood

**Fig. 5.7** Fick principle for measuring pulmonary blood flow. Fick theorized that the difference in oxygen content between pulmonary venous blood and pulmonary arterial blood must be due to uptake of oxygen in the pulmonary capillaries, therefore the pulmonary blood flow can be calculated.

returning to the pulmonary capillary bed $[O_2]_{pv}$ and arterial blood leaving the heart $[O_2]_{pa}$ must be caused by uptake of oxygen within the lungs. This uptake must be equal to the body's consumption of oxygen (see Fig. 5.7).

## Distribution of blood within the lung

Blood flow within the normal, healthy upright lung is not uniform. Blood flow at the base of the lung is greater than at the apex. Why is this the case?

Because the lungs are vertical in an upright human, they are under the influence of gravity and the pulmonary vessels at the lung base will therefore have a greater hydrostatic pressure than vessels at the apex.

The hydrostatic pressure exerted by a vertical column of fluid is given by the relationship:

$$P = \rho \cdot g \cdot h$$

where $\rho$ = density of the fluid, $h$ = height of the column and $g$ = acceleration due to gravity.

From the equation above, it can be seen that:
• Vessels at the lung base are subjected to a higher hydrostatic pressure (therefore, increased driving force for flow)
• In addition, the increase in hydrostatic pressure will distend these vessels lowering the the resistance to blood flow. Thus, pulmonary

blood flow in the bases will be greater than in the apices.

Ventilation also increases from apex to base, but is less affected than blood flow because the density of air is much less than blood. In diastole, the hydrostatic pressure in the pulmonary artery is $11\,cmH_2O$. The apex of each lung is approximately 15cm above the right ventricle, and the hydrostatic pressure within these vessel is lowered or even zero. Vessels at the apex of the lung are therefore narrower or even collapse because of the lower hydrostatic pressure within them.

### Pattern of blood flow
The distribution of blood flow within the lung can be described in three zones (Fig. 5.8).

### Zone 1 (at the apex of the lung)
In zone 1, arterial pressure is less than alveolar pressure: capillaries collapse and no flow occurs. Note that under normal conditions, there is no zone 1 because there is sufficient pressure to perfuse the apices.

### Zone 2
In zone 2, arterial pressure is greater than alveolar pressure, which is greater than venous pressure. Postcapillary venules open and close depending on

hydrostatic pressure (i.e. hydrostatic pressure difference in systole and diastole). Flow is determined by the arterial–alveolar pressure difference (transmural pressure).

### Zone 3 (at the base of the lung)
In zone 3, arterial pressure is greater than venous pressure, which is greater than alveolar pressure. Blood flow is determined by arteriovenous pressure difference as in the systemic circulation.

## Control of pulmonary blood flow
We have already mentioned how the pulmonary circulation adapts to changes of hydrostatic pressure and how it can recruit capillaries during exercise. These effects are passive and caused by changes in hydrostatic pressure. The pulmonary blood flow can also be controlled by other local mechanisms to improve efficiency of gaseous exchange. Like the systemic circulation, other mediators such as thromboxane, histamine and prostacylin also alter pulmonary vascular tone.

Contraction and relaxation of smooth muscle contained within the walls of arteries, arterioles and veins is the mechanism for active control of pulmonary blood flow.

An important mechanism of control, particularly in disease, is hypoxic vasoconstriction.

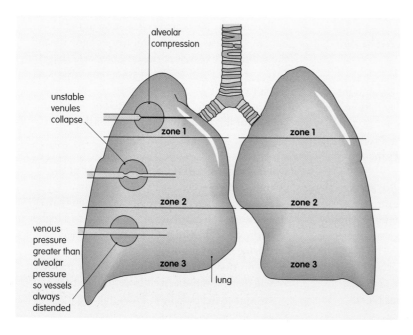

**Fig. 5.8** Zones of pulmonary blood flow.

## Hypoxic vasoconstriction

The aim of breathing is to oxygenate the blood sufficiently. This is achieved by efficient gaseous exchange between alveolar gas and the bloodstream. If an area of lung is poorly ventilated and the alveolar partial pressure of oxygen (alveolar oxygen tension) is low, perfusion of this area with blood will lead to inefficient gaseous exchange. It would be more beneficial to perfuse an area that is well ventilated. This is the basis behind hypoxic vasoconstriction. Small pulmonary arteries and arterioles are in close proximity to the gas exchange surface, and vessels in and around the alveolar wall are surrounded by alveolar gas. Oxygen passes through the alveolar walls into the smooth muscle of the blood vessel by diffusion. The extremely high oxygen tension to which these smooth muscles are normally exposed acts to dilate the pulmonary vessels. In contrast, if the alveolar oxygen tension is low, pulmonary blood vessels are constricted, which leads to reduced blood flow in the area of lung which is poorly ventilated and diversion to other regions where alveolar oxygen tension is high.

It should be noted that it is the partial pressure of oxygen in the alveolus ($P_AO_2$) and not in the pulmonary artery ($P_aO_2$) that causes this response.

The actual mechanism and the chemical mediators involved in hypoxic vasoconstriction are not known. Many mediators have been investigated and nitric oxide has been shown to reverse the vasoconstriction. Factors that regulate pulmonary vascular tone are shown in Fig. 5.9.

In summary:
- The aim of ventilation is to oxygenate blood sufficiently and blow off carbon dioxide
- High levels of alveolar oxygen dilate pulmonary vessels
- Low levels of alveolar oxygen constrict pulmonary blood vessels
- This aims to produce efficient gaseous exchange.

Higher than normal alveolar carbon dioxide partial pressures also cause pulmonary blood vessels to constrict, thus reducing blood flow to an area that is not well ventilated.

## Pulmonary water balance

Figure 5.10 shows the structure of the alveolar–capillary membrane. Note that on one side there is the interstitial space whilst on the other the epithelial and endothelial membranes are fused and there is only a tiny membrane between pulmonary capillary blood and the alveolus. It is essential for gas exchange that this surface is kept dry; the mechanisms by which liquid is prevented from entering are discussed below.

Fluids in the pulmonary capillary and interstitial spaces obey Starling's forces (Fig. 5.11). In addition, surfactant lowers the surface tension of the alveolar

| Factors that regulate vascular tone | |
| --- | --- |
| **Vasodilation** | **Vasoconstriction** |
| Nitric oxide | Histamine |
| Prostacyclin | Serotonin |
| Prostaglandin | Thromboxane |
| Bradykinin | Leukotrienes |
| Acetylcholine | Platelet activating factor |
| | Angiotensin II |

**Fig. 5.9** Factors that regulate vascular tone.

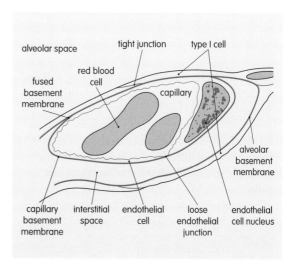

**Fig. 5.10** The alveolar–capillary membrane. Note that the basement membranes of the alveolus and capillary are fused on one side; on the other is the interstitial space. (Adapted with permission from *Crofton and Douglas's Respiratory Diseases* 5e, Blackwell Science 2000, Vol. 1.)

**Fig. 5.11** Comparison of Starling's forces between pulmonary and systemic capillary beds. The resorptive force is positive and hence fluid is reabsorbed into the pulmonary capillary. Without surfactant in the alveoli the tissue hydrostatic pressure could be −23 mmHg and the reabsorptive force would be −10 mmHg causing transudation of fluid into the alveolus.

**pulmonary capillary**

arterial                                                    venous

fluid                          fluid

| hydrostatic pressure 10 mmHg | colloid oncotic pressure 28 mmHg | hydrostatic pressure 7 mmHg |

(= intrapleural pressure)

| tissue hydrostatic pressure | −4 mmHg | −4 mmHg |
| colloid oncotic pressure | 5 mmHg | 5 mmHg |

| net hydrostatic pressure | 10 − (−4) = 14 mmHg | 7 − (−4) = 11 mmHg |
| net colloid oncotic pressure | 28 − 5 = 23 mmHg | 28 − 5 = 23 mmHg |

**reabsorptive force 23 − 14 = 9 mmHg**        **reabsorptive force 23 − 11 = 12 mmHg**

**systemic capillary**

arterial                                                    venous

fluid                          fluid

| hydrostatic pressure 30 mmHg | colloid oncotic pressure 28 mmHg | hydrostatic pressure 10 mmHg |

| tissue hydrostatic pressure | −6 mmHg | −6 mmHg |
| colloid oncotic pressure | 5 mmHg | 5 mmHg |

| net hydrostatic pressure | 30 − (−6) = 36 mmHg | 10 − (−6) = 16 mmHg |
| net colloid oncotic pressure | 28 − 5 = 23 mmHg | 28 − 5 = 23 mmHg |

**ultrafiltration force = 13 mmHg**        **reabsorptive force = 7 mmHg**

lining fluid, thus reducing the transudation of liquid into the alveolus by increasing the interstitial pressure from −23 mmHg to −4 mmHg. Hydrostatic pressure within the capillary tends to force fluid out into the interstitial space. The colloid osmotic pressure difference between interstitial space and capillary tends to force fluid into the capillary.

The resultant fluid flow from capillary to interstitial space is small and normally fluid drains to lymphatics and the perivascular space. Under pathological conditions, fluid can reside either in the interstitial space (interstitial oedema) or in the alveoli (alveolar oedema). This may be due to an increase in:

- Hydrostatic pressure in the pulmonary capillaries
- Permeability of the capillaries.

Adult respiratory distress syndrome (ARDS) is non-cardiogenic pulmonary oedema caused by capillaries which have become acutely inflamed and 'leaky'.

## The ventilation:perfusion relationship

### Basic concepts

To achieve efficient gaseous exchange, it is essential that the flow of gas (ventilation: $\dot{V}$) and the flow of blood (perfusion: $\dot{Q}$) are closely matched.

The ideal situation would be where:

- All alveoli are ventilated equally with gas of identical composition and pressure

• All pulmonary capillaries in the alveolar wall are perfused with equal amounts of mixed venous blood.

Unfortunately, this is not the case. Ventilation is not uniform throughout the lung; neither is perfusion.

The partial pressure of oxygen in the alveoli determines the amount of oxygen transferred to the blood. Two factors affect the partial pressure of oxygen in the alveoli: the amount of ventilation (i.e. the addition of oxygen to the alveolar compartment) and the perfusion of blood through pulmonary capillaries (i.e. the removal of oxygen from the alveolar compartment).

It is the ratio of ventilation to perfusion that determines the concentration of oxygen in the alveolar compartment.

## Ventilation:perfusion ratio

By looking at the ventilation:perfusion ratio, we can see how well ventilation and perfusion are matched.

By definition, ventilation:perfusion ratio $= \dot{V}_A/\dot{Q}$

where $\dot{V}_A$ = alveolar minute ventilation (usually about 4.2 L/min); $\dot{Q}$ = pulmonary blood flow (usually about 5.0 L/min).

Thus, normal $\dot{V}_A/\dot{Q} = 0.84$ (i.e. approximately 1)

This is an average value across the lung. Different ventilation:perfusion ratios are present throughout the lung from apex to base (Fig. 5.12).

## Extremes of ventilation:perfusion ratio

Looking at the ventilation:perfusion ratio, it can be seen that there are two extremes to this relationship. These extremes were introduced in Chapter 1. Either there is:
• No ventilation (a shunt): $\dot{V}_A/\dot{Q} = 0$
• No perfusion (dead space): $\dot{V}_A/\dot{Q} = \infty$

## Right-to-left shunt

A right-to-left shunt is described when the pulmonary circulation bypasses the ventilation process (Fig. 5.13), either by:
• Bypassing the lungs completely (e.g. transposition of great vessels, see Chapter 3)
• Perfusion of an area of lung that is not ventilated.

The shunted blood will not have been oxygenated or been able to given up its carbon dioxide. Therefore, its levels of $PO_2$ and $PCO_2$ are those of venous blood. When added to the systemic circulation, this blood will proportionately decrease arterial $PO_2$; it is called the venous admixture.

A right-to-left shunt may cause a low arterial $PO_2$ but a normal $PCO_2$—how can this be explained? The venous admixture has a low arterial $PO_2$ and high $PCO_2$. This initially causes the arterial $PO_2$ to be lowered and the arterial $PCO_2$ to be increased. This high $PCO_2$ causes an increase in ventilation, which reduces $PCO_2$ in those areas of lung that are well

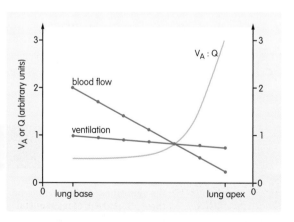

**Fig. 5.12** Distribution of ventilation ($V_A$) and perfusion (Q). Blood flow and ventilation are both higher at the lung base but the difference in blood flow is more striking. (Adapted from *Respiratory Physiology* 2e by J. Widdicombe and A. Davies. Edward Arnold, 1991.)

**Fig. 5.13** Shunted blood. The shunted blood has a low oxygen concentration (i.e. of venous blood) and is known as the venous admixture.

ventilated, giving them a lower than normal $PCO_2$. This reduction in $PCO_2$ lowers the arterial $PCO_2$ to its normal value. This additional ventilation in well-ventilated areas, however, has very little effect on the arterial oxygen content because of the shape of the oxyhaemoglobin dissociation curve (i.e. haemoglobin is already saturated in the well-ventilated areas). Only a small increase in oxygen content is seen because of increased dissolved oxygen from the overventilated areas. This small increase in $PO_2$ from overventilated areas is unable to increase the arterial $PO_2$ to its normal value. Thus, the mixed blood has a lower $PO_2$ and normal $PCO_2$.

In normal subjects, there is only a very small amount of shunt (about 1%). However, right-to-left shunt makes a significant contribution to abnormal gas exchange in some disease states, notably:

- Cyanotic congenital heart disease
- Pulmonary oedema
- Severe pneumonia.

Giving oxygen to patients with shunt does not increase arterial oxygen tension. This makes sense because:
- Shunted blood is not actually exposed to the oxygen.
- Haemoglobin is already saturated in well-ventilated areas.

## Effect of V/Q mismatch on blood gases

The easiest way to imagine how the ventilation:perfusion ratio affects the arterial oxygen concentration is to look at the extremes of ventilation:perfusion.

### Ventilation but no perfusion

If a unit of lung is ventilated but not perfused, that unit will have a $PO_2$ and $PCO_2$ of inspired gas, because no gas exchange with the blood has taken place (Fig. 5.14C). If the perfusion of the unit increases (lowering the ventilation:perfusion ratio), $PCO_2$ will rise and the $PO_2$ will fall (an example of lung normally perfused is shown in Fig. 5.14A).

### Perfusion but no ventilation

If the perfusion is increased further and the ventilation reduced until the unit of lung is perfused but not ventilated, the gas within that unit will be in equilibrium with the blood perfusing the alveolar capillaries (venous blood), because no gas exchange has taken place (Fig. 5.14B). This relationship is also described in Fig. 5.15; read the caption to work through the figure.

It should be noted that:

- $PO_2$ varies to a much greater extent than $PCO_2$ with small changes in ventilation:perfusion ratio
- Overall, variation in $PO_2$ is much greater than that of $PCO_2$

**Fig. 5.14** The effect of altering the ventilation:perfusion ratio on the $P_AO_2$ and $P_ACO_2$ in a lung unit. (A) normal lung. (B) lung unit is not ventilated; $O_2$ falls and $CO_2$ rises within lung unit. (C) lung unit is not perfused; $O_2$ is not taken up and $CO_2$ does not diffuse into the alveolus.

**Fig. 5.15** The effect of altering the ventilation:perfusion ratio on both $PO_2$ and $PCO_2$. Point A represents normal arterial values of $PO_2$ and $PCO_2$ at a value of ventilation: perfusion ratio of 0.84. Increasing ventilation:perfusion ratios reduces $PCO_2$ but causes a corresponding rise in $PO_2$. Eventually point I is reached, where $PCO_2$ is zero and $PO_2$ is equal to that of inspired gas; this relates to a point of infinite ventilation:perfusion (i.e. there is no perfusion). Point V represents the opposite end of the ventilation: perfusion spectrum where the lung is not ventilated at all. The alveolar end capillary blood partial pressures of oxygen and carbon dioxide are of venous values. Thus values of ventilation:perfusion ratio greater than normal are to the right of point A and those that are less are to the left. (Adapted from *Physiology* 3e by R.M. Berne and M.N. Levy. Mosby Year Book, 1993.)

- $PCO_2$ cannot rise above that of mixed venous blood, assuming the ventilation:perfusion ratio applies to a small area of lung.

## Regional variation of ventilation and perfusion

Both ventilation and perfusion increase towards the lung base because of the effects of gravity.

Because the blood has a greater density than air, the gravitational effects on perfusion are much greater than on ventilation. This leads to a regional variation (see Fig. 5.12) in ventilation:perfusion ratio from lung apex (high $\dot{V}/\dot{Q}$) to lung base (low $\dot{V}/\dot{Q}$).

These regional variations in ventilation:perfusion ratio are caused by the lung being upright; thus, changes in posture will alter the ventilation: perfusion ratio throughout the lung. For example, when lying down, the posterior area of the lung has a low ventilation:perfusion ratio and the anterior area has a high ventilation:perfusion ratio.

The effect of high and low ventilation:perfusion ratios on carbon dioxide and oxygen in the alveolus and blood is highlighted in Fig. 5.16 and described below.

### At low ventilation:perfusion ratios (e.g. at the lung base)
#### Effect on carbon dioxide concentrations
Carbon dioxide diffuses from the blood to alveoli; however, because ventilation is low, carbon dioxide is not taken away as rapidly. Thus, carbon dioxide tends to accumulate in the alveolus until a new, higher steady-state $P_ACO_2$ is reached.

Diffusion occurs only until equilibrium is achieved, when $P_aCO_2$ is equal to $P_ACO_2$. If there were no ventilation, the $P_ACO_2$ of this lung unit would rise quickly to meet mixed venous $P_vCO_2$, and no diffusion could take place.

Assuming that the overall lung function is normal, this regional variation in $P_ACO_2$ will not affect overall $P_vCO_2$. Thus, reducing the ventilation:perfusion ratio will not increase $P_aCO_2$ above the mixed venous value.

#### Effect on oxygen concentrations
Oxygen diffuses from the alveolus into the blood; however, because ventilation is low, oxygen taken up by the blood and metabolized is not replenished fully by new air entering the lungs. Oxygen in the alveolus is depleted until a new, lower steady-state $P_AO_2$ is reached. Because diffusion continues until equilibrium is achieved, the $P_aO_2$ of this unit will also be low (Fig. 5.16A).

### At high ventilation:perfusion ratios (e.g. at the lung apex)
#### Effect on carbon dioxide concentrations
The carbon dioxide diffusing from the blood is nearly all removed; carbon dioxide in the alveolus is depleted until a new, lower steady-state $P_ACO_2$ is reached. Diffusion continues until equilibrium is achieved: $P_aCO_2$ will also be low.

If we take this to the extreme, then as ventilation: perfusion ratios tend to zero, $P_ACO_2$ tends to zero.

#### Effect on oxygen concentrations
Oxygen diffusing from the alveolar gas is not taken away by the blood in such large amounts because the relative blood flow is reduced; in addition, oxygen is replenished with each breath. Thus, oxygen tends to accumulate in the alveolus until a new steady-state concentration is reached (Fig. 5.16B).

**Fig. 5.16** Ventilation and perfusion at lung base (A) and apex (B). At the lung base perfusion is high and the V/Q ratio is low. This reduces alveolar $O_2$ and raises $CO_2$. At the apex the V/Q ratio is higher, leading to a high alveolar $O_2$ and more $CO_2$ blown off.

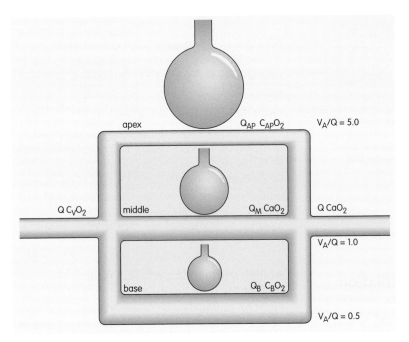

**Fig. 5.17** Ventilation and perfusion at the lung apex, middle and base.

Diffusion occurs until a new higher equilibrium is achieved; thus, $P_aO_2$ is also higher.

## How do regional variations in V/Q affect overall gas exchange?

As mentioned previously, a normal healthy lung is not ventilated or perfused uniformly and ventilation: perfusion ratios vary (Fig. 5.17). The actual difference between gaseous exchange in a healthy lung and in an ideal lung is perhaps smaller than one

might expect. The ideal lung is capable of only 2–3% more gaseous exchange.

However, if the ventilation:perfusion inequality from lung apex to base becomes more severe, the transfer of oxygen and carbon dioxide will be significantly affected. The majority of the blood will come from poorly ventilated areas at the lung base, where $P_AO_2$ is low; thus $P_aO_2$ will be low. $P_aCO_2$ will similarly be raised at the base of the lung.

**Fig. 5.18** Normal human ventilation:perfusion curves. Note that ventilation and perfusion are matched in health. At the average V/Q ratio of 0.8, blood flows to the areas that are well ventilated. (Adapted from *Respiratory Physiology* 5e by J. West. Lippincott Williams & Wilkins, 1995.)

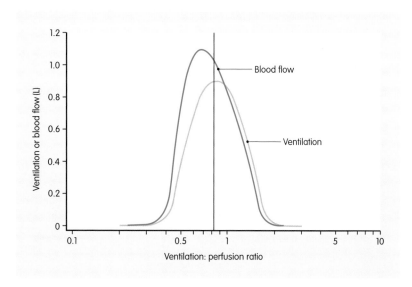

The non-linear shape of the oxyhaemoglobin dissociation curve does not allow areas with high ventilation:perfusion ratios to compensate for areas of low ratio.

### Ventilation: perfusion distributions

If we look at the variation in ventilation and blood flow in relation to $\dot{V}/\dot{Q}$ in the normal lung (Fig. 5.18), it should be noted that:

- Where the ventilation:perfusion ratio is high, absolute values of ventilation are low
- Where the ventilation:perfusion ratio is low, absolute values of blood flow are also low.

Thus, the majority of blood flow and ventilation go to areas of lung that have a ventilation:perfusion ratio that is close to the average value. In the diseased lung, this might not be the case and blood may flow to areas where ventilation:perfusion ratios are extremely low; this is effectively a shunt.

Areas with extremely high ventilation:perfusion ratios may be ventilated to high absolute values and receive very poor blood flow. This is effectively wasted ventilation (Fig. 5.19).

## Measurement of ventilation and perfusion

### Ventilation:perfusion scans

In clinical practice, ventilation:perfusion ratios are assessed primarily by means of radioisotope scans.

Ventilation is detected by inhalation of a gas or aerosol labelled with the radioisotope, $Xe^{133}$. The distribution of pulmonary blood flow is tested with an intravenous injection of $Tc^{99m}$-labelled macro-aggregated albumin (MAA). These radioactive particles are larger than the diameter of the pulmonary capillaries and they remain lodged for several hours. A gamma camera is then used to detect the position of the MAAs.

The two scans are then assessed together for 'filling defects', or areas where ventilation and perfusion are not matched. The technique is primarily used to detect pulmonary emboli. Spiral CT scans are now superseding this technique. Figure 5.20 shows a lung scan following pulmonary embolism.

### Multiple inert gas procedure

As noted above, radioisotope scans can allow only a broad comparison to be made between areas of ventilation and perfusion in the lungs. The multiple inert gas procedure measures the actual ratio of ventilation:perfusion, but is a much more complicated technique. In the multiple inert gas procedure, six inert gases are infused into the venous blood stream. Each gas has a different partition coefficient in gas and blood (i.e. different solubility in gas and blood).

Steady state is reached by a constant rate of infusion and expiration. From component balances

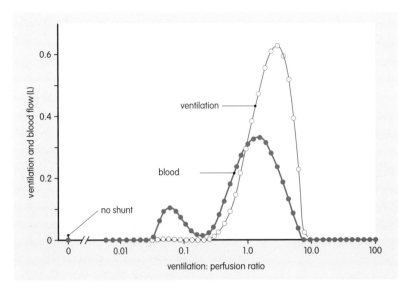

**Fig. 5.19** Ventilation:perfusion curves for patient with chronic bronchitis. (Redrawn with permission from *Respiratory Physiology* 5e by J. West. Lippincott Williams & Wilkins, 1995.)

**Fig. 5.20** Ventilation:perfusion scan following pulmonary embolus. (Courtesy by Ivor Jones and the Nuclear Medicine staff, Derriford Hospital, Plymouth).

for each gas of amount infused and amount expired the ventilation:perfusion distribution is calculated.

Amount infused = $Pin \cdot S \cdot Q$

Amount expired = $Pex \cdot V$

where S = solubility of the gas.

Thus, ventilation and perfusion can be calculated giving a ventilation:perfusion distribution.

## Gas transport in the blood

### Oxygen transport

Oxygen is carried in the blood in two forms:
- Dissolved in plasma
- Bound to haemoglobin.

### Dissolved oxygen

To meet the metabolic demands of the body, large amounts of oxygen must be carried in the blood. We have seen that the amount of gas dissolved in solution is proportional to the partial pressure of the gas (Henry's law). The solubility of oxygen in the blood is low: 0.000225 mL of oxygen per kilopascal per millilitre of blood. With normal arterial $P_aO_2$ (100 mmHg; 13.3 kPa), for each 100 mL of blood there is only 0.003 mL of dissolved oxygen.

Normal cardiac output is 5.0 L/min; it is therefore capable of supplying:

$5 \times 1000 \times 0.003 = 15$ mL of oxygen per minute

At rest, the body requires approximately 250 mL of oxygen per minute. Thus, if all the oxygen in the blood was carried in the dissolved form, cardiac output would meet only 6% of the demand.

In fact, in contrast to the tiny amounts calculated above, the oxygen content of blood is approximately 200mL of oxygen per litre of arterial blood. Therefore, most of the oxygen must be carried in chemical combination, not in simple solution. Oxygen is combined with haemoglobin.

## Haemoglobin

Haemoglobin (Hb) is found in red blood cells and is a conjugate protein molecule, containing iron within its structure. The molecule consists of four polypeptide subunits, two $\alpha$ and two $\beta$. Associated with each polypeptide chain is a haem group that acts as a binding site for oxygen (Fig. 5.21).

The haem group consists of a porphyrin ring containing iron and is responsible for binding of oxygen:

• Haemoglobin contains iron in a ferrous ($Fe^{2+}$) or ferric ($Fe^{3+}$) state
• Only haemoglobin in the ferrous form can bind oxygen
• Methaemoglobin (containing iron in a ferric state) cannot bind oxygen.

The quaternary structure of haemoglobin determines its ability to bind oxygen.

In its deoxygenated state, haemoglobin (known as reduced haemoglobin) has a low affinity for oxygen.

The binding of one oxygen molecule to haemoglobin causes a conformational change in its protein structure; this positive cooperativity allows easier access to the other oxygen-binding sites, thus increasing haemoglobin's affinity for further binding of oxygen. Haemoglobin is capable of binding up to four molecules of oxygen.

$$Hb + 4O_2 \rightarrow Hb(O_2)_4$$

It should be noted that during this reaction the iron atom of the haem group remains in the ferrous $Fe^{2+}$ form. It is not oxidized to the ferric $Fe^{3+}$ form. The interaction of oxygen with haemoglobin is oxygenation *not* oxidation.

The main function of haemoglobin is to take up oxygen in the blood at the alveolar capillary membrane and to transport oxygen within the blood and release it into the tissues. However, haemoglobin also has other functions:

• Buffering of $H^+$ ions
• Transport of $CO_2$ as carbamino compounds.

## Haemoglobin binding

Haemoglobin has four binding sites; the amount of oxygen carried by haemoglobin in the blood depends on how many of these binding sites are occupied. Therefore, the haemoglobin molecule can be said to be saturated or partially saturated:

• Saturated—all four binding sites are occupied by $O_2$
• Partially saturated—some oxygen has bound to haemoglobin, but not all four sites are occupied.

If completely saturated, each gram of haemoglobin can carry 1.34mL of oxygen. There are 150g of haemoglobin per litre of the blood; therefore, the maximum binding of oxygen to haemoglobin we could expect is:

$$150 \times 1.34 = 201\,mL \text{ of oxygen per litre of blood}$$

In addition, there is approximately 10mL of $O_2$ in solution. The total (211mL) is called the oxygen capacity; the haemoglobin is said to be 100% saturated ($SO_2 = 100\%$). The actual amount of oxygen bonded to haemoglobin and dissolved in the blood at any one time is called the oxygen content.

The oxygen saturation ($SO_2$) of the blood is defined as the amount of oxygen carried in the blood, expressed as a percentage of oxygen capacity:

$$SO_2 = O_2 \text{ content} \div O_2 \text{ capacity} \times 100$$

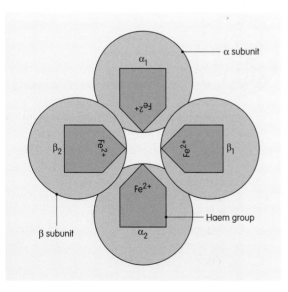

**Fig. 5.21** Schematic diagram of haemoglobin: $\alpha$ subunit consists of a polypeptide chain of 141 amino acids and one haem group; $\beta$ subunit consists of a polypeptide chain of 146 amino acids and one haem group.

## Cyanosis

Haemoglobin absorbs light of different wavelengths depending on whether it is in the reduced or oxygenated form. Oxyhaemoglobin appears bright red, whereas reduced haemoglobin appears purplish, giving a blueish pallor to skin. This is called cyanosis, which can be described as either central or peripheral. Cyanosis depends on the absolute amount of deoxygenated haemoglobin in the vessels, not the proportion of deoxygenated:oxygenated haemoglobin. In central cyanosis, there is more than 5g/dL deoxygenated haemoglobin in the blood and this can be seen in the peripheral tissues (e.g lips, tongue). Peripheral cyanosis is due to a local cause (e.g. vascular obstruction of a limb).

It follows that an anaemic patient with low haemoglobin may become dangerously desaturated without appearing cyanosed!

## Oxygen dissociation curve

How much oxygen binds to haemoglobin is dependent upon the partial pressure of oxygen in the blood. This relationship is represented by the oxygen dissociation curve (Fig. 5.22A); this is an equilibrium curve at specific conditions:
- 150g of haemoglobin per litre of blood
- pH 7.4
- Temperature 37°C.

You will need to be able to reproduce this curve in your exams. The easiest way to remember it is by using four points. Values at 25%, 50%, 75%, and 100% are useful markers and the curve is easily drawn from the origin through these points. You will also need to remember arterial and mixed venous blood partial pressures of oxygen.

### Factors affecting the oxygen dissociation curve

The shape of the curve, and therefore oxygen delivery to the tissues, is affected by a number of factors including:
- pH
- $CO_2$

- Temperature
- Other forms of haemoglobin.

These factors shift the oxygen dissociation curve to the right or to the left:
- A shift to the right allows easier dissociation of oxygen (i.e. lower oxygen saturation at any particular $PO_2$) and increases the oxygen release from oxyhaemoglobin
- A shift to the left makes oxygen binding easier (i.e. higher oxygen saturation at any particular $PO_2$) and increases the oxygen uptake by haemoglobin.

The following factors shift the curve to the right (Fig. 5.22B):
- Increased $PCO_2$ and decreased pH (increased hydrogen ion concentration), known as the Bohr shift
- Increased temperature
- Increase in 2,3-diphosphoglycerate (2,3-DPG), which binds to the β chains.

2,3-Diphosphoglycerate is a product of anaerobic metabolism. Red blood cells possess no mitochondria and therefore carry out anaerobic metabolism to produce energy. 2,3-DPG binds more strongly to reduced haemoglobin than to oxyhaemoglobin. Concentrations of 2,3-diphosphoglycerate increase in chronic hypoxia, e.g. in patients with chronic lung disease, or at high altitude.

If you cannot remember how the above factors affect the oxygen dissociation curve, it is helpful to think of exercising muscle. It would be useful if its blood supply gave up oxygen more easily (right shift of the curve). An exercising muscle produces carbon dioxide (increased carbon dioxide), which forms carbonic acid in the blood, which in turn dissociates to form hydrogen ions (lowers the pH). Exercising muscle is hot (increased temperature) and uses up oxygen forming more reduced haemoglobin in red blood cells (increased 2,3-DPG concentration).

**Fig. 5.22** (A) Oxyhaemoglobin dissociation curve. (B) The effect of temperature, $PCO_2$, pH and 2,3-DPG on the oxyhaemoglobin dissociation curve.

A

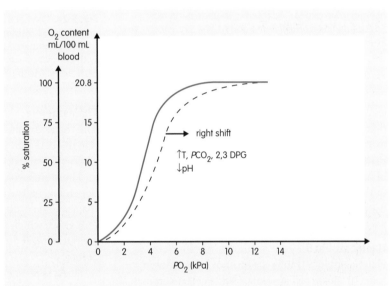

B

## Other forms of haemoglobin
### Myoglobin

Myoglobin is an iron-containing molecule found within skeletal muscle and cardiac muscle. It consists of a single polypeptide chain with a haem group:

- Myoglobin is capable of binding oxygen
- It acts as a temporary storage of oxygen within skeletal muscle
- Myoglobin has a higher affinity for oxygen than does normal adult haemoglobin (HbA), seen as a shift to the left of the dissociation curve (Fig. 5.23)

- Myoglobin is unsuitable for oxygen transport, because it binds oxygen at partial pressures below those of mixed venous blood (<40mmHg) and so could not readily release $O_2$ to the tissues.

### Fetal haemoglobin (HbF)

Fetal haemoglobin differs from adult haemoglobin by having two γ chains instead of two β chains (Fig. 5.23).

Fetal haemoglobin has a higher affinity for oxygen because its γ chains bind 2,3-DPG less avidly than the β chains of adult haemoglobin and are therefore able to bind oxygen at lower partial pressures (maternal venous $P_vO_2$ is low: <40mmHg).

**Fig. 5.23** Comparison of oxygen dissociation curves for myoglobin, fetal haemoglobin (HbF) and adult haemoglobin (HbA). (Adapted with permission from *Physiology* 3e, by R.M. Berne and M.N. Levy. Mosby Year Book, 1993.)

**Fig. 5.24** Oxyhaemoglobin curve showing effects of anaemia and carbon monoxide poisoning (50% HbCO and anaemia compared with normal haemoglobin). (Adapted with permission from *Physiology* 3e, by R.M. Berne and M.N. Levy. Mosby Year Book, 1993.)

Release of carbon dioxide from fetal haemoglobin causes a shift to the left of the fetal oxyhaemoglobin dissociation curve, thus increasing its affinity for oxygen. This released carbon dioxide binds to maternal haemoglobin, causing a shift to the right of maternal haemoglobin, thus reducing the affinity of the latter for oxygen. Oxygen is therefore released by maternal haemoglobin and bound by fetal haemoglobin. This is known as the double Bohr shift.

### Haemoglobin S
Haemoglobin S (HbS) is a form of haemoglobin found in sickle cell anaemia. Sickle cell anaemia is an autosomal recessive disorder in which there is a defect in the β-globulin chain of the haemoglobin molecule.

There is a substitution of the amino acid valine for glutamine at position 6 of the β chain, forming HbS. The heterozygote has sickle cell trait and the homozygote sickle cell anaemia. The abnormal HbS molecules polymerize when deoxygenated and cause the red blood cells containing the abnormal haemoglobin to sickle. The fragile sickle cells haemolyse and may block vessels, leading to ischaemia and infarction.

The heterozygous patient may have painful crises with bone and abdominal pain; there may also be intrapulmonary shunting.

### Thalassaemia
The thalassaemias are autosomal recessive disorders due to decreased production of either the α or the β chain of haemoglobin.

There are two genes for the β chain and, depending on the number of normal genes, the thalassaemia is quoted as major or minor. There are four genes which code for the α chain, leading to various clinical disorders depending on the genetic defect.

HbA$_2$ is present in a small amount in the normal population and consists of two α and two δ chains. It is markedly raised in β thalassaemia minor.

### Carboxyhaemoglobin (carbon monoxide poisoning)
Carbon monoxide (CO) displaces oxygen from oxyhaemoglobin because the affinity of haemoglobin for carbon monoxide is more than 200 times that for oxygen. This changes the shape of the oxyhaemoglobin dissociation curve. Note that in Fig. 5.24, showing the effects of carbon monoxide poisoning:

- In this instance, oxygen capacity is 50% of normal (i.e. 50% HbO$_2$ and 50% HbCO). The actual value will depend on the partial pressure of CO (e.g. with a $P$CO of 16mmHg, 75% of Hb will be in the form of HbCO)

- Saturation is achieved at a $PO_2$ of <40mmHg (below venous $PO_2$)
- HbCO causes a shift to the left for the oxygen dissociation curve (i.e. HbCO has a higher affinity for oxygen than normal $HbO_2$)
- Carbon monoxide binds to two of the four available haem groups
- Carbon monoxide takes a long time to be cleared, but this can be speeded up by ventilation with 100% oxygen
- The patient is not cyanosed, because HbCO is cherry-red.

## Carbon dioxide transport

There are three ways in which carbon dioxide can be transported in the blood:
- Dissolved in plasma
- As bicarbonate ions
- As carbamino compounds.

### Dissolved carbon dioxide

The solubility of carbon dioxide in the blood is much greater than that of oxygen (20 times greater); so, unlike oxygen, a significant amount (approximately 10%) of carbon dioxide is carried in solution.

The solubility of carbon dioxide = 5.2mL of carbon dioxide per kilopascal per litre of blood.

Normal $P_aCO_2 = 5.3$kPa.

So, the normal dissolved carbon dioxide = 27.4mL of carbon dioxide per litre of blood.

### Bicarbonate ions

Approximately 60% of carbon dioxide is transported as bicarbonate ions. Dissolved carbon dioxide interacts with water to form carbonic acid as follows:

$$CO_2 + H_2O \leftrightarrow H_2CO_3 \qquad (1)$$

Carbonic acid rapidly dissociates into ions:

$$H_2CO_3 \leftrightarrow H^+ + HCO_3^- \qquad (2)$$

The total reaction being:

$$CO_2 + H_2O \leftrightarrow H_2CO_3 \leftrightarrow H^+ + HCO_3^-$$

The first reaction is very slow in plasma, but within the red blood cell is dramatically speeded up by the enzyme, carbonic anhydrase. Reaction (2) is very fast, but if allowed to proceed alone, a large amount of $H^+$ ions would be formed, slowing down or halting the reaction. Haemoglobin has the property that it can bind $H^+$ ions and act as a buffer, thus allowing the reaction to proceed rapidly.

$$H^+ + HbO_2^- \leftrightarrow HHb + O_2$$

$$H^+ + Hb^- \leftrightarrow HHb$$

Reduced Hb can bind $H^+$ more actively; this is because reduced Hb is less acidic. The buffering capacities of haemoglobin and oxyhaemoglobin are conferred by the imidazole groups of the 36 histidine residues in the haemoglobin molecule. The imidazole groups dissociate less readily in the deoxygenated form of haemoglobin, which is therefore a weaker acid and so a better buffer. This action reduces $H^+$ ions in the plasma and also pulls the second reaction to the right.

The bicarbonate produced in the red blood cells diffuses down its concentration gradient into the plasma in exchange for chloride ions ($Cl^-$). This process is known as the chloride shift (see Fig. 5.25).

### Carbamino compounds

Carbon dioxide is capable of combining with proteins, interacting with their terminal amine groups to form carbamino compounds (Fig. 5.25). The most important protein involved is haemoglobin, as it is the most abundant in the blood. It is also important to note that:
- The interaction of carbon dioxide and haemoglobin is rapid
- No enzyme is involved
- Haemoglobin binds carbon dioxide in its deoxygenated state (reduced haemoglobin)
- Approximately 30% of carbon dioxide is carried as carbamino compounds.

### Haldane effect

Carriage of carbon dioxide is increased in deoxygenated blood because of two factors:
- Reduced haemoglobin has a greater affinity for carbon dioxide than oxyhaemoglobin
- Reduced haemoglobin is less acidic (i.e. a better proton acceptor: $H^+$ buffer) than oxyhaemoglobin.

The Haldane effect minimizes changes in pH of the blood when gaseous exchange occurs. The decrease in pH due to the oxygenation of Hb is offset by the increase that results from the loss of $CO_2$ to the alveolar air. The reverse occurs in the tissues.

This is an important effect because:

**Fig. 5.25** Binding of $CO_2$. Bicarbonate produced in the red blood cell diffuses out into the plasma down its concentration gradient. Chloride diffuses into the red blood cell to maintain electrical equilibrium pulling water with it. (Adapted with permission from *Physiology* 3e, by R.M. Berne and M.N. Levy. Mosby Year Book, 1993.)

- In peripheral capillaries, the unloading of oxygen from haemoglobin aids the binding of carbon dioxide to haemoglobin
- In pulmonary capillaries, the loading of oxygen on haemoglobin reduces the binding of carbon dioxide to haemoglobin.

This allows efficient gaseous exchange of carbon dioxide in the tissues and the lungs.

### Carbon dioxide dissociation curve

The carriage of carbon dioxide is dependent upon the partial pressure of carbon dioxide in the blood. This relationship is described by the carbon dioxide dissociation curve (Fig. 5.26). Compared with the oxygen dissociation curve:

- The carbon dioxide curve is more linear
- The carbon dioxide curve is much steeper than the oxygen curve (between venous and arterial partial pressure of respiratory gases)
- The carbon dioxide curve varies according to oxygen saturation of haemoglobin.

Two main carbon dioxide dissociation curves, for mixed venous and arterial blood, can be drawn (Fig. 5.26).

### Stores of oxygen and carbon dioxide

There are only small stores (approximately 1550mL) of oxygen in body tissues as follows:
- Lungs—450mL
- Blood—850mL

**Fig. 5.26** Ventilation effects on oxygen and carbon dioxide levels in the blood.

- Myoglobin—200mL
- Tissue fluids—50mL.

On the other hand, carbon dioxide has vast stores (approximately 120L):
- Blood carbonates
- Bone carbonates
- Tissue carbonates (including fat tissue).

A change in ventilation will affect both $P_aO_2$ and $P_aCO_2$. Because oxygen stores are small in comparison with those of carbon dioxide, a short-term variation in ventilation will affect $P_aO_2$. A

**Fig. 5.27** Differences between hyperventilation and hypoventilation.

| Comparison of hyperventilation and hypoventilation | |
| --- | --- |
| **Hyperventilation** | **Hypoventilation** |
| **Causes** | **Causes** |
| anxiety<br>brainstem lesion<br>drugs | obstruction:<br>  asthma<br>  chronic obstructive airways disease<br>  foreign body (e.g. peanut)<br>brainstem lesion<br>pneumothorax or lung collapse<br>trauma (e.g. fractured rib)<br>drugs, notably opioids |
| **Consequences** | **Consequences** |
| ventilation too great for metabolic demand<br>too much $CO_2$ blown off from lungs<br>$P_aCO_2$ <40 mmHg | ventilation is too low for metabolic demand<br>not enough $CO_2$ is blown off at the lungs<br>$P_aCO_2$ >40 mmHg |

persistent change in ventilation will be shown by a change in $P_aCO_2$. Clinically, ventilation is assessed by measurement of $P_aCO_2$.

## Hypoventilation and hyperventilation

If $P_aCO_2$ is a measure of ventilation, it is appropriate in a review of carbon dioxide transport to consider two key concepts in respiratory medicine: hypoventilation and hyperventilation.

For the body to function normally, ventilation must meet the metabolic demand of the tissues (Fig. 5.27).

Thus, metabolic tissue consumption of oxygen must be equal to the oxygen taken up in the blood from alveolar gas. Or, metabolic tissue production of carbon dioxide must be equal to the amount of carbon dioxide blown off at the alveoli.

### Hypoventilation

The term hypoventilation refers to a situation when ventilation is insufficient to meet metabolic demand.

### Hyperventilation

The term hyperventilation refers to a situation where ventilation is excessive to metabolic demand.

The alveolar ventilation equation (see Fig. 5.28 for derivation) states that if carbon dioxide produced in the tissues equals carbon dioxide exhaled (as is usual at rest) then alveolar $PCO_2$ (i.e. $P_ACO_2$) is inversely proportional to the alveolar ventilation:

$$P_ACO_2 = K \times \dot{V}CO_2 / \dot{V}_A$$

where $\dot{V}CO_2$ is the volume of $CO_2$ exhaled, $\dot{V}_A$ is the alveolar ventilation and K is a constant.

We can see that this makes sense: increasing alveolar ventilation increases the concentration of $CO_2$ blown off from the lungs.

Because alveolar gas is in equilibrium with the blood, $P_ACO_2$ can be estimated as $P_aCO_2$. Thus, it can be seen how ventilation will affect partial pressures of carbon dioxide and that hypoventilation and hyperventilation can be shown clinically by the partial pressure of carbon dioxide in the blood.

In order to relate $P_ACO_2$ to $P_AO_2$ so that we can see how hyperventilation and hypoventilation affect alveolar oxygen, we use the alveolar gas equation:

$$P_AO_2 = P_IO_2 - (P_ACO_2/R) + K$$

where $P_IO_2$ = partial pressure of oxygen in inspired air and $R$ = respiratory exchange ratio (or the ratio of $CO_2$ production to $O_2$ consumption: normally about 0.8).

Mild or moderate exercise in a normal subject does not cause hyperventilation: the depth of breathing is increased (hyperpnoea) to balance the increased metabolic demand in exercise.

## Hypercapnia and hypocapnia
### Hypercapnia

A high partial pressure (concentration) of carbon dioxide in the blood ($P_aCO_2$ >45 mmHg) is termed hypercapnia (Fig. 5.29).

### Hypocapnia

A low partial pressure of carbon dioxide in the blood ($P_aCO_2$ <40 mmHg) is termed hypocapnia.

The alveolar ventilation equation: states that the alveolar $PCO_2$ is inversely proportional to the alveolar ventilation (as long as $CO_2$ production is constant).

$$P_ACO_2 = K \cdot \dot{V}CO_2/\dot{V}_A$$

$\dot{V}CO_2$ = the volume of $CO_2$ exhaled
$\dot{V}_A$ is alveolar ventilation
K is a constant.

$CO_2$ exhaled ($\dot{V}CO_2$) = minute ventilation ($\dot{V}E$) × the fractional concentration of $CO_2$ in the expired air ($F_ECO_2$).
$CO_2$ produced in the tissues = exhaled $CO_2$

$$\dot{V}CO_2 = \dot{V}_E \cdot F_ECO_2$$

$CO_2$ expired = the amount of $CO_2$ released at the alveoli, so:

$$\dot{V}CO_2 = \dot{V}_A \cdot F_ACO_2$$

where $\dot{V}_A$ = alveolar ventilation; $F_ACO_2$ = fractional concentration of $CO_2$ at the alveoli.

$$F_ACO_2 = \dot{V}CO_2/V_A$$

Using Dalton's law, relating the partial pressure to fractional concentration:

$$P_ACO_2 \propto \dot{V}CO_2/\dot{V}_A$$

Or:

$$P_ACO_2 = K \cdot \dot{V}CO_2/\dot{V}_A$$

Fig. 5.28 The alveolar ventilation equation.

Fig. 5.29 Clinical signs of hypercapnia.

## Respiratory failure

Hypercapnia and hypocapnia are important concepts in the assessment of respiratory failure (see Chapter 8). Respiratory failure is defined as a $P_aO_2 < 8\,kPa$ (60 mmHg) and is divided into type I and type II depending on the $P_aCO_2$.

In type I respiratory failure, $P_aCO_2 < 6.5\,kPa$. $P_aO_2$ is low (hypoxaemic), but $P_aCO_2$ may be normal or low; this represents a ventilation : perfusion mismatch.

In type II respiratory failure, $P_aCO_2 > 6.5\,kPa$. Both $P_aO_2$ and $P_aCO_2$ indicate that the lungs are not well ventilated.

The significance of this classification is that in type II respiratory failure the patient may have developed tolerance to increased levels of $P_aCO_2$; in other words, the drive for respiration no longer relies on hypercapnic drive (high $P_aCO_2$) but on hypoxic drive (low $P_aO_2$). Thus, if the patient is given high-concentration oxygen therapy the hypoxic drive for ventilation may decrease and the patient may stop breathing and die!

# Acid–base balance

## Normal pH

The pH of the intracellular and extracellular compartments must be tightly controlled for the body to function efficiently, or at all. The normal arterial pH lies within a relatively narrow range: 7.35–7.45 ([H$^+$] range, 45–35 mmol/L). An acid–base disturbance arises when arterial pH lies outside this range. If the blood pH is less than 7.35, an acidosis is present; if pH is greater than 7.45, the term alkalosis is used. Although a larger variation in pH can be tolerated (pH 6.8–7.8) for a short time, recovery is often impossible if blood remains at pH 6.8 for long.

Such a tight control on blood pH is achieved by a combination of blood buffers and the respiratory and renal systems which make adjustments to return pH towards its normal levels.

Before we review the mechanism of compensation, and discuss the acid–base disturbances, it is useful to revise some key concepts.

## Key concepts in acid–base balance
### Metabolic production of acids
Products of metabolism (carbon dioxide, lactic acid, phosphate, sulphate etc.) form acidic solutions, thus increasing the hydrogen ion concentration and reducing pH. We also have an intake of acids in our diet (approximately 50–100mmol $H^+$ per day).

We rely on three methods to control our internal hydrogen ion concentration:
- Dilution of body fluids
- The physiological buffer system
- Excretion of volatile and non-volatile acids.

### Buffers
A buffer is a substance that can either bind or release hydrogen ions, therefore keeping the pH relatively constant even when considerable quantities of acid or base are added. There are four buffers of the blood:
- Haemoglobin
- Plasma proteins
- Phosphate
- Bicarbonate.

It is the bicarbonate system that acts as the principal buffer and which is of most interest in respiratory medicine.

We have already seen that $CO_2$ dissolves in water and reacts to form carbonic acid and that this dissociates to form bicarbonate and protons:

$$CO_2 + H_2O \leftrightarrow H_2CO_3 \leftrightarrow H^+ + HCO_3^-$$

This equilibrium tells us that changes in either $CO_2$ or $HCO_3^-$ will have an effect on pH. For example, increasing $CO_2$ will drive the reaction to the right, increasing hydrogen ion concentration.

 Remember that increasing the hydrogen ion concentration makes a solution more acid, i.e. it *reduces* pH.

As changes in $CO_2$ and bicarbonate can alter pH, controlling these elements allows the system to control acid–base equilibrium. This is why the bicarbonate buffer system is so useful; the body has control over both elements:
- Carbon dioxide is regulated through changes in ventilation
- Bicarbonate concentrations are determined by the kidneys.

### The Henderson–Hasselbalch equation
We can calculate the pH resulting from the dissociation of carbonic acid by using the Henderson–Hasselbalch equation. In its simplest form this states:

$$[H^+] \propto PCO_2/[HCO_3^-]$$

The effect on pH of changing carbon dioxide or bicarbonate is now even clearer: if carbon dioxide rises, and there is no change in bicarbonate, then the hydrogen ion concentration will rise.

## Acid–base disturbances
As noted above, blood pH can either be higher than normal (alkalosis) or lower (acidosis). From the Henderson–Hasselbalch equation we can see that an acidosis could be caused by either of:
- A rise in $PCO_2$
- A fall in $HCO_3^-$.

Similarly alkalosis could occur through:
- A fall in $PCO_2$
- A rise in $HCO_3^-$.

Where the primary change is in $CO_2$ we term the disturbance *respiratory*, and where it is in bicarbonate, *metabolic*. This allows us to classify four types of disturbance:
- Respiratory alkalosis
- Respiratory acidosis
- Metabolic alkalosis
- Metabolic acidosis.

The disturbance was described as *primary* because the kidneys and lungs may try to return the acid–base disturbance towards normal values. This is called compensation and means that even in respiratory disturbances it may not be just $CO_2$ that is abnormal, bicarbonate may have altered too. Similarly $CO_2$ may be abnormal in a metabolic disturbance. The ways in which the two systems compensate are:

- The respiratory system alters ventilation; this happens quickly
- The kidney alters excretion of bicarbonate; this takes 2–3 days.

It is now clear that lung disease that affects gas exchange and therefore $PCO_2$ will have major effect on the body's acid–base status. It is also clear that whilst the respiratory system can act quickly to compensate for metabolic disturbances, it will take time for compensation to take place in respiratory disease; the renal system cannot act as quickly. We see this in clinical practice: a change in bicarbonate is characteristic of chronic lung disease, rather than acute.

## Assessing acid–base disturbances

Assessing acid–base disorders is relatively simple if you appoach the problem in stages (Fig. 5.30).
1. Start with the pH—is it outside the normal range?
2. If there is an acidosis or alkalosis, can it be explained by a change in $CO_2$?
3. If it can, then the primary disturbance is respiratory.
4. Now look at bicarbonate—has this moved to return the ratio to normal?
5. If it has, it is a respiratory disorder with metabolic compensation.

## Davenport diagram

The Davenport diagram (Fig. 5.31) demonstrates the relationship between plasma $[HCO_3^-]$, pH and $PCO_2$ in a graphical form.

## Respiratory acidosis

Respiratory acidosis results from an increase in $PCO_2$ caused by:
- Hypoventilation (less $CO_2$ is blown off)
- Ventilation:perfusion mismatch.

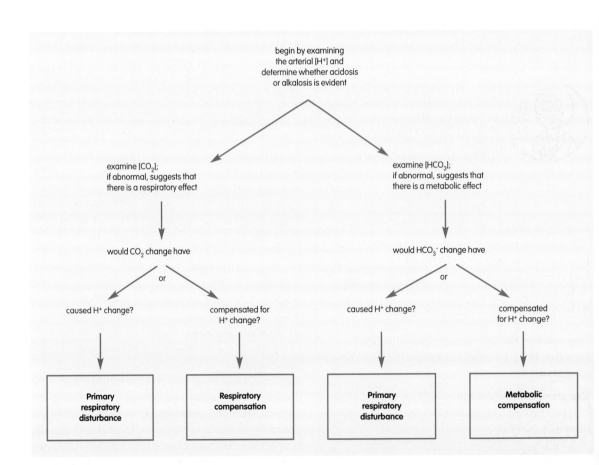

**Fig. 5.30** Assessing acid–base disorders.

**Fig. 5.31** The relationship between plasma $[HCO_3^-]$, pH and $PCO_2$. A buffer line runs from points A to B. Any change in $PCO_2$ will have an equivalent rise or fall in $[HCO_3^-]$ because of bicarbonate buffering of hydrogen ions; this can be shown by moving up and down the buffer line. Point N shows the normal plasma pH and $[HCO_3^-]$. Lines running perpendicular to the buffer line are of constant $PCO_2$.

From the Henderson–Hasselbach equation, we see that an increase in $PCO_2$ causes an increase in hydrogen ion concentration (i.e. a reduction in pH). Thus, plasma bicarbonate concentration increases to compensate for the increased hydrogen ion concentration (Fig. 5.32).

Throughout the following text, it is easiest to follow the principles of acid–base balance by using the Davenport diagram.

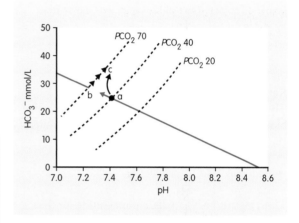

**Fig. 5.32** Respiratory acidosis causes increases in $PCO_2$, $HCO_3^-$ and reduction in pH shown as a move from a to b. The kidneys compensate by increasing $HCO_3^-$ reabsorption and production shown from point b to point c. Arrows a–c show a real-life situation.

## Renal compensation

The increase in hydrogen ion concentration in the blood results in increased filtration of hydrogen ions at the glomeruli, thus:

- Increasing $HCO_3^-$ reabsorption
- Increasing $HCO_3^-$ production.

Thus, plasma $HCO_3^-$ rises compensating for the increased $[H^+]$, i.e. renal compensation raises pH towards normal.

## Causes of respiratory acidosis

Mechanisms reducing ventilation or causing V:Q mismatch include:

- COPD
- Asthma
- Blocked airway (by tumour or foreign body)

- Spontaneous lung collapse, brainstem lesion
- Injury to the chest wall.

Drugs that reduce respiratory drive (ventilation) including morphine, barbiturates and general anaesthetics.

## Respiratory alkalosis

Respiratory alkalosis results from a decrease in $PCO_2$ generally caused by alveolar hyperventilation (more carbon dioxide is blown off). This causes a decrease in hydrogen ion concentration and thus an increase in pH (Fig. 5.33).

**Fig. 5.33** Respiratory alkalosis causes reduced $PCO_2$, $HCO_3^-$ and increases the pH. Shown as a move from point a to point b. The kidneys compensate by reducing the rate of renal excretion of $H^+$ so that less $HCO_3^-$ is reabsorbed or produced by the kidney. This is shown as a move from point b to point c. The real-life situation is shown from point a to c.

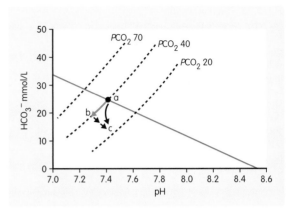

**Fig. 5.34** Metabolic acidosis causes a rise in $H^+$, reduced $HCO_3^-$ and reduced pH. Shown as a move from point a to point b. The lungs compensate by blowing off $CO_2$ and therefore increasing the pH, shown as a move from point b to point c. The arrows a–c show the real-life situation.

### Renal compensation

The reduction in hydrogen ion concentration in the blood results in decreased hydrogen ion filtration at the glomeruli, thus:

- Reducing $HCO_3^-$ reabsorption
- Reducing $HCO_3^-$ production.

Thus, plasma $HCO_3^-$ falls, compensating for the reduced $[H^+]$; i.e. renal compensation reduces pH towards normal.

### Causes of respiratory alkalosis

The causes of respiratory alkalosis include:

- Increased ventilation—caused by hypoxic drive in pneumonia, diffuse interstitial lung diseases, high altitude etc
- Hyperventilation—brainstem damage, infection causing fever, drugs (e.g. aspirin), hysterical overbreathing.

## Metabolic acidosis

Metabolic acidosis results from an excess of hydrogen ions in the body, which reduces bicarbonate concentration (shifting the equation below to the left). Respiration is unaffected; therefore, $PCO_2$ is initially normal (Fig. 5.34).

### Respiratory compensation

$$CO_2 + H_2O \leftrightarrow H_2CO_3 \leftrightarrow H^+ + HCO_3^-$$

The reduction in pH is detected by the peripheral chemoreceptors. This causes an increase in ventilation, which lowers $PCO_2$. Also:

- The above equation is driven further to the left, reducing hydrogen ion concentration and bicarbonate
- The decrease in hydrogen ion concentration raises pH towards normal.

Respiratory compensation cannot fully correct the values of $PCO_2$, $[HCO_3^-]$ and $[H^+]$, as there is a limit to how far $PCO_2$ can fall with hyperventilation. Correction can be carried out only by removing the excess hydrogen ions from the body or restoring the lost bicarbonate (i.e. correcting the metabolic fault).

### Causes of metabolic acidosis

Causes of metabolic acidosis are:

- Ingestion of acid
- Loss of $HCO_3^-$ from the kidneys
- Metabolic production of hydrogen ions. The kidneys may not be able to excrete the excess hydrogen ions immediately, or at all (as in renal failure).

## Metabolic alkalosis

Metabolic alkalosis results from an increase in bicarbonate concentration or a fall in hydrogen ion

**Fig. 5.35** Metabolic alkalosis due to loss of H$^+$ ions and increase in HCO$_3^-$ with increase in pH shown as a move from point a to point b. The lungs compensate by reducing ventilation and increase $PCO_2$, shown as a move from point b to point c. The arrow from point a to point c shows the real situation.

concentration. Removing hydrogen ions from the right of the equation (below) drives the reaction to the right, increasing bicarbonate concentration. Decrease in hydrogen ion concentration raises pH; initially, $PCO_2$ is normal (Fig. 5.35).

## Respiratory compensation

$$CO_2 + H_2O \leftrightarrow H_2CO_3 \leftrightarrow H^+ + HCO_3^-$$

The increase in pH is detected by the peripheral chemoreceptors. This causes a decrease in ventilation which raises $PCO_2$. Also:

- The above equation is driven further to the right, increasing hydrogen ion and bicarbonate concentrations
- The decrease in hydrogen ion concentration raises pH towards normal.

Respiratory compensation is through alveolar hypoventilation but ventilation cannot reduce enough to correct the disturbance. This can only be carried out by removing the problem either of reduced hydrogen ion concentration or increased bicarbonate concentration. This is done by reducing renal hydrogen ion secretion.

More bicarbonate is excreted because more is filtered at the glomerulus and less is reabsorbed in combination with hydrogen ions.

## Causes of metabolic alkalosis

The causes of metabolic alkalosis include:

- Vomiting (hydrochloric acid loss from the stomach)
- Ingestion of alkaline substances
- Increased plasma bicarbonate.

- What are the normal diastolic and systolic pressures in the pulmonary circulation?
- Describe recruitment and distension. How do these affect pulmonary vascular resistance?
- Outline what factors affect pulmonary blood flow and resistance of the pulmonary vasculature.
- Describe the pattern of blood flow through the lungs in terms of three zones.
- Explain the term hypoxic vasoconstriction and its importance.
- Describe what is meant by the ventilation:perfusion ratio.
- State the two extremes of ventilation:perfusion ratio.
- Define venous admixture.
- Describe with the aid of a diagram how disease might affect the ventilation:perfusion ratio distribution.
- Describe the structure of haemoglobin and its ability to bind oxygen.
- Draw and explain the oxygen dissociation curve for haemoglobin. What factors affect the curve?
- Describe how fetal haemoglobin differs from adult haemoglobin and the double Bohr shift.
- Explain the terms hypoventilation and hyperventilation.
- State the normal blood pH range.
- What is a buffer? Give four examples of buffers in the blood and their relative importance.
- Draw a Davenport diagram.
- Explain what is meant by an acid–base disturbance. Explain the four deviations.
- List the causes for respiratory acidosis and alkalosis.
- List the causes for metabolic acidosis and alkalosis.

# 6. Control of Respiratory Function

## Control of ventilation

### Basics of control

Every control system needs certain key elements for it to function correctly. These are:

- A control variable—a variable to be kept within certain limits (e.g. $P_aCO_2$ or $P_aO_2$)
- A desired value for that control variable, often quoted as normal physiological range (e.g. $P_aCO_2$ of around 40mmHg)
- A measured value for the control variable (e.g. actual $P_aCO_2 = 46$mmHg, 35mmHg etc.)
- Sensors to detect the measured value or a difference from the desired value (e.g. muscle spindle stretch receptors or chemoreceptors)
- Effectors (e.g. respiratory muscles, which alter ventilation and thus change $P_aCO_2$)
- A controller that relates the measured value to the desired value and changes output to the effectors (respiratory muscles), altering ventilation.

There are two types of control system: feedback and feed-forward:

- Feedback control—the system detailed below (Fig. 6.1), in which the controller looks at the measured value of the control variable (e.g. $P_aCO_2$) and relates this to the desired value. Adjustments to the system are then made
- Feed-forward control—the system detailed below (Fig. 6.2), which anticipates the effects of external factors to the system and makes adjustments to the system in an attempt to control their effect. An example of this is behavioural control of breathing when we sing.

### Control within the respiratory system

When considering control of breathing, the main control variable is $P_aCO_2$ (we try to control this value near to 40mmHg). This can be carried out by adjusting the respiratory rate, the tidal volume, or both.

By controlling $P_aCO_2$ we are effectively controlling alveolar ventilation (see Chapter 3) and thus $P_ACO_2$.

Note that we move between $P_aO_2$ and $P_AO_2$ here and throughout the chapter. Remember that these are different—if you are unclear, the abbreviations are explained on p. 69.

Although $P_aCO_2$ is the main control variable, $P_aO_2$ is also controlled, but normally to a much lesser extent than $P_aCO_2$. However, the $P_aO_2$ control system can take over and become the main controlling system when the $P_aO_2$ drops below 50mmHg.

Control can seem to be brought about by:
- Metabolic demands of the body (*metabolic control*)—tissue oxygen demand and acid–base balance
- Behavioural demands of the body (*behavioural control*)—singing, coughing, laughing (i.e. control is voluntary).

These are essentially feedback and feed-forward control systems, respectively. The behavioural control of breathing overlays the metabolic control. Its control is derived from higher centres of the brain. The axons of neurons whose cell bodies are situated in the cerebral cortex bypass the respiratory centres in the brainstem and synapse directly with lower motor neurons that control respiratory muscles. This system will not be dealt with within this text; we shall deal only with the metabolic control of respiration.

### Metabolic control of breathing

Metabolic control of breathing is a function of the brainstem (pons and medulla). The controller can be considered as specific groups of neurons (previously called respiratory centres).

#### Pontine neurons

Those located in the pons are the pontine respiratory group and consist of two groups of neurons:

**Fig. 6.1** Example of feedback control in the respiratory system. $P_aCO_2$ is used as the control variable.

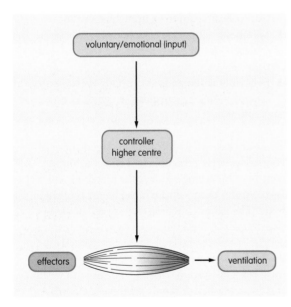

**Fig. 6.2** Example of feed-forward control in the respiratory system. Higher centres predict the effect of external changes (e.g. emotion or singing) and alter the output to the effectors (respiratory muscles) to achieve the required ventilation.

- Expiratory neurons in the nucleus parabrachialis medialis
- Inspiratory neurons in the lateral parabrachial nucleus and Kölliker's fuse nucleus.

The role of the pontine respiratory group (PRG) is to regulate (i.e. affect the activity of) the dorsal respiratory group (DRG) and possibly the ventral respiratory group (VRG, neuron groups in the medulla).

## Medullary neurons

It is believed that the medulla is responsible for respiratory rhythm.

Three groups of neurons associated with respiratory control have been identified in the medulla:

- The dorsal respiratory group, situated in the nucleus of tractus solitarius
- The ventral respiratory group, situated in the nucleus ambiguus and the nucleus retroambigualis
- The Bötzinger complex, situated rostral to the nucleus ambiguus.

These groups receive sensory information, which is compared with the desired value of control; adjustments are made to respiratory muscles to rectify any deviation from ideal.

The dorsal respiratory group (Fig. 6.3) contains neuron bodies of inspiratory upper motor neurons. These inhibit the activity of expiratory neurons in the ventral respiratory group and have an excitatory effect on lower motor neurons to the respiratory muscles, increasing ventilation.

Ventral respiratory group neurons in the nucleus ambiguus (Fig. 6.4) are again inspiratory upper motor neurons.

Ventral respiratory group neurons in the rostral part of the nucleus retroambigualis (Fig. 6.5) contain inspiratory upper motor neurons which go on to supply through their lower motor neurons external intercostal muscles and accessory muscles.

Ventral respiratory group neurons in the caudal part of the nucleus retroambigualis (Fig. 6.6) are expiratory upper motor neurons.

The Bötzinger complex (Fig. 6.7) contains only expiratory neurons. Its sensory input is through the nucleus tractus solitarius. It has two functions:

- Inhibition of inspiratory neurons of the dorsal and ventral respiratory groups
- Excitation of expiratory neurons in the ventral respiratory group.

Two main theories exist as to how the medulla influences respiratory rhythm:

**Fig. 6.3** Dorsal respiratory group. Note the output to respiratory muscle and inhibition of expiratory neurons in the ventral respiratory group. UMN = upper motor neuron; LMN = lower motor neuron; VRG = ventral respiratory group; DRG = dorsal respiratory group.

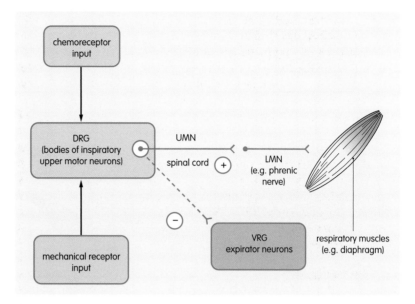

**Fig. 6.4** Ventral respiratory group in the nucleus ambiguus. LMN = lower motor neuron; UMN = upper motor neuron; VRG = ventral respiratory group.

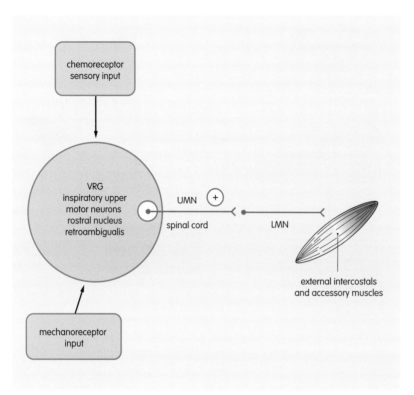

**Fig. 6.5** Ventral respiratory group located in rostral nucleus retroambigualis. UMN = upper motor neuron; LMN = lower motor neuron; VRG = ventral respiratory group.

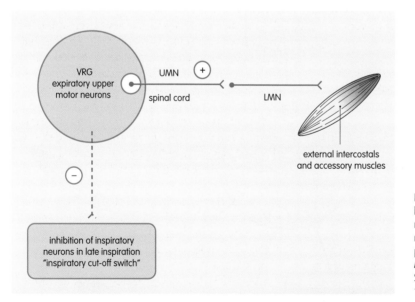

**Fig. 6.6** Ventral respiratory group located in caudal nucleus retroambigualis (expiratory neurons). (Adapted with permission from *Consultation in Diagnostic Imaging*, by W.W. Scott and P.P. Scott. BC Decker, 1985.)

- Dorsal respiratory group inspiratory pacemaker—neurons discharge in a phasic manner, inhibiting expiratory neurons
- Neural networks—local re-excitation causes phasic firing in both inspiratory and expiratory neurons with reciprocal inhibition.

## Effectors (muscles of respiration)

The muscles involved in respiration have been described in Chapter 4. The major muscle groups involved are the diaphragm, internal and external intercostals, and abdominal muscles.

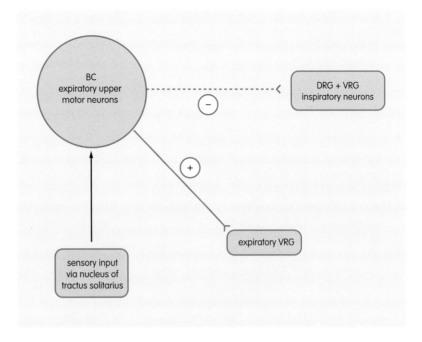

**Fig. 6.7** Bötzinger complex (BC); located first rostral to nucleus ambiguus and comprised entirely of expiratory neurons. PRG = pontine respiratory group; DRG = dorsal respiratory group. (Adapted with permission from *Decision Making in Medicine*, by H.L. Green and W.P. Johnson. Mosby Year Book, 1993.)

Effectors carry out the control action for the central controller. Thus, the strength of contraction and coordination of these muscles is set by the central controller. If the muscles are not coordinated, this will result in abnormal breathing patterns.

## Sensors (receptors)

Sensors report current values or discrepancies from ideal values for the various variables being controlled (e.g. $P_aCO_2$, $P_aO_2$ and pH) to the central controller.

There are many types of sensors and receptors involved with respiratory control:
- Chemoreceptors—central and peripheral
- Lung receptors—irritant, pulmonary stretch and juxtapulmonary
- Receptors in the chest wall—muscle spindles and Golgi tendon organs
- Other receptors—nasal, tracheal and laryngeal receptors, arterial baroreceptors, pain receptors.

### Chemoreceptors

Chemoreceptors monitor blood gas tensions, $P_aCO_2$, $P_aO_2$ and pH, and help keep minute volume appropriate to metabolic demands of the body. Therefore, chemoreceptors respond to:
- Hypercapnia
- Hypoxia
- Acidosis.

There are both central and peripheral chemoreceptors.

### Central chemoreceptors

Central chemoreceptors are tonically active and vital for maintenance of respiration;80% of the drive for ventilation is a result of stimulation of the central chemoreceptors. When they are inactivated, respiration ceases. These receptors are readily depressed by drugs (e.g. opiates and barbiturates).

The receptors are located in the brainstem on the ventrolateral surface of the medulla, close to the exit of cranial nerves IX and X. They are anatomically separate from the medullary respiratory control centre.

Central chemoreceptors respond to hydrogen ion concentration within the surrounding brain tissue and cerebrospinal fluid.
- Raised hydrogen ion concentration increases ventilation
- Lowered hydrogen ion concentration decreases ventilation.

Diffusion of ions across the blood–brain barrier is poor. Blood levels of hydrogen ions and bicarbonate have little effect in the short term on the concentrations of hydrogen ions and bicarbonate in the cerebrospinal fluid and thus have little effect on the central chemoreceptors.

Carbon dioxide, however, can pass freely by diffusion across the blood–brain barrier. On entering the cerebrospinal fluid, the increase in carbon dioxide increases the free hydrogen ion concentration. This increase in hydrogen ion concentration stimulates the central chemoreceptors. Thus:

- Central chemoreceptors are sensitive to $P_aCO_2$ not arterial hydrogen ion concentration
- Central chemoreceptors are not sensitive to $P_aO_2$
- Because there is less protein in the cerebrospinal fluid (<0.4g/L) than in the plasma (60–80g/L), a rise in $P_aCO_2$ has a larger effect on pH in the cerebrospinal fluid than in the blood (CSF has lower buffering capacity).

Long-standing raised $P_aCO_2$ causes the pH of the cerebrospinal fluid to return towards normal. This is because prolonged hypercapnia alters production of bicarbonate by the glial cells and allows bicarbonate to cross the blood–brain barrier. It can therefore diffuse freely into the CSF and alter the CSF pH.

### Peripheral chemoreceptors

Figure 6.8 shows the location of chemoreceptors around the carotid sinus and aortic arch. These are the carotid bodies and aortic bodies, respectively. Stimulation of peripheral chemoreceptors has both cardiovascular and respiratory effects. Of the two receptor groups, the carotid bodies have the greatest effect on respiration.

### Carotid bodies

The carotid bodies contains two different types of cells: type I (glomus) cells and type II (sustentacular) cells. Type I cells are stimulated by hypoxia; they connect with afferent nerves to the brainstem. Type II cells are supportive (structural and metabolic), similar to glial cells of the central nervous system.

There is a rich blood supply to the carotid bodies (blood flow per mass of tissue far exceeds that to the brain); venous blood flow, therefore, remains saturated with oxygen.

The exact mechanism of action of the carotid bodies is not known. It is believed that type I (glomus) cells are activated by hypoxia and release transmitter substances that stimulate afferents to the brainstem.

Peripheral chemoreceptors are sensitive to:

- $P_aO_2$
- $P_aCO_2$
- pH
- Blood flow
- Temperature.

The carotid bodies are supplied by the autonomic nervous system, which appears to alter their sensitivity to hypoxia by regulating blood flow to the chemoreceptor:

- Sympathetic action vasoconstricts, increasing sensitivity to hypoxia
- Parasympathetic action vasodilates, reducing sensitivity to hypoxia.

The relationship between $P_aO_2$ and the response from the carotid bodies is not a linear one. At a low $P_aO_2$ (<50mmHg), a further decrease in arterial oxygen tension significantly increases ventilation (Fig. 6.9). However, at levels of oxygen tension close to 100mmHg, changes have little effect on ventilation. If $P_aO_2$ increases above 100mmHg (achieved when breathing high-concentration oxygen), ventilation is only slightly reduced.

Unlike central chemoreceptors, peripheral chemoreceptors are directly stimulated by blood pH. Although peripheral chemoreceptors are stimulated by $P_aCO_2$, their response is much less than that of central chemoreceptors (less than 10% of the effect).

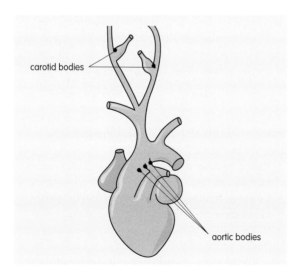

**Fig. 6.8** Peripheral chemoreceptors. Carotid bodies are situated around the carotid sinus and are sensitive both to $P_aCO_2$ and $P_aO_2$. Aortic bodies are situated around the aortic arch and are sensitive only to $P_aCO_2$.

carotid bodies

aortic bodies

**Fig. 6.9** Response of ventilation to $P_aO_2$. The response to a lowered $P_aO_2$ is small until the $P_aO_2$ falls below a value of 50mmHg, after which point the response increases dramatically.

In summary:
- Lowered $P_aO_2$ (especially below 50mmHg) increases ventilation
- Increased $P_aCO_2$ increases ventilation (but this is <10% of the effect of central receptors)
- Raised hydrogen ion concentration increases ventilation (however, aortic bodies do not respond)
- The response of these receptors is very fast and can oscillate within a respiratory cycle.

It is the peripheral chemoreceptors that are responsible for the ventilatory response to hypoxaemia that occurs at high altitude (see p. 111).

## Receptors in the lung
The receptors in the lung monitor mechanical activity. There are three types of receptors in the lung:
- Pulmonary stretch receptors—slowly and rapidly adapting
- Pulmonary and bronchial C fibre receptors—formerly juxtapulmonary, J receptors
- Irritant receptors.

### Stretch receptors
These receptors are situated in the smooth muscle of the bronchial walls and respond to changes in transmural pressure. They are classified into two types: slowly adapting, which produce a maintained response to a maintained stimulus; and rapidly adapting, which produce a transient response to a maintained stimulus.

### Slowly adapting
With slowly adapting stretch receptors, a maintained stimulus leads to a maintained response. Primarily, these receptors are concerned with physiological control and regulatory reflexes. They are stimulated by inflation (which stretches the lungs):
- Inflation leads to decreased respiration (inflation reflex or Hering–Breuer reflex)
- Deflation leads to increased respiration (deflation reflex).

These reflexes are active in the first year of life, but are weak in adults. Therefore, they are not thought to determine the rate and depth of breathing in adults. However, these reflexes are seen to be more active if the tidal volume increases above 1.0L and therefore might have a role in exercise.

Afferent fibres travel to the respiratory centres through the vagus nerve. The functions of these receptors are:
- The termination of inspiration
- Regulation of the work of breathing
- Reinforcement of respiratory rhythm in the first year of life.

However, if the nerve is blocked by anaesthesia there is no change seen in the rate and depth of breathing.

### Pulmonary and bronchial C fibre receptors
These receptors are stimulated by:
- Large inflation
- Forced deflation
- Pulmonary vascular congestion
- Oedema—interstitial fluid in the alveolar wall
- Chemical mediators—histamine and capsacin.

The receptors are thought to be situated in the alveolar wall close to pulmonary capillaries and in the bronchial mucosa. Afferent fibres travel to respiratory centres through the vagus nerve (non-myelinated C fibres).

When stimulated they cause:
- Closure of the larynx
- Rapid, shallow breathing
- Bradycardia
- Hypotension.

They also contribute to the breathlessness of heart failure.

### Irritant receptors

These receptors are scattered through the airways and lie between epithelial cells. They are stimulated by inhaled particles, noxious gases, increased airflow, pulmonary congestion and mechanical deformation. Chemical mediators of allergic reactions also stimulate these receptors which in part account for an increase in ventilation in asthma.

Stimulation of these receptors in the trachea causes a cough reflex, thereby eliminating the particles from the airways. Receptors in lower areas cause bronchoconstriction, laryngeal constriction and rapid, shallow breathing. This is an attempt to limit how far a particle is inhaled.

In the nose and upper airways, there are irritant receptors (Chapter 2), which act to protect the lower airway.

### Receptors in the chest wall

Receptors in the chest wall consist of:
- Joint receptors—measure the velocity of rib movement
- Golgi tendon organs—found within the muscles of respiration (e.g. diaphragm and intercostals) and detect the strength of muscle contraction
- Muscle spindles—monitor the length of muscle fibres both statically and dynamically (i.e. detect muscle length and velocity).

These receptors help to minimize changes to ventilation imposed by an external load (e.g. lateral flexion of the trunk). They achieve this by modifying motor neuron output to the respiratory muscles. The aim is to achieve the most efficient respiration in terms of tidal volume and frequency. Thus, reflexes from muscles and joints stabilize ventilation in the face of changing mechanical conditions.

It is thought that stimulation of mechanoreceptors in the chest wall, along with hypercapnia and hypoxaemia, leads to increased respiratory effort in a patient with sleep apnoea. It is this sudden respiratory effort that then wakes the patient up.

### Arterial baroreceptors

Hypertension stimulates arterial baroreceptors, which inhibit ventilation. Hypotension has the opposite effect.

### Pain receptors

Stimulation of pain receptors causes a brief apnoea, followed by a period of hyperventilation.

## Coordinated responses of the respiratory system

### Response to carbon dioxide

Carbon dioxide is the most important factor in the control of ventilation. Under normal conditions $P_aCO_2$ is held within very tight limits and ventilatory response is very sensitive to small changes in $P_aCO_2$.

The response of ventilation to carbon dioxide has been measured by inhalation of mixtures of carbon dioxide, raising the $P_aCO_2$ and observing the increase in ventilation (Fig. 6.10).

Note that a small increase in $P_ACO_2$ causes a significant increase in ventilation. The response to $P_ACO_2$ is also dependent upon the arterial oxygen tension. At lower values of $P_aO_2$ the ventilatory response is more sensitive to changes in $P_aCO_2$ (steeper slope) and ventilation is greater for a given $P_aCO_2$. If the $P_aCO_2$ is reduced, this causes a significant reduction in ventilation.

Factors that affect ventilatory response to $P_aCO_2$ are:
- $P_aO_2$
- Blood pH
- Genetics
- Age
- Psychiatric state

**Fig. 6.10** The response of ventilation to $CO_2$. Note that at higher levels of $P_aO_2$ an increase in $P_ACO_2$ has less effect on ventilation (the curve is less steep).

**Fig. 6.11** The response of ventilation to $P_AO_2$ at three values of $P_ACO_2$. Lowered $P_AO_2$ has a much greater effect on ventilation when increased values of $P_ACO_2$ are present.

- Fitness
- Drugs (e.g. opiates, such as morphine and diamorphine, reduce respiratory and cardiovascular drive).

## Response to oxygen

As mentioned above, the response to reduced $P_aO_2$ is by stimulation of the peripheral chemoreceptors. This response, however, is not significant until the $P_aO_2$ drops to around 50mmHg. The relationship between $P_aO_2$ and ventilation has been studied by measuring changes in ventilation while a subject breathes hypoxic mixtures (Fig. 6.11). It is assumed that end expiratory $P_AO_2$ and $P_ACO_2$ are equivalent to arterial gas tensions.

The response to $P_AO_2$ is also seen to change with different levels of $P_ACO_2$.

- The greater the carbon dioxide tension, the earlier the response to low oxygen tension
- Therefore, at high $P_ACO_2$, a decrease in oxygen tension below 100mmHg causes an increase in ventilation.

Under normal conditions, $P_aO_2$ does not fall to values of around 50mmHg and, therefore, daily control of ventilation does not rely on hypoxic drive. However, under conditions of severe lung disease, or at high altitude, hypoxic drive becomes increasingly important. A patient with COPD may rely almost entirely on hypoxic drive alone, having lost ventilatory response to carbon dioxide (described above). Central chemoreceptors have become

unresponsive to carbon dioxide; in addition, ventilatory drive from the effects of reduced pH on peripheral chemoreceptors is also lessened by renal compensation for the acid–base abnormality. Administration of high-concentration oxygen therapy (e.g. 100% $O_2$) may abolish any hypoxic drive the patient was previously relying upon, depressing ventilation and worsening the patient's condition.

## Response to pH

From earlier in the chapter you should remember that hydrogen ions do not cross the blood–brain barrier and therefore affect only peripheral chemoreceptors. It is difficult to separate the response from increased $P_aCO_2$ and decreased pH. Any change in pH may be compensated in the long term by the kidneys and therefore has less effect on ventilation than might be expected.

An example of how pH may drive ventilation is seen in the case of metabolic acidosis. The patient will try to achieve a reduction in hydrogen ion concentration by blowing off more carbon dioxide from the lungs. This is achieved by increasing ventilation.

## Response to exercise

As human beings, we are capable of a huge increase in ventilation in response to exercise: approximately 15 times the resting level. In moderate exercise, the carbon dioxide output and oxygen uptake are well matched. The increase in respiratory rate and tidal volume do not cause hyperventilation, and the subject is said to be hyperpnoeic:

- $P_aCO_2$ does not increase, but may fall slightly
- $P_aO_2$ does not decrease
- In moderate exercise, arterial pH varies very little.

Hyperpnoea is an increased depth of breathing and occurs in exercise. Tachypnoea is an abnormally high respiratory rate (over 20 breaths per minute) often seen in patients with pneumonia. Both are responses to increased metabolic demand, and are therefore different from hyperventilation (defined as ventilation that is too great for metabolic needs).

So where does the drive for ventilation come from? There have been many possible causes of the increase in ventilation seen during exercise, but none is completely satisfactory:

- Carbon dioxide load within venous blood returning to the lungs affects ventilation
- Change in pattern of oscillations of $P_aCO_2$ (Fig. 6.12)

- Central control of $P_aCO_2$ is reset to a lower value and held constant during exercise
- Movement of limbs activates joint receptors, which contribute to increased ventilation
- Increase in body temperature during exercise may also stimulate ventilation
- The motor cortex stimulates respiratory centres
- Adrenaline released in exercise also stimulates respiration.

### The possible role of oscillations of $P_aCO_2$

It is suggested that there are cyclical changes of $P_aCO_2$, with inspiration and expiration. Although mean $P_aCO_2$ does not change during moderate exercise, the amplitude of these oscillations may increase, providing the stimulus for ventilation.

In heavy exercise, there can be measurable changes in $P_aO_2$ and $P_aCO_2$, which stimulate respiration. In addition, the pH falls because anaerobic metabolism leads to production of lactic acid (blood lactate levels increase 10-fold). This lactic acid is not oxidized because the oxygen supply cannot keep up with the demands of the exercising muscles (i.e. an 'oxygen debt' is incurred). Rises in potassium ion concentration and temperature may also contribute to the increase in ventilation.

When exercise stops, respiration does not immediately return to basal levels. It remains elevated to provide an increased supply of oxygen to the tissues to oxidize the products of anaerobic metabolism ('repaying the oxygen debt').

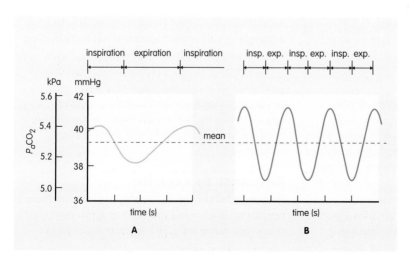

**Fig. 6.12** Cyclical changes of $P_aCO_2$ with inspiration and expiration, (A) at rest, (B) during exercise. Larger oscillations are thought to alter ventilation.

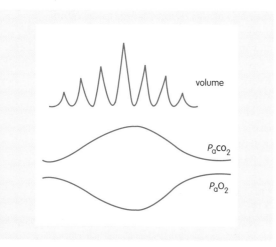

**Fig. 6.13** Cheyne–Stokes respiration. (Adapted with permission from *Physiology* 3e, by R.M. Berne and M.N. Levy. Mosby Year Book, 1993.)

## Abnormalities of ventilatory control
### Cheyne–Stokes respiration

In Cheyne–Stokes respiration, ventilation alternates between progressively deeper breaths and then progressively shallower breaths, in a cyclical manner. Ventilatory control is not achieved and the respiratory system appears to become unstable:

* Arterial carbon dioxide and oxygen tensions vary significantly
* Tidal volumes wax and wane (Fig. 6.13)
* There are short periods of apnoea separated by periods of hyperventilation.

Cheyne–Stokes breathing is observed at various times:

* At altitude—often when asleep
* During sleep
* During periods of hypoxia
* After voluntary hyperventilation
* During disease, particularly with combined right and left heart failure and uraemia
* Secondary to brainstem lesions or compression.

## Respiratory response to extreme environments

## Response to high altitude

At high altitude, the barometric pressure is much lower than at sea level; for example, at the top of Mount Everest (8848m), the barometric pressure is only 250mmHg compared with 760mmHg at sea level. Hence, the partial pressure of oxygen is lower. Dalton's law of partial pressures states that 'The pressure exerted by a mixture of nonreacting gases is equal to the sum of the partial pressures of the separate components.' Thus:

$$P_{atm} = PO_2 + PN_2 + PCO_2 + PH_2O$$

In addition, the partial pressure of water vapour is constant, because inspired air is saturated at body temperature. Therefore, the partial pressure of oxygen in the alveoli (and in the blood) is significantly lower than at sea level.

The carriage of oxygen in the blood is dependent on:

* Partial pressure of oxygen in the blood
* Haemoglobin concentration
* The oxyhaemoglobin dissociation curve.

At altitude the partial pressure of oxygen in the blood is lowered. This would tend to limit the amount of oxygen carriage. To combat this problem the body can:

* Hyperventilate in an attempt to decrease the partial pressure of carbon dioxide in the alveoli and therefore increase the partial pressure of oxygen
* Increase the amount of haemoglobin in the blood, thereby increasing oxygen carriage (oxygen capacity)
* Shift the oxygen dissociation curve
* Alter the circulation
* Increase anerobic metabolism in tissues, increase cytochrome oxidase activity, and increase myoglobin in muscle tissue.

### Hyperventilation

It can be seen by looking at the alveolar gas equation (see p. 67) that if we hyperventilate, thereby reducing $P_ACO_2$, it is possible to bring the partial pressure of oxygen in the alveolar gas much closer to the partial pressure of inspired gas.

$$P_AO_2 = P_IO_2 - (P_ACO_2/R) + K$$

This is very advantageous at altitude—at 5000ft, the partial pressure of oxygen is about 130mmHg. Thus, for saturated air entering the lungs:
$P_IO_2 = 130 - 47 = 93$mmHg.

If a subject's $P_ACO_2$ was 40mmHg and $R = 0.8$, then from the alveolar gas equation:

$P_AO_2 = 93 - (40/0.8) = 43\,mmHg$

If the $P_ACO_2$ were reduced to 10mmHg, then the $P_AO_2$ would be 80.5mmHg.

At higher altitudes, because of the shape of the oxyhaemoglobin dissociation curve, the effect on oxygen carriage in the blood is more dramatic.

Hyperventilation is stimulated by the effect of hypoxia on peripheral chemoreceptors.

## Polycythaemia

The function of the polycythaemia that is experienced by those living at altitude is not to give a rosy-cheeked complexion, but to increase the haemoglobin concentration and therefore the oxygen-carrying capacity of the blood. The $P_aO_2$ and oxygen saturation of the haemoglobin is unchanged, but the total amount of oxygen per unit volume of blood is increased towards normal levels.

Hypoxaemia stimulates the kidney to release the hormone erythropoietin, which increases red-cell production. This leads to a higher oxygen capacity, but has the adverse effect of increasing blood viscosity and therefore increasing the tendency for thrombus formation.

## Shifting of the oxyhaemoglobin dissociation curve

It would be extremely advantageous if we as humans could significantly shift the oxyhaemoglobin dissociation curve to the left when loading haemoglobin with oxygen, and to the right when unloading oxygen. At altitude, there is a shift to the right, which aids unloading. This is caused by an increase in 2,3-diphosphoglycerate as a result of respiratory alkalosis.

## Adverse effects of altitude

Low oxygen tensions in the alveoli cause vasoconstriction of the pulmonary vasculature. This leads to hydrodynamic pulmonary hypertension and increased work for the right heart. Because this alters the Starling forces affecting the pulmonary vessels, pulmonary oedema may occur (reducing gaseous exchange). The permeability of capillaries is increased and a high-protein transudate forms.

## Diving

Increased pressure applies in underwater situations. When diving, pressure increases because of the weight of the column of water above. The pressure rises by 1atm (760mmHg) for every 10m descended. Solids and liquids are incompressible, and any increased pressure has little effect on these. Gases, however, are compressible and gas contained within a cavity or in solution (Henry's law) is affected by pressure changes.

Thus, on descent, the pressure increases and a gas is:

• Compressed
• Forced into solution.

On ascent gas may:
• Expand (which if enclosed in a cavity or sinus could rupture the surrounding structure)
• Come out of solution.

The different types of dive are discussed briefly below.

## Single-breath dive

A single-breath dive is short enough to be accomplished on the air inhaled at the surface. The diver holds his breath and submerges. The air in the diver's lung is subjected to increased pressure, increasing the $PO_2$ and $PCO_2$. Oxygen supply is increased, but so is carbon dioxide, stimulating the chemoreceptors: the diver soon must return to the surface. The dive can be prolonged by hyperventilation before submerging, but this can be dangerous on ascent because, as the ambient pressure falls, so the $PO_2$ falls to levels at which the diver may become unconscious. Standard advice is that four maximum breaths are allowed.

The ratio of total lung volume to residual volume limits the depth of the dive (6.0/1.5 = 4atm—i.e. 40m).

## Snorkel dive

A snorkel dive is carried out at a shallow depth, so that connection with the air can be maintained by a tube. The maximum lung pressure that the inspiratory muscles can generate is about 100mmHg, equivalent to a depth of about 1.2m. This pressure cannot be maintained for more than a few minutes, thus the length of the snorkel is reduced to approximately 40cm, reducing the dead space in the tube.

## Conventional and SCUBA dives

Conventional dives involve being enclosed within a chamber while breathing compressed gases.

During SCUBA (self-contained underwater breathing apparatus) dives, gas is breathed through a regulated valve system from a pressure tank carried by the diver. The pressure of gas breathed is ambient, eliminating problems of lung mechanics. There are problems with conventional and SCUBA dives at depths over 50m (5atm) because of:

- Increased density of the inhaled gas, increasing the work of breathing
- Nitrogen narcosis
- Decompression sickness.

### Nitrogen narcosis

Nitrogen has high solubility in fat and this solubility increases with increasing pressure. Nitrogen acts like a general anaesthetic, expanding the lipid components of cell membranes, leading to the destruction of membrane proteins, including ion channels that are responsible for neural signalling. It is believed this property leads to narcosis. Symptoms of nitrogen narcosis include:

- Euphoria
- Mental confusion
- Impaired neuromuscular coordination (clumsiness)
- Loss of consciousness.

Effects are detectable at 4atm; serious impairment of performance occurs at 10atm; full surgical anaesthesia occurs at 30atm.

### Decompression sickness

Under normal atmospheric pressure, the solubility of nitrogen is low and body tissues contain little nitrogen in solution: 9mL nitrogen dissolved per litre of body water; 50mL of nitrogen dissolved per litre of body fat. As we descend during a dive, ambient pressure increases, thus increasing the partial pressure of nitrogen and forcing nitrogen into solution (especially in adipose tissue).

On ascending, the nitrogen comes out of solution. If ascent is rapid, there is inadequate time for the nitrogen to reach the lungs and be blown off. Instead it comes out of solution and forms bubbles (like formation of bubbles on opening a bottle of lemonade). Bubbles obstruct the circulation, especially in tissues with a high fat content, leading to bends (bubble formation in the joints) and chokes (bubble formation in the pulmonary vessels).

## Drugs and the respiratory system

### Overview

Many drugs are used to treat diseases of the respiratory system. Some are considered under the relevant diseases in Chapter 7; however, some important categories of drugs are introduced here. These categories are:

- Drugs used in asthma
- Respiratory stimulants
- Drugs used in allergies and anaphylaxis
- Mucolytics
- Cough preparations
- Drugs used in smoking cessation.

We have not included a review of antibiotics here. You should ensure that you understand the mechanisms of action and main indications of common antibiotics used in respiratory medicine.

In addition, a number of drugs have side effects upon the respiratory system; those drugs that cause respiratory depression are considered below.

### Drugs used in the treatment of asthma

Drugs used in the treatment of asthma can be split into two main categories:
- Relievers (bronchodilators)
- Preventers (corticosteroids, leukotriene receptor antagonists, sodium cromoglycate).

The 'step-wise' approach to using these drugs to treat asthma is described in Chapter 7.

### Relievers
#### Bronchodilators

Bronchodilators can be split into four groups:
- Short-acting $\beta_2$ agonists
- Anticholinergics
- Long-acting $\beta_2$ agonists
- Xanthines.

**Fig. 6.14** Mechanisms of action of $\beta_2$ agonists—relaxation of bronchial muscle (which leads to bronchodilation) and inhibition of mast-cell degranulation ($\beta$ receptors on mast cell).

## Short-acting $\beta_2$ agonists

Bronchial smooth muscle contains numerous $\beta_2$ receptors, which act through an adenylate cyclase/cAMP second-messenger system to cause smooth muscle relaxation and hence bronchodilation (Fig. 6.14).

Examples of short-acting $\beta_2$ agonists are:
- Salbutamol
- Terbutaline.

These drugs are usually inhaled, either as an aerosol, a powder, or as a nebulized solution. They can also be given intravenously, intramuscularly and subcutaneously. They are used for acute symptoms and act within minutes, producing effects lasting 4–5 hours.

The $\beta_2$ agonists are not completely specific and have some $\beta_1$ agonistic effects, especially in high doses.

Side effects of $\beta_2$ agonists include:
- Tachycardia
- Fine tremor
- Nervous tension
- Headache.

At the doses given by aerosol, these side effects seldom occur. Tolerance may occur with high repeated doses.

## Anticholinergics

Anticholinergics are competitive antagonists of muscarinic acetylcholine receptors. They therefore block the vagal control of bronchial smooth muscle tone in response to irritants and reduce the reflex bronchoconstriction. Ipratropium bromide and oxitropium bromide are both anticholinergics; they have two mechanisms of action:
- Reduction of reflex bronchoconstriction (e.g. from dust or pollen)
- Reduction of mucous secretions.

These drugs reach their maximum effect within 60–90 minutes and act for between 4–6 hours. They are poorly absorbed orally; they must, therefore, be given by aerosol.

As anticholinergics only affect the vagally mediated element of bronchoconstriction, they are not the first choice bronchodilator in asthma treatment. There is some evidence that these drugs are effective when given together with a $\beta_2$ agonist in severe asthma. However, their main use is in COPD that does not respond to $\beta_2$ agonists.

Side effects are rare, but include:
- Dry mouth
- Urinary retention
- Constipation.

## Long-acting $\beta_2$ agonists

Like the short-acting $\beta_2$ agonists, these drugs also relax bronchial smooth muscle. They differ from the short-acting drugs in that their:
- Effect lasts for much longer (up to 12 hours)
- Full effect is only achieved after regular administration of several doses and generally less desensitization occurs.

For these reasons long-acting $\beta_2$ agonists should be used on a regular basis rather than to treat acute attacks.

The main long-acting $\beta_2$ agonists are:
- Salmeterol
- Eformoterol
- Bambuterol.

## Xanthines

Xanthines appear to work by inhibiting phosphodiesterase, thereby preventing the breakdown of cAMP (Fig. 6.15). The amount of cAMP within the bronchial smooth muscle cells is therefore increased, which causes bronchodilation in a similar way to $\beta_2$ agonists.

These drugs are metabolized in the liver and there is a considerable variation in half life between individuals. This has important implications because there is a small therapeutic window. Factors altering theophylline clearance are shown in Fig. 6.16.

Tobacco shortens the half-life of theophylline (due to enzyme induction) and clearance can remain enhanced for up to 3 months after a patient has stopped smoking.

Theophylline can be given intravenously in the form of aminophylline (theophylline with ethylenediamine), but must be administered very slowly (over 20 minutes to administer dose). Aminophylline is given in cases of severe asthma attacks that do not respond to $\beta_2$ agonists and in acute asthma.

$\beta_2$ receptor

$G_s$ | adenyl cyclase

PDE → 5 AMP

ATP    cAMP

inhibition by xanthines thus increasing the amount of cAMP

**Fig. 6.15** Xanthines. The inhibition of phosphodiesterase (PDE) leads to an increase in cellular cyclic AMP which is believed to lead to bronchodilation as in Fig. 6.1.

# Preventers
## Glucocorticosteroids

Steroids reduce the formation, release and action of many different chemicals involved in inflammation. Their mode of action is complex and involves gene-modulation (Fig. 6.17) after binding to steroid receptors in the cytoplasm of cells. This has a number of effects including:
- Down-regulation of pro-inflammatory cytokines
- Production of anti-inflammatory proteins.

One of these anti-inflammatory proteins is thought to reduce the activity of phospholipase $A_2$ which itself plays a role in the production of arachidonic acid (Fig. 6.18).

Steroids in treatment of asthma may be topical (inhaled) or systemic (oral or parenteral).

### Inhaled steroids
These include:
- Beclomethasone
- Budesonide
- Fluticasone.

Side effects of inhaled steroids in adults are relatively minor (primarily hoarseness and oral candidiasis). They may have a short-term effect on growth in children.

### Oral steroids
The primary oral steroid is prednisolone. Side effects of systemic steroids include:
- Adrenal suppression
- Effects on bones (including growth retardation)
- Diabetes mellitus
- Increased susceptibility to infection
- Weight gain
- Effects on skin (e.g. bruising and atrophy)
- Mood changes.

| Factors altering theophylline clearance | |
|---|---|
| **Increased clearance** | **Decreased clearance** |
| Smoking | Liver disease |
| Alcohol | Pneumonia |
| Rifampicin | Cimetidine |
| Childhood | Clarythromycin (erythromycin etc.) |
| | Old age |
| i.e. P450 enzyme induction | i.e. P450 enzyme inhibition |

**Fig. 6.16** Factors altering theophylline clearance.

115

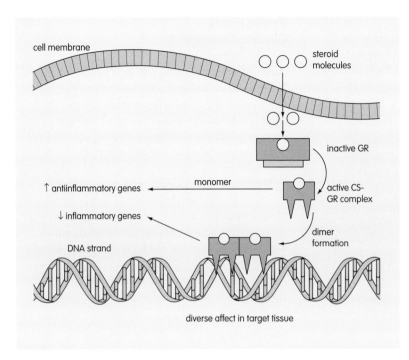

**Fig. 6.17** Mechanism of action of steroids. Steroid molecules diffuse across cell membrane and bind to steroid receptors forming CS-GR complexes. These complexes may bind to DNA as dimers and modulate the output of many different gene products. Alternatively, CS-GR monomers may block induction of inflammatory genes by erogenous stimuli.

## Leukotriene receptor antagonists

Cysteinyl leukotrienes are eicosanoids that cause bronchoconstriction. Their pro-inflammatory actions (Fig. 6.19) centre on their ability to:
• Increase vascular permeability
• Cause influx of eosinophils.

Leukotriene receptor antagonists (or 'leukotriene modifiers') therefore have anti-inflammatory and bronchodilatory effects. The exact mode of action is unclear.

The two key leukotriene receptor antagonists are montelukast and zafirlukast. Montelukast is used in prophylaxis of exercise-induced asthma and in patients with mild–moderate asthma whose symptoms are not well controlled by other asthma drugs.

## Sodium cromoglycate

The mode of action of sodium cromoglycate is not completely understood. It is known to stabilize mast cells, possibly by blocking transport of calcium ions, and has no bronchodilator effect. It cannot be used to treat an acute attack, but is given for prophylaxis, especially in patients with

atopy. The route of administration is by inhalation.

Its mechanism of action is to:
• Prevent mast-cell degranulation and hence mediator release
• Reduce C fibre response to irritants therefore reducing bronchoconstriction
• Inhibit platelet-activating factor (PAF) induced bronchoconstriction.

In addition to its use in allergen-mediated asthma, sodium cromoglygate is effective in non-allergen mediated bronchoconstriction (e.g. in exercise-induced asthma) and continued use results in reduced bronchial hyperactivity. It is often used in paediatrics. Nedocromil sodium is a drug with similar actions.

## Respiratory stimulants

A respiratory stimulant (analeptic) such as doxapram can be used for patients with chronic obstructive pulmonary disease in type II respiratory failure. However, mechanical ventilation and a high incidence of side effects have reduced their use. Doxapram stimulates

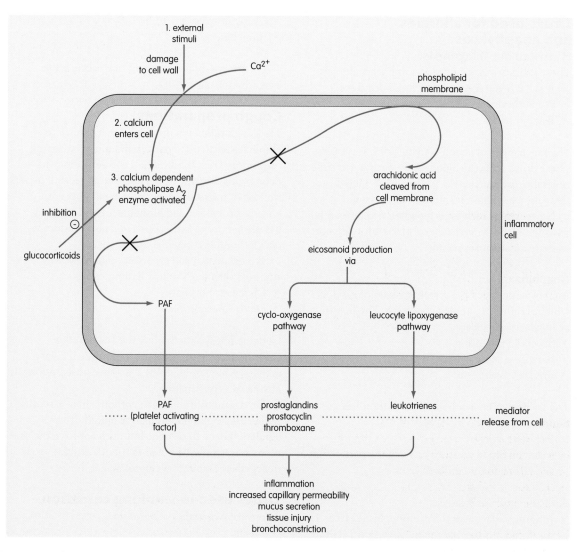

**Fig. 6.18** Inhibition of inflammatory mediator cascade (i.e. cross through pathways to show that they are no longer active). (From D. Seaton in *Crofton and Douglas's Respiratory Diseases* Se. 2000, Blackwell Science Ltd., Vol. 1, p. 261.)

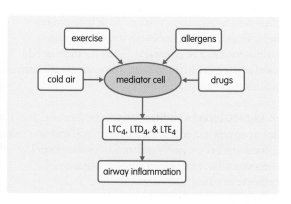

**Fig. 6.19** Overview of cysteinyl leukotriene release.

carotid body chemoreceptors and must be given intravenously.

Side effects of doxapram are:

- Tachycardia
- Palpitations
- Nausea
- Sweating
- Tremor.

Contraindications of doxapram are:

- Epilepsy
- Hypertension
- Hyperthyroidism.

# Drugs used for allergies and anaphylaxis

## H₁ Histamine antagonists

These drugs are used in the treatment of allergies, such as hayfever. Examples of these drugs are:

- Promethazine
- Trimeprazine.

The mechanism of action is to block $H_1$ receptors. These drugs cross the blood–brain barrier and have a general depressant action (sedative); in high doses, this action can cause respiratory depression.

Newer drugs such as terfenadine do not readily cross the blood–brain barrier and therefore do not cause respiratory depression.

## Anaphylaxis

Anaphylactic shock is a systemic allergic reaction which is a life-threatening condition. The features of anaphylactic shock are:

- Severe hypotension
- Laryngeal spasm
- Bronchoconstriction.

The treatment of anaphylaxis must therefore be rapid:

- Secure the airway
- Maintain blood pressure by lying the patient flat and raising his or her legs.

Drug therapy is as follows:

- Intramuscular adrenaline (epinephrine) (0.5–1.0 mg, 0.5–1.0mL of adrenaline injection 1:1000), repeated at 10-minute intervals depending on the blood pressure
- 100% oxygen
- Chlorpheniramine (antihistamine) 10–20mg intravenously, continued for 24–48 hours
- Salbutamol can be given intravenously for those patients not responsive to adrenaline
- Hydrocortisone 200–300mg intravenously may be given as a second-line drug to reduce further deterioration.

# Mucolytics

Mucolytics (e.g. carbocisteine and methyl cysteine hydrochloride) are designed to reduce the viscosity of sputum, thereby aiding expectoration. The indications for use have been in:

- Chronic bronchitis
- Chronic asthma
- Cystic fibrosis
- Bronchiectasis.

These drugs may be of benefit in treating acute exacerbations in COPD.

# Cough preparations

The cough reflex is a protective mechanism to eliminate particulate matter and mucus from the respiratory tree. Inhibition of this reflex may have a deleterious effect, causing build up of secretions and the risk of infection, especially in patients with chronic bronchitis and bronchiectasis. They may have some use in a dry cough or a non-productive cough found in bronchial carcinoma.

Typical drugs used are weak opioids, which suppress the cough reflex. Examples are:

- Codeine phosphate
- Dextromethorphan.

Codeine phosphate inhibits the cough reflex centrally. A side effect is the inhibition of ciliary activity, which reduces the clearance of secretions. It also causes constipation.

Dextromethorphan is a synthetic, non-narcotic, nonanalgesic and non-addictive opioid. It has a similar efficacy to codeine but does not have the side effects. It should be noted that both drugs in large doses cause respiratory depression.

# Drugs used in smoking cessation

There are two main classes of drugs used in smoking cessation:

- Nicotine replacement therapy (NRT)
- Bupropion (amfebutamone).

NRT products (gums, patches and nasal sprays) are classified as over-the-counter medicines and have been shown to be effective in treating tobacco withdrawal and dependence. They should not be used in patients with severe cardiovascular disease (including immediately after myocardial infarction).

Bupropion is an antidepressant also licensed for use as an adjunct to smoking cessation. The main side effects are a dry mouth and difficulty sleeping. The drug should not be used if there is a history of epilepsy or eating disorders.

In addition to pharmacological methods, a number of other interventions have been shown to be effective in helping smokers quit:

- Simple advice and/or brief counselling from GPs
- Group counselling at smoking cessation clinics
- Mass media campaigns (e.g. No Smoking Day)
- Helplines providing one-to-one telephone support.

## Respiratory depressants

If a drug has a depressant action on the central nervous system, large enough doses of it will cause respiratory depression. The most notable of the drugs which cause respiratory depression are the opioid analgesics.

Other drugs that may also cause respiratory depression are listed below:

- Barbiturates
- Benzodiazepines
- $H_1$ histamine antagonists
- Alcohol.

Opioids and barbiturates depress central chemoreceptor activity and this contributes to the respiratory depression they cause.

## Opioid analgesics

These drugs are in very common use in clinical medicine, and include:

- Morphine
- Diamorphine (heroin)
- Pethidine.

In high doses, these drugs cause respiratory and cardiovascular depression, which can be lethal. These drugs bind to opioid receptors in the spinal cord, pons and midbrain, and mimic the action of endogenous opioid.

Overdose is usually iatrogenic in origin or from illicit drug abuse (heroin). The effects of overdose can be reversed by administration of an opioid-receptor antagonist (e.g. naloxone).

Overdose may occur in the newborn if the mother has been given opioids during a caesarean section because the drug crosses the placenta. This can cause respiratory depression in the neonate. The infant is injected with naloxone and resuscitation commenced immediately.

Signs of overdose are varied state of consciousness, respiratory depression and pin-point pupils.

Other main side effects of opioids are:

- Nausea and vomiting
- Constipation

- Difficulty in micturition
- Drowsiness.

Contraindications to opioid analgesics are respiratory depression and acute alcoholism.

### Barbiturates

All barbiturates have a depressant activity on the central nervous system. They are used as induction agents for general anaesthesia (thiopentone), for treatment of grand mal epilepsy (phenobarbitone), and for sedation.

The mechanism of action of barbiturates is enhancement of GABA-mediated inhibition of the central nervous system. These drugs prolong the opening of individual chloride channels by a given GABA stimulus.

Barbiturates cause respiratory and cardiovascular depression when administered at 10–100 times the clinical dose.

### Benzodiazepines

Benzodiazepines are extensively used as anxiolytics, hypnotics, and for sedation. Their use has become unfashionable because of tolerance and withdrawal effects, which develop after about 2–4 weeks of use.

Their mechanism of action is the same as that of the barbiturates, although benzodiazepines bind to a different site on the $GABA_A$ receptor complex.

Normally, even high orally administered doses of benzodiazepines do not cause severe respiratory depression. However, intravenous administration or oral administration either to elderly patients or to patients with underlying pulmonary disease can cause respiratory depression.

## Respiratory support

Patients with respiratory disease who are hypoxaemic and/or hypercapnic will often require a form of respiratory support. This support may range from oxygen given briefly via a face mask in a patient with mild hypoxaemia to mechanical ventilation in respiratory failure. The two basic categories of respiratory support are considered below and include:

- Oxygen therapy
- Assisted ventilation (non-invasive or mechanical).

# Oxygen therapy

Oxygen therapy aims to correct hypoxaemia. Progress is monitored, and the amount of oxygen adjusted, according to pulse oximetry and arterial blood gas analysis.

Oxygen can be delivered either by:
- Nasal prongs
- Face mask.

## Nasal prongs

These allow the patient to talk and eat whilst receiving oxygen. Air is humidified to avoid discomfort from nasal crusting. Oxygen is delivered at rates of 1–4 L/min, which, when diluted with inspiratory air, equates to oxygen concentrations of between 25 and 30%.

Delivery through nasal prongs is also used in long term oxygen therapy (LTOT), for example in patients with COPD who have a domiciliary oxygen supply.

## Face masks

These fit over the nose and mouth and are used with higher flow oxygen (e.g. 6 L/min or an oxygen concentration of 60%). Remember that high concentrations of oxygen should not be given to patients with acute-on-chronic respiratory failure (see p. 94).

# Assisted ventilation

In some cases even high flow oxygen is not sufficient to restore blood gases to adequate levels. A patient with COPD for example, may maintain near normal blood gases until an infection adds to the workload; some form of ventilatory support is then indicated in order to:
- Offload the respiratory muscles and reduce the work of breathing
- Improve gas exchange.

Remember that excessive load is a major problem in acute-on-chronic respiratory failure. Taking away some of the work with assisted ventilation will help correct the vicious circle in which lung disease increases work which consumes oxygen which increases work requirement.

# Non-invasive ventilation (NIV)

In non-invasive ventilation, respiratory support is given via the patient's upper airway and intubation is avoided. This method is therefore only suitable if a patient can protect their own airway, but has the advantage of reducing the risks of a hospital acquired infection. The patient breathes spontaneously and the lungs are expanded by a volume of gas delivered, usually at a positive pressure. This decreases the work of the respiratory muscles, particularly the diaphragm.

NIV is particularly effective in patients with acute hypercapnic respiratory failure, particularly in COPD. Lung volumes in these patients do not return to baseline after expiration so that greater pressures are needed to expand the lungs (i.e. there is an intrinsic positive end expiratory pressure or iPEEP). The positive pressure of the gas given via the mask therefore reduces the extra work generated by air trapping.

Two basic types of non-invasive ventilation are considered here:
- Continuous positive airway pressure (CPAP)
- Bilevel positive airway pressure (BiPAP).

As the name implies, CPAP delivers a continuous positive air pressure throughout the respiratory cycle. BiPAP is an example of intermittent positive pressure ventilation (IPPV). BiPAP also reduces the work of breathing but differs in that it senses when inspiration is occurring and delivers a higher pressure during the inspiratory part of the cycle.

Non-invasive ventilation may be used in acute situations or on a long-term basis in patients with COPD; it is also used in weaning from conventional, intubated ventilators.

# Mechanical ventilation

True mechanical ventilation links the patient to the ventilator by means of an endotracheal tube (usually inserted via the nose) or, if ventilation is likely to be prolonged, via tracheostomy. An airtight seal is created and gas is delivered either at constant pressure or at PEEP. Indications for mechanical ventilation include:
- Protection of airway in unconscious patients
- Severe hypoxaemia (e.g. in ARDS)
- Controlling hypercapnia in ventilatory failure (i.e. Type 2 respiratory failure) when NIV is inappropriate.

# Complications of respiratory support

There are several important complications of respiratory support; most, including those presented by intubation and difficulties in weaning the patient, are outside the scope of this book.

## Oxygen toxicity

The use of high-concentration oxygen therapy can have adverse effects on the respiratory system. This is especially evident after prolonged use.

Oxygen intoxication was first recognized by Paul Bert in 1878. He noticed that breathing oxygen at 1 atm for as little as 12 hours can lead to pulmonary congestion (reducing vital capacity), pulmonary oedema, exudation (reducing gaseous exchange) and damage to the pulmonary epithelium.

In the premature infant, administration of high-concentration oxygen can also cause retrolental fibroplasia. Fibrous tissue forms behind the lens and can lead to permanent blindness. This is thought to be caused by vasoconstriction, secondary to a high partial pressure of oxygen. This can be avoided by keeping a low $PO_2$.

Respiratory distress can occur because of absorption atelectasis.

## Absorption atelectasis

Absorption atelectasis is the collapse of an alveolus due to blockage (Fig. 6.20). When breathing 100% $O_2$, the oxygen in the alveolus is quickly absorbed because there is a huge partial pressure difference between the alveolar gas (about 760 mmHg) and the partial pressure of gases in the venous blood. This results in collapse of the alveolus. It is then difficult to open the collapsed alveoli because of high surface tension effects.

**Fig. 6.20** Absorption atelectasis. The sum of the partial pressures (in mmHg) of alveolar gas far exceeds those in the mixed venous blood. Oxygen is taken up rapidly by the blood causing collapse of the alveoli. (Adapted from *Respiratory Physiology* 5e, by J. West. Lippincott Williams & Wilkins, 1995.)

Absorption atelectasis also occurs in airway occlusion when breathing a normal air mixture. The rate of absorption is much slower as the driving force (the partial pressure difference between venous blood and alveolar gas) is much lower. There is still a partial pressure difference driving diffusion because the fall in oxygen tension from arterial to venous blood is greater than the rise in carbon dioxide tension. Collapse can be avoided by adding even small concentrations of nitrogen. Nitrogen is poorly absorbed because of its poor solubility and therefore remains in the alveoli delaying or preventing collapse.

121

- Describe what is meant by feedback and feed-forward control.
- Discuss the central control of breathing with reference to the pontine respiratory group, and the dorsal and ventral respiratory groups of the medulla.
- List the different types of receptors involved in control.
- What factors stimulate central and peripheral chemoreceptors?
- Outline the responses of the respiratory system to changes in carbon dioxide concentration, oxygen concentration and pH.
- Discuss the mechanisms thought to influence the control of ventilation in exercise.
- Discuss the changes that occur in response to high altitude.
- What types of respiratory support might a patient with COPD receive?
- Outline the treatment of a patient with an acute asthma attack.
- Explain the mechanism of action of the $\beta_2$ agonists.
- Outline the drugs used to prevent asthma attacks.
- List the classes of drugs used to treat diseases of the respiratory system.
- List the treatment measures for management of anaphylaxis.
- Describe the drugs that have an adverse effect on the respiratory system.
- Describe absorption atelectasis.

# 7. Disorders of the Lungs

## Introduction

A large number of lung disorders are covered in this chapter; they are grouped mainly according to the 'surgical sieve' approach, that is in categories reflecting the type of disorder (e.g. congenital) or underlying pathology (e.g. infection). The aim is to provide a clear structure for revision, allowing the disorders to be worked through in a logical fashion. However, this may make it difficult to see which are the common or important diseases. Therefore, set out below is a list of key disorders; this is necessarily brief but includes some of the diseases commonly seen in clinical practice plus others that illustrate an important pathological process.

The surgical sieve can be a tool for fomulating a differential diagnosis, making sure that no possible cause has been forgotten. A number of mnemonics exist for the categories. One is: TIN CAN BED PAN. This is short for: **T**rauma **I**nflammatory **N**eoplastic **C**ongenital **A**rteriovenous **N**eurological **B**lood **E**ndocrine **D**rugs **P**sychogenic **A**llergic **N**ot known.

## The key disorders
### Asthma
- A chronic inflammatory disorder of the airways, characterized by symptoms that are intermittent and have a diurnal variation (p. 137).

### Chronic obstructive pulmonary disease (COPD)
- Chronic bronchitis and emphysema in the same patient, who is almost always a smoker (p. 133).

### Lung cancer
- Accounts for 20% of all cancers; the risk is directly related to tobacco exposure (p. 156).

### Pneumonia
- An infection of peripheral lung tissue associated with significant morbidity and mortality worldwide (p. 126).

### Pulmonary embolism
- The most serious complication of venous thrombosis; prophylaxis is important in high risk patients (p. 146).

### Bronchiectasis
- Permanent dilatation of the bronchi secondary to chronic infection (p. 141).

### Cystic fibrosis
- An autosomal recessive condition predisposing to chronic lung infection and bronchiectasis (p. 142).

### Pneumothorax
- Air in the pleural space; the tension type is a medical emergency (p. 165).

### Pleural effusion
- Fluid in the pleural space; a complication of several common lung disorders (p. 163).

### Pulmonary fibrosis
- End point of many different lung diseases and an example of the basic pathology of restrictive disorders (p. 149).

### Sarcoidosis
- A multisystem disorder; pulmonary features include bilateral hilar lymphadenopathy (p. 152).

## Occupational lung diseases
Certain disorders with common themes are dealt with separately under the surgical sieve approach. One category that is important, and that you should consider as a whole, is that of occupational lung disorders. More details on this group of diseases is given in Chapter 9 (Fig. 9.1, p. 183).

**Fig. 7.1** Radiograph of a bronchogenic cyst. There is a right paratracheal mass (arrows). Courtesy of Dr D. Sutton and Dr J.W.R. Young.

## Congenital abnormalities

### Congenital cysts

The respiratory system is an outgrowth of the ventral wall of the foregut. Bronchogenic cysts may result from abnormal budding of the tracheobronchial tree. They are lined by bronchial elements: cartilage, smooth muscle and ciliated respiratory epithelium. Cysts are classified according to position:
- Central (mediastinal)—85%
- Peripheral (intrapulmonary)—15%.

Cysts are usually single, spherical or oval, unilocular masses. They are mainly asymptomatic and can present at any age, although they are more common in men. Surgical excision is recommended. Radiologically, it is impossible to differentiate between a bronchogenic cyst and malignancy (Fig. 7.1).

### Lobar sequestrations

Lobar sequestrations are masses of pulmonary tissue that do not communicate anatomically with the tracheobronchial tree (Fig. 7.2).

### Vascular abnormalities

Vascular abnormalities include absent pulmonary artery trunk, absent unilateral pulmonary artery,

| B | Comparison between intralobular and extralobular sequestrations | |
| --- | --- | --- |
| | **Intralobular** | **Extralobular** |
| incidence | more common | less common |
| male-to-female ratio | 1 : 1 | 4 : 1 |
| side of thorax | 60% left | 90% left |
| arterial supply | 70% thoracic aorta | 40% thoracic aorta |
| venous drainage | pulmonary veins | systemic |
| position | within normal lung and its pleural covering | separate from normal lung in its own pleural cover |
| other congenital defects | uncommon | frequent |

**Fig. 7.2** (A and B) Differences between extralobular and intralobular sequestrations.

pulmonary artery stenosis, pulmonary arteriovenous malformations, anomalous origin of the left pulmonary artery and anomalous pulmonary venous drainage.

### Congenital lobar emphysema

Lobar emphysema is an overdistension of a lobe (usually an upper lobe) caused by intermittent bronchial obstruction. Symptoms in early life are caused by pressure effects. Pathogenesis includes defects in the bronchial cartilage, mechanical causes of bronchial obstruction and idiopathic causes. Prognosis is good.

### Agenesis and hypoplasia
#### Agenesis
Agenesis is a complete absence of one or both lungs with no trace of bronchial or vascular supply.

## Hypoplasia

In hypoplasia, the bronchus is fully formed, but reduced in size; there is failure of alveolar development. Hypoplasia is associated with other congenital abnormalities such as Potter's syndrome and diaphragmatic hernia.

## Abnormalities of trachea or bronchi

Abnormalities of trachea or bronchi include tracheal agenesis, tracheo-oesophageal fistula, tracheal stenosis, tracheal narrowing caused by extrinsic pressure, tracheomalacia and tracheobronchomegaly.

## Atelectasis

Atelectasis (from the Greek *ateles* imperfect + *ektasis* expansion) is classified as primary or secondary:
- Primary—lung fails to expand at birth
- Secondary—caused by obstruction or compression (Fig. 7.3).

### Obstructive atelectasis

Obstruction is the commonest cause of atelectasis; this is also known as resorptive atelectasis (Fig. 7.4).

Obstructive atelectasis follows an acute and complete obstruction of a large bronchus. Air in the collapsed area of the lung is absorbed and secretions distal to the obstruction accumulate; subsequently, these bronchial secretions become infected and suppurate. Distal to the blockage, the bronchi mechanically distend.

If the collapse has been present for some time, irreversible pulmonary fibrosis occurs. Pulmonary artery branches may have narrowed lumens.

### Compressive atelectasis

In compressive atelectasis, bronchial obstruction does not occur; therefore, bronchial secretions are free to drain up the bronchial tree. As such, the collapsed lung does not become seriously infected.

Compressive atelectasis results from external compression of the lung. Causes of compression include pleural effusion, haemothorax, empyema, pneumothorax, space-occupying intrathoracic lesion and abdominal distension.

Haemodynamic and vascular changes occur. High inflation pressures on inspiration are required to

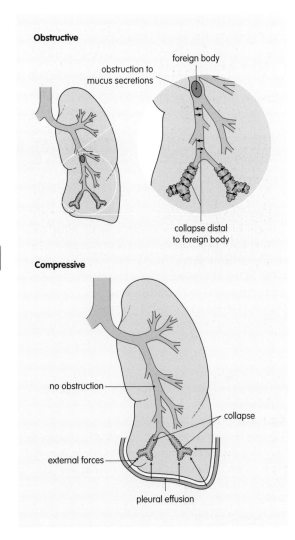

**Fig. 7.3** Obstructive and compressive atelectasis.

| Comparison of acute and chronic obstruction | |
|---|---|
| **Acute** | **Chronic** |
| inhalation and impaction of foreign bodies | tumours |
| mucus plugging of bronchi (e.g. after anaesthesia) | lymphadenopathy |
| after tracheostomy | aneurysm |
| lung infections | |

**Fig. 7.4** Causes of acute and chronic obstruction.

overcome retractive forces. Re-expansion of the lung usually occurs after compression is resolved.

## Patchy atelectasis

Depending on the cause, atelectasis may occur in a patchy or diffuse distribution.

## Infections of the lung

## Pneumonia

Pneumonia is defined as an infection of peripheral lung parenchyma (as opposed to infection of the central conducting airways—bronchitis). Clinically, pneumonia is an acute illness in which there are signs of consolidation in the chest or new changes on chest X-ray. In the UK, pneumonia is responsible for approximately 60000 deaths a year.

Pneumonia can be classified on the basis of:
- The setting or circumstances in which it originated (community or hospital acquired or pneumonia in immunocompromised hosts)
- Anatomy (lobar or bronchopneumonia)
- Organisms (bacterial, atypical, viral, fungal, protozoal).

It is now common to use the first classification as this has more clinical significance (whilst the anatomical site is of limited use in guiding treatment and the organism may never be known).

The anatomical classification for pneumonia is not used here, but if you come across it elsewhere: lobar pneumonia occurs when organisms widely colonize alveolar spaces, whereas bronchopneumonia occurs when organsims colonize bronchi and extend into alveoli.

## Community acquired pneumonia (CAP)
### Pathogenesis of CAP

Organisms enter the lungs usually having been inhaled from the environment or nasopharynx. These organisms may be eliminated by the lung's defence mechanisms (see Chapter 3 ) or they may survive and multiply. Factors that undermine the lung's defences will therefore increase the risk of pneumonia. These factors include:
- Alcohol excess
- Cigarette smoking
- Chronic heart and lung diseases
- Bronchial obstruction
- Immunosuppression
- Drug abuse.

The pathogen stimulates host defences and alveolar airspaces become filled with eosinophilic oedematous fluid containing neutrophil polymorphs. The oedema transports organisms through the pores of Kohn into the alveoli.

In days 2–4, a red hepatization occurs; there is accumulation in alveolar spaces of polymorphs, lymphocytes and macrophages. The alveolar exudate contains a fine network of fibrin and large numbers of extravasated red cells. The lung is red, solid and airless. Red hepatization corresponds to an area of oedema and haemorrhage.

In days 4–8, a grey hepatization occurs. Fibrinous pleurisy is present. Alveolar spaces are microscopically distended and filled by a dense network of fibrin-containing neutrophil polymorphs. Grey hepatization represents a zone of advanced consolidation with destruction of red and white blood cells. The lung is grey or brown and solid.

Resolution occurs after 8–10 days in untreated cases. When bacteria have been eliminated, macrophages enter and replace granulocytes. The exudate is liquefied by fibrinolytic enzymes and coughed up or absorbed. There is preservation of the underlying alveolar wall architecture.

### Aetiology

Figure 7.5 shows the key pathogens in CAP. S. pneumoniae is the causative organsim in 55–75% of cases. Note, however, that in around a third of cases, no cause is found.

Community acquired pneumonia is usually caused by Gram-positive bacteria, whereas hospital acquired pneumonias are mainly caused by Gram-negative bacteria.

| Causes and features of community acquired pneumonia | | |
| --- | --- | --- |
| Organism | Features of pneumonia | % cases |
| Streptococcus pneumoniae | Gram +ve alpha-haemolytic; polysaccharide capsule determines virulence and is detectable serologically; responsible for a high mortality (especially in the setting of bacteraemia) unless treated appropriately; vaccine available | 55–75 |
| Mycoplasma pneumoniae | epidemics every 3–4 years usually in young patients; 50% have cold agglutinins; associated with many extrapulmonary manifestations; penicillin ineffective as no bacterial cell wall | 5–18 |
| Influenza | epidemics common; affects patients with underlying lung disease; can be severe; S. aureus, S. pneumoniae, H. influenzae occur secondarily; a vaccine is available | 8 |
| Legionella pneumophila | gram – ve; found in cooling towers and air-conditioning; causes very severe pneumonia with high mortality and is frequently associated with extrapulmonary features; antigen may help in diagnosis | 2–5 |
| Chlamydia pneumoniae | headache very common; usually serological diagnosis | 2–5 |
| Haemophilus influenzae | gram –ve rod; more commonly associated with exacerbations of COPD | 4–5 |
| Viruses other than influenza | | 2–8 |
| Staphylococcus aureus | gram +ve coccus; often follows flu; alcoholics and patients with mitral valve disease are susceptible; often causes severe, often cavitating pneumonia; commonly fatal | 1–5 |
| Klebsiella pneumoniae | gram –ve; seen in alcoholics; severe and often cavitates | 1 |

**Fig. 7.5** Organisms causing community acquired pneumonia.

## Clinical features

The common respiratory symptoms are shown in Fig. 7.6. Note that the presence of confusion is a poor prognostic factor (see below).

On examination the patient is typically pyrexial, tachycardic and tachypnoeic. Lung expansion is reduced and signs of consolidation are found (see Chapter 9). Coarse crackles may be heard as the infection resolves.

If you suspect pneumonia, ask about alcohol intake and comorbidities (especially chronic heart and lung disease and diabetes mellitus); foreign travel (i.e. risk of legionella) and upper respiratory tract infection are so common that positive answers are unlikely to narrow down the list of possible organisms.

## Complications

The key complications are:
- Respiratory failure
- Parapneumonic effusions
- Empyema
- Lung abscess
- Pulmonary fibrosis, after resolution.

## Investigations

- Sputum—culture and Gram stain
- Blood—full blood count, blood culture (low sensitivity, high specificity)
- Pleural fluid—culture and Gram stain
- Chest radiography
- Bronchoscopy with BAL if diagnosis uncertain
- Assessment of oxygenation
- Other specific tests—mycoplasma, legionella and chlamydia antibodies; pneumococcal antigen testing by counter-immunoelectrophoresis (CIE) of the sputum, urine and serum.

| Typical clinical features of bacterial pneumonia | |
|---|---|
| Clinical feature | Incidence (%) |
| respiratory features | |
| cough | 90 |
| sputum | 70 |
| dyspnoea | 70 |
| chest pain | 65 |
| upper respiratory tract symptoms | 33 |
| haemoptysis | 13 |
| nonrespiratory features | |
| vomiting | 20 |
| confusion | 15 |
| diarrhoea | 15 |
| rash | 5 |
| abdominal pain | 5 |
| signs | |
| fever | 80–90 |
| tachypnoea | 80–90 |
| tachycardia | 80–90 |
| abnormal chest signs | 80–90 |
| hypotension | 20 |
| confusion | 15 |
| herpes labialis | 10 |

**Fig. 7.6** Typical clinical features of bacterial pneumonia.

## Management
Antibiotic treatment should be started immediately, without waiting for microbiology results.
For most cases use:
- Combined oral treatment with amoxicillin and a macrolide (erythromycin or clarithromycin).
For severe cases, admit to hospital and start:
- IV combination of broad spectrum antibiotic or cephalosporin, together with a macrolide as above.

In addition, pleuritic pain should be relieved with simple analgesia and oxygen therapy administered if appropriate.

## Prognosis
It is important to assess the severity of CAP as this impacts on prognosis and therefore treatment planning. British Thoracds Society guidelines state the key adverse prognostic features are:
- New mental confusion
- Urea >7 mmol/L
- Respiratory rate ≥30/min
- Systolic blood pressure <90mmHg or diastolic ≤60mmHg.

Patients with two or more of these features are at high risk of mortality and should be managed aggressively.

# Hospital acquired pneumonia
Hospital acquired or nosocomial pneumonia refers to a new lower respiratory tract infection at least two days after hospital admission. It occurs in 1–5% of admissions and is a serious cause of morbidity and mortality.

## Aetiology
In addition to the risk factors discussed above, factors predisposing to hospital acquired infections are:
- Intubation
- Suppressed cough leading to aspiration (e.g. postoperatively)
- Reduced host defences
- Long stays in hospital, with associated exposure to pathogens.

## Pathogens
Gram-negative bacteria (e.g. *Escherichia*, *Klebsiella* and *Pseudomonas*) are the cause of hospital acquired pneumonia in many cases, although *Staph. aureus* (particularly drug resistant strains) is also common.

## Clinical features and investigations
These are similar to those described above under CAP.

## Management
Good Gram-negative coverage is achieved with an aminoglycoside plus anti-pseudomonal penicillin or a third generation cephalosporin. Most hospital acquired pneumonia is serious and these drugs are frequently given intravenously.

# Pneumonia in the immunocompromised
### *Pneumocystis carinii* pneumonia
*Pneumocystis carinii* pneumonia (PCP) is a fungal infection that is largely confined to the lung. It is the commonest opportunistic infection in the immunocompromised.

Infection occurs by inhalation of the organism. The patient presents with an insidious or abrupt onset of dry cough, fever and dyspnoea.
Pleural effusions are rare.

## Pathology

There is an interstitial infiltrate of mononuclear cells and alveolar airspaces are filled with foamy eosinophilic material.

## Diagnosis

Bilateral pneumonia in an immunocompromised patient should raise suspicion of PCP.

Diagnosed in 90% of cases by staining using Giemsa, methanamine–silver, papanicocoau, or Gram–Weigert stains with monoclonal antibodies.

Chest radiography shows diffuse bilateral alveolar and interstitial shadowing, beginning in peripheral regions and spreading in a butterfly pattern.

## Treatment

High-dose co-trimoxazole is given, intravenously at first. Prophylaxis is recommended in patients with low CD4 counts or where previous infection has occurred.

Mortality of untreated patients is 100%; in treated patients, mortality is 20–50%.

## Cytomegalovirus

Cytomegalovirus (CMV) is a DNA virus in the herpes group. Of patients with AIDS, 90% are infected with CMV. CMV also occurs in recipients of bone marrow and solid organ transplants. Only occasionally does CMV cause pneumonia.

Usual symptoms are a non-productive cough, dyspnoea and fever. Disseminated infection occurs, causing encephalitis, pneumonitis, retinitis and diffuse involvement of the gastrointestinal tract.

## Pathology

Features in the pathology of CMV infection include:
- Interstitial inflammatory infiltrate of mononuclear cells
- Scattered alveolar hyaline membranes
- Protein-rich fluid in alveoli
- Intranuclear inclusion bodies found in alveolar epithelial cells.

## Diagnosis

CMV infection can be diagnosed by the identification of characteristic intranuclear owl's eye inclusions in tissues and by direct immunofluorescence.

## Treatment

Treatment is by ganciclovir 5 mg/kg daily for 14–21 days.

## Aspergillus

Four pulmonary diseases are caused by the fungus *Aspergillus fumigatus*:
- Allergic aspergillosis
- Mucoid impaction
- Aspergilloma
- Invasive aspergillosis.

### Invasive aspergillosis

Invasive aspergillosis occurs in immunocompromised individuals with severe neutropenia or T-lymphocyte deficiency. It is confined to the lungs and may present as a necrotizing pneumonia, lung abscess, or solitary granuloma. Microabscesses contain the characteristic fungal filaments.

Recovery may occur after vigorous treatment with intravenous amphotericin. Prognosis is generally poor.

## Cryptococcus

Cryptococcus is a budding, yeast-like fungus that may disseminate to all organs. Pulmonary lesions commonly involve the lower lobes, are nodular, and may simulate carcinoma. Other pulmonary manifestations include:
- Cavitation within lung nodules
- Calcification
- Pneumonitis
- Pleural effusions
- Intrathoracic lymph node enlargement.

Meningeal involvement is the commonest form of cryptococcosis.

## Varicella zoster

Varicella zoster is an uncommon cause of pneumonia. The associated pustular rash confirms diagnosis. Treatment is with aciclovir.

## Kaposi's sarcoma

Kaposi's sarcoma is included here because may be a differential diagnosis in the immunocompromised host. It is a multifocal neoplastic condition typically seen in patients with AIDS. Lesions of the pleura, parenchyma, lymph nodes and airways occur. Overall prognosis is poor.

## Lung abscess

Lung abscess is a localized area of infected parenchyma, with necrosis and suppuration.

## Aetiology

A lung abscess may occur due to:

- Aspiration of infected material (e.g. in alcoholism, unconscious patients)
- Complications of pneumonia
- Infection of cavities in bronchiectasis or TB
- Bronchial obstructions (e.g. tumours or foreign body)
- Pulmonary infarction.

## Clinical features

Onset may be acute or insidious, depending on the cause of the abscess. Acute symptoms include malaise, anorexia, fever and a productive cough. Copious foul-smelling sputum is present, caused by the growth of anaerobic organisms.

In large abscesses there may be dullness to percussion. Pallor is common, caused by anaemia. Clubbing is a late sign.

## Complications

Abscesses can heal completely leaving a small fibrous scar. Complications include empyema, bronchopleural fistula, pyopneumothorax, pneumatoceles, haemorrhage caused by erosion of a bronchial or pulmonary artery, meningitis and cerebral abscess.

## Investigations

- Investigations must exclude necrosis in a malignant tumour or cavitation caused by tuberculosis; bronchosopy may be indicated to sample cells or exclude an obstruction. Chest radiography shows a walled cavity with fluid level
- Sputum culture may identify a causative organism
- Blood culture and full blood count show that the patient is often anaemic with high erythrocyte sedimentation rate. Patients usually have mild to moderate leucocytosis.

## Treatment

Follow disease carefully with regular chest radiographs and sputum collections. Resolution of disease is prompt after institution of appropriate antibiotics. Postural drainage should be used. Surgery is not usually indicated.

# Tuberculosis

Tuberculosis is the world's leading cause of death from a single infectious disease. It is a notifiable disease and the prevalence is on the increase, primarily due to the arrival of the human immunodeficiency virus (HIV). In the UK, 6000 new cases occur per year, with the highest incidence among immigrants, who are 40 times more likely to develop the disease than the native Caucasian population. Their UK-born children are regarded as being at high risk and as such are immunized soon after birth. The discussion below deals only with pulmonary tuberculosis, and does not consider the extra-pulmonary effects.

The causative agent in most cases of tuberculosis is *Mycobacterium tuberculosis*. Patients with pre-existing lung disease or the immunosuppressed may also be infected by opportunistic mycobacteria. These are also known as atypical mycobacteria or non-tuberculous mycobacteria and include:

- *Mycobacterium kansasii*
- *Mycobacterium avium* complex (MAC).

## Transmission and dissemination

Transmission is through the air or from direct contact. The pulmonary or bronchial focus ulcerates into an airway. A cough, sneeze or exhalation then discharges droplets of viable mycobacterium. The droplet nuclei are then inhaled by an uninfected person and can lodge anywhere in the lungs or airways. Initial infection usually occurs in childhood.

## Primary tuberculosis

The initial lesion is usually solitary, 1–2cm in diameter, and subpleural in the middle or upper zones of the lung. The focus of primary infection is called a Ghon complex. The primary infection has two components:

- The initial inflammatory reaction
- Resultant inflammation in lymph nodes draining the area.

Within 3–8 weeks, the process becomes a tubercle, a granulomatous form of inflammation. The granulomatous lesion commonly undergoes necrosis in a process called caseation and is surrounded by multinucleated giant cells and epithelioid cells (both derived from macrophage). The caseous tissue may liquefy, empty into an airway, and be transmitted to other parts of the lung. Lymphatic spread of mycobacterium occurs. The combination of tuberculous lymphadenitis and the Ghon complex is termed the primary complex.

In most cases, the primary foci will organize and form a fibrocalcific nodule in the lung with no clinical sequelae.

## Secondary tuberculosis (postprimary tuberculosis)

Secondary tuberculosis results from reactivation of a primary infection or re-infection. Any form of immunocompromise may allow reactivation. The common sites are posterior or apical segments of the upper lobe or the superior segment of the lower lobe. Tubercle follicles develop and lesions enlarge by formation of new tubercles. Infection spreads by lymphatics and a delayed hypersensitivity reaction occurs.

In secondary tuberculosis, the lesions are often bilateral and usually cavitated. Most lesions are connected to fibrocalcific scars.

## Progressive tuberculosis

Progressive tuberculosis may arise from a primary lesion or may be caused by reactivation of an incompletely healed primary lesion or re-infection. Tuberculosis progresses to widespread cavitation, pneumonitis and lung fibrosis. Early symptoms are seldom diagnostic.

## Miliary tuberculosis

In miliary tuberculosis, an acute diffuse dissemination of tubercle bacilli occurs through the bloodstream. Numerous small granulomas form in many organs, with the highest numbers found in the lungs. These granulomas often contain numerous mycobacteria and are usually the result of a delay in diagnosis or commencement of treatment.

Miliary tuberculosis may be a consequence of either primary or secondary tuberculosis and is universally fatal without treatment.

The pathology of tuberculosis is shown in Fig. 7.7; complications are shown in Fig. 7.8.

## Clinical features

Primary tuberculosis is usually asymptomatic but may cause a mild febrile illness, with or without erythema nodosum. If the illness follows the progressive course, other symptoms then appear either immediately or gradually over weeks or months. Symptoms range from tiredness, anorexia and malaise to bronchopneumonia with fever, cough, dyspnoea and respiratory distress. Sputum is purulent, mucoid or blood-stained.

A pleural effusion or pneumonia may be the presenting complaint; often the disease is discovered due to an abnormal chest radiograph in an asymptomatic patient.

## Diagnosis

Chest radiographs show upper zone shadows and fibrosis. Sequential sputum samples are taken:
- Stain with Ziehl–Neelson stain for acid-fast and alcohol-fast bacilli
- Culture on Lowenstein–Jensen medium, which takes up to 8 weeks.

Bronchoscopy is useful if no sputum is available. Biopsies from pleura, lymph nodes and solid lesions within the lung may be necessary.

## Prevention

BCG (bacille Calmette–Guérin) vaccination is a vaccine made from non-virulent tubercle bacilli. The BCG vaccination is offered to schoolchildren at 12–13 years in the UK and to newborns of high-risk groups (e.g. Asians). It is given to individuals who are tuberculin negative (Mantoux, Heaf or tuberculin test). A positive tuberculin test indicates prior infection and those testing positive are screened with a chest X-ray. A 0.1 mL intradermal dose of the vaccine (chosen dilution is usually 1:1000) is given to children and adults. Immunization decreases the risk of developing tuberculosis by up to 70%. Once an individual has been vaccinated, subsequent tuberculin tests are positive.

## Treatment

Most patients are treated on an outpatient basis with combination therapy, involving four drugs: isoniazid, rifampicin, pyrazinamide and ethambutol.

Treatment lasts 6 months and is in two phases:
- Initial phase lasting 2 months (rifampicin, isoniazid, pyrazinamide plus streptomycin or ethambutol)
- Continuation phase lasting 4 months (isoniazid and rifampicin).

The fourth drug (streptomycin or ethambutol) may be omitted in the initial phase except in drug resistant strains. In adults the daily doses in the initial phase are: rifampicin 600 mg (taken 30 min before breakfast), isoniazid 300 mg, pyrazinamide 1.5–2.0 g.

Patients should be regularly followed up because lack of compliance is a major reason for treatment

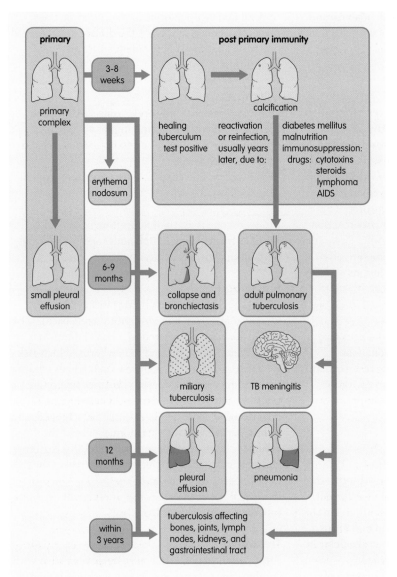

**Fig. 7.7** Pathology of tuberculosis. Note the different routes from primary systems (via progression, reactivation or re-infection). (From *Clinical Medicine* 3e, by P. Kumar and M. Clark. Baillière Tindall, 1994.)

| Early and late complications of tuberculosis | |
|---|---|
| **Early** | **Late** |
| pneumonia | bronchiectasis |
| empyema | mycetomas in cavities |
| haemoptysis | colonization of fibrotic lung with a non-tuberculous mycobacterium |
| laryngitis | extra-pulmonary disease |
| pneumothorax | |

**Fig. 7.8** Complications of tuberculosis.

failure. Drug toxicity is a problem in a minority of cases.

## Disorders of the airways

### Obstructive and restrictive defects

#### Obstructive defects

Airway obstruction and resultant airflow limitation may be caused by local or diffuse lesions; examples include asthma and COPD. Airways are widened distal to the diseased airway. Symptoms include coughing, wheezing and dyspnoea.

Pulmonary function tests show the following results:

- Increased residual volume and total lung capacity
- Reduced vital capacity, $FEV_1$, peak expiratory flow rate and $FEV_1$:FVC ratio.

## Restrictive defects

Examples of defects that restrict normal lung movement during respiration include pulmonary fibrosis, pleural disease and consolidation. Patients' breathing is shallow and rapid.

Characteristically, all lung volumes are reduced. $FEV_1$:FVC ratio is normal, but vital capacity is decreased.

# Chronic obstructive pulmonary disease

Chronic obstructive pulmonary disease (COPD) is a gradually progressive disease of the lungs involving airway obstruction. Unlike in asthma, the airway obstruction does not change over several months and is only partially reversible (e.g. with a bronchodilator). COPD is a very common disease and is a leading cause of death in the UK (30000 deaths per year). The disease is strongly associated with cigarette smoking.

Two disorders comprise COPD—chronic bronchitis and emphysema. Although by definition these are both present in a patient with COPD, they differ in pathology and site and are dealt with separately below. Clinical presentation varies widely, depending on which of the two diseases predominates; two clinical groups of patient can be identified, although these represent the two ends of a spectrum of illness and in practice most patients will fall between the two (Fig. 7.9).

## Aetiology

Cigarette smoking is the major aetiological factor; all others are minor in comparison. Cigarette smoking has three major effects:

- Impairs ciliary movement
- Causes mucus gland hypertrophy
- Alters the structure and function of alveolar macrophages.

Atmospheric pollution, occupational exposure and recurrent bronchial infections are also implicated. Recurrent bronchial infections are frequent causes of acute exacerbations; their role in development rather than progression of the condition is less clear.

| 'Pink puffers' and 'blue bloaters' | | |
|---|---|---|
| | **Pink puffer** | **Blue bloater** |
| body size | thin | obese |
| chest hyperinflation | marked | present |
| predominant disease | emphysema | chronic bronchitis |
| postmortem finding | panacinar emphysema | centrilobular emphysema |
| cor pulmonale | absent | present |
| secondary polycythaemia | absent | present |
| cyanosis | absent | centrally |
| blood gases | low $P_aCO_2$ | raised $P_aCO_2$ |

**Fig. 7.9** 'Pink puffers' and 'blue bloaters'.

Genetic abnormalities play a small role in the aetiology of emphysema (see below) but a genetic component of COPD is likely since only 15% of smokers will develop the disease.

## Diagnosis

A diagnosis of COPD is based on:

- History of chronic symptoms, without intervening periods when the patient is well
- Exposure to risk factors (primarily smoking)
- Evidence of airways obstruction (preferably using spirometry) that is not completely reversible.

Clinical features depend on the severity of the disease (Fig. 7.10) but can be summarized as:

- Productive cough
- Breathlessness, with or without wheeze
- Recurrent low-grade infective exacerbations.

Typical signs found on examination are shown in Chapter 9 (Fig. 9.42, p. 199).

## Complications of COPD
### Exacerbations

An acute worsening of the patient's condition is usually due to infection, which can be viral (e.g. influenza) or bacterial (commonly *H. influenzae*). A mild exacerbation may only require an increase in

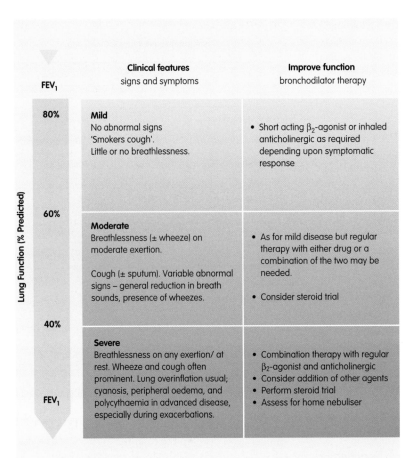

**Fig. 7.10** Clinical features and management of COPD. (Redrawn with permission from, Clinical Features and Management of COPD, *Thorax*; 52: suppl 5. British Thorax Society, 1997)

medication at home. If the exacerbation is severe, the patient may deteriorate rapidly and require hospitalization.

## Respiratory failure

In severe exacerbations the patient may be unable to maintain normal blood gases. This state is known as respiratory failure and is discussed in more detail elsewhere. Respiratory failure is the leading cause of death in patients with COPD and is often hypercapnic (type II).

## Cor pulmonale

Mortality increases in those patients with COPD who develop cor pulmonale, or right ventricular enlargement secondary to disorders affecting the lungs. In COPD it is pulmonary hypertension that causes the right ventricle to hypertrophy and eventually fail. Further details are found under pulmonary hypertension below.

## Investigations

Lung function tests show an obstructive pattern. Transfer factor/diffusing capacity is low (note that it is normal in asthma). Exercise testing assesses the extent of disability.

Chest radiography typically shows hyperinflation or flat hemidiaphragms, reduced peripheral vascular markings, and bullae. Alternatively, radiographs may appear normal.

Full blood counts may show secondary polycythaemia, but blood gas tests are often normal. $\alpha_1$ Antitrypsin levels should be measured.

## Treatment

The most important intervention is to encourage smoking cessation, thus reducing the rate of deterioration. Self-administration of inhaled drugs is the key to management of COPD: patients must be taught correct inhaler technique. Treatment options are summarized in Fig. 7.10 and include:

- Bronchodilators—combining drugs may be useful (N.B. anticholinergics are more effective than in asthma)
- Xanthines—e.g. theophylline (but remember narrow therapeutic window)
- Corticosteroids—only if there is a documented spirometric response or if $FEV_1$ is <50% of predicted or best. Combination therapies may again be more useful
- Antibiotics—shorten exacerbations and should always be given in acute episodes
- Vaccine—annual flu vaccine
- Long-term domiciliary oxygen therapy—if necessary, administer for 19 hours per day at a flow rate of 1–3 L/min. Arterial oxygen saturation needs to be above 90%
- Surgery—may be indicated to remove emphysematous lung.

In addition, severe exacerbations may be treated by:
- Oxygen (24–28% by mask at 2 L/min)
- Ventilatory support if pH < 7.6 and $P_aCO_2$ is rising (intubation or NIV).

# Chronic bronchitis

Chronic bronchitis is defined clinically as a persistent cough with sputum production for at least 3 months of the year for 2 consecutive years.

## Pathology

Hyperplasia and hypertrophy occur to the mucus-secreting glands found in the submucosa of the large cartilaginous airways. Mucous gland hypertrophy is expressed as gland–wall ratio or by the Reid index (normally, <0.4). Hyperplasia of the intraepithelial goblet cells occurs at the expense of ciliated cells in the lining epithelium. Regions of epithelium may undergo squamous metaplasia.

Small airways become obstructed by intraluminal mucus plugs, mucosal oedema, smooth muscle hypertrophy and peribronchial fibrosis. Secondary bacterial colonization of retained products occurs (Fig. 7.10).

The effect of these changes is to cause obstruction, increasing resistance to airflow. A mismatch in ventilation:perfusion occurs, impairing gas exchange.

# Emphysema

Emphysema is a permanent enlargement of the air spaces distal to the terminal bronchiole accompanied by destruction of their walls. As alveolar walls are destroyed, bullae form which may rupture causing pneumothorax. Destruction of the parenchyma increases compliance of the lung and causes a mismatch in ventilation:perfusion.

Classification of emphysema is based on anatomical distribution (Fig. 7.11). The two main types are: centriacinar and panacinar.

## Centriacinar (centrilobular) emphysema

This is the form of emphysema that is associated with chronic bronchitis in COPD ('blue bloater') (Fig. 7.9); it occurs predominantly in male smokers. As the name suggests, damage (i.e. septal destruction and dilatation) is limited to the centre of the acinus, around the terminal bronchiole. The upper lung lobes are affected more commonly than the lower lobes. Respiratory bronchiolitis is frequently present.

## Panacinar (panlobular) emphysema

Panacinar (panlobular) emphysema is a characteristic lesion of $\alpha_1$ antitrypsin deficiency. Loss of lung parenchyma, including pulmonary capillaries, occurs. The whole of the acinus is involved distal to the terminal bronchioles. Panacinar emphysema usually affects the lower lobes.

Enlarged air spaces may become cystic and form bullae. This form of emphysema is not usually associated with chronic bronchitis (Fig. 7.12C).

## Irregular emphysema

Irregular emphysema is associated with scarring and damage affecting lung parenchyma, commonly found around old healed tuberculosis scars in the lung apices. Air trapping caused by fibrosis is thought to be the pathogenesis.

Irregular emphysema overlaps clinically with paraseptal emphysema (Fig. 7.12D).

## Paraseptal (distal acinar) emphysema

In paraseptal (distal acinar) emphysema, alveolar wall destruction is restricted to the periphery of the acinus, with the upper lobes more frequently

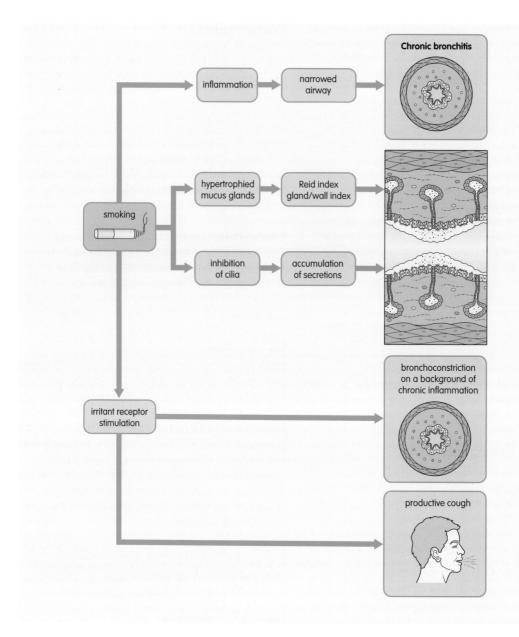

**Fig. 7.11** Pathogenesis of chronic bronchitis.

affected. If dilated airspace measures more than 10mm in diameter, the condition is termed bullous (Fig. 7.12E).

## $\alpha_1$ **Antitrypsin deficiency**

$\alpha_1$ Antitrypsin is an acute-phase serum protein produced in the liver, which functions as an antiprotease and inhibits the action of:

- Neutrophil elastase—an enzyme released during an inflammatory response, which is capable of destroying alveolar cell wall tissue
- Trypsin
- Collagenase.

In $\alpha_1$ antitrypsin deficiency, serum levels of the enzyme are reduced. This is an autosomal dominant

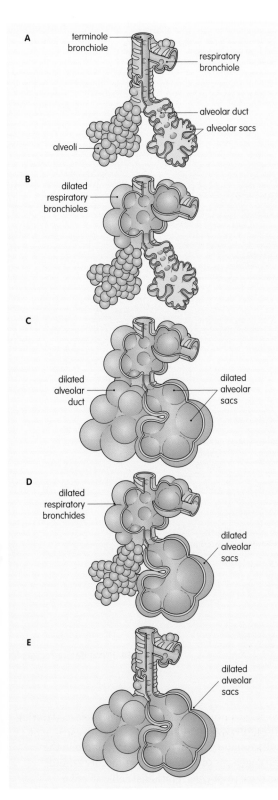

**Fig. 7.12** Main types of emphysema. (A) Normal distal lung acinus; (B) centriacinar emphysema; (C) panacinar emphysema; (D) irregular emphysema; (E) paraseptal emphysema.

condition, where homozygous individuals develop severe panacinar emphysema.

$\alpha_1$ Antitrypsin deficiency develops at an early age (before 40 years of age) with equal distribution between sexes. The homozygous state has an incidence of 1:3630 in Caucasians, but is rarer in dark-skinned people.

## Asthma

Asthma is a chronic inflammatory disorder of the lungs characterized by variability in symptoms and lung function.

### Prevalence

Five per cent of the adult population are receiving therapy for asthma at any one time. Prevalence of asthma in the Western world is rising, particularly in children; up to 20% have symptoms at some time in their childhood.

### Classification

Bronchial asthma may be categorized into two groups on the basis of atopy: extrinsic or intrinsic (Fig. 7.13). Precipitating factors are described in Fig. 7.14.

Occupational asthma is increasing; currently there are over 200 materials encountered at the workplace that are implicated (Fig. 7.15). Occupational asthma may be classified as:

- Allergic (immunologically mediated with a latent period between exposure and symptoms)
- Non-allergic (immediate response after exposure, e.g. to toxic gases).

Take a full history, including occupational history. Do symptoms improve at the weekend or on holiday? If so, there may be an occupational cause.

### Pathogenesis of asthma

Pathogenesis of asthma is very complex. Airway inflammation (Fig. 7.16) causes:

- Smooth muscle constriction
- Thickening of the airway wall (smooth muscle hypertrophy and oedema)
- Basement membrane thickening
- Mucus and exudate in the airway lumen.

Fig. 7.13 Classification of asthma.

| Asthma | | |
|---|---|---|
| | **Extrinsic asthma** | **Intrinsic asthma** |
| underlying abnormality | immune reaction (atopic) | abnormal autonomic regulation of airways |
| onset | childhood | adulthood |
| distribution | 60% | 40% |
| allergens | recognized | none identified |
| family history | present | absent |
| predisposition to form IgE antibodies | present | absent |
| association with chronic obstructive pulmonary disease | none | chronic bronchitis |
| natural progression | improves | worsens |
| eosinophilia | sputum and blood | sputum |
| drug hypersensitivity | absent | present |

| Precipitating factors for asthma | | | | | |
|---|---|---|---|---|---|
| **Allergens** | **Occupational sensitizers** | **Viral infections** | **Atmospheric factors** | **Drugs** | **Other factors** |
| house dust mite (*Dermatophagoides pteronyssius*) | colophony fumes (from soldering) | para influenza | cigarette smoke | β-blockers | cold air |
| flour | isocyanates (from polyurethane varnishes) | respiratory syncytial virus | ozone | nonsteroidal anti-inflammatory drugs | emotion |
| animal danders | acid anhydrides (from industrial coatings) | rhinovirus | sulphur dioxide | | fumes |
| grain | | | | | exercise |

Fig. 7.14 Precipitating factors for asthma.

Microscopically, the viscid mucus contains:
- Desquamated epithelial cells
- Whorls of shed epithelium (Curshmann's whorls)
- Charcot Leyden crystal (eosinophil cell membranes)
- Infiltration of inflammatory cells, particularly CD4+ T lymphocytes.

## Inflammatory mediators

Inflammatory mediators play a vital role in the pathogenesis of asthma. Inflammatory stimuli activate mast cells, epithelial cells, alveolar macrophages and dendritic cells resident within the airways, causing the release of mediators that are chemotactic for cells derived from the circulation—

**Fig. 7.15** Factors implicated in occupational asthma. (Adapted from *Pulmonary Physiology* by G. Criner and G. D'Alonzo. Fence Creek Publishing, 1999, pp. 213 and 398.)

| Factors implicated in occupational asthma | |
| --- | --- |
| **Agents** | **Workers at risk include:** |
| **High-molecular weight agents** | |
| cereals | bakers, millers |
| animal-derived allergens | animal handlers |
| enzymes | detergent users, pharmaceutical workers, bakers |
| gums | carpet makers, pharmaceutical workers |
| latex | health professionals |
| seafoods | seafood processors |
| **Low-molecular weight agents** | |
| isocynates | spray painters, insulation installers etc. |
| wood dusts | forest workers, carpenters |
| anhydrides | users of plastics, expoxy resins |
| fluxes | electronic workers |
| chloramine | janitors, cleaners |
| acrylate | adhesive handlers |
| drugs | pharmaceutical workers, health professionals |
| metals | solderers, refiners |

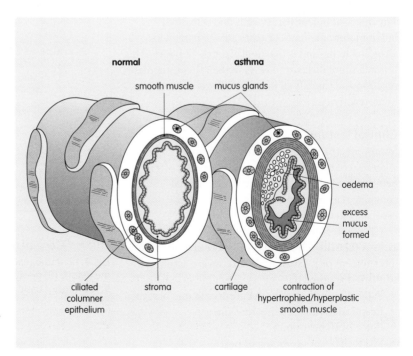

**Fig. 7.16** Mechanisms of airway narrowing in asthma. (From *Pulmonary Physiology* by G. Criner and G. D'Alonzo. Fence Creek Publishing, 1999, p. 213.)

139

secondary effector cells (eosinophils, neutrophils and platelets).

Mediators that are thought to be involved in asthma include (Fig. 7.17):

- Preformed mediators—present in cytoplasmic granules ready for release. Associated with human lung mast cells and include histamine, neutral proteases and chemotactic factors for neutrophils and eosinophils
- Newly generated mediators—manufactured secondary to the initial triggering stimulus after release of preformed mediators. Some of these mediators are derived from the membrane phospholipid and are associated with the metabolism of arachidonic acid (e.g. prostaglandins and leukotrienes). The production of inflammatory cytokines and chemokines is important in the activation and recruitment of inflammatory cells.

### Early and late responses

Two patterns of response can be considered; in practice most asthmatics show evidence of both responses, although either may be absent.

### Immediate (early) reaction

The release of preformed mediators causes maximal airway narrowing within 10–15 minutes of challenge with a return to baseline within 1–2 hours.

### Late reaction

The influx of inflammatory cells and release of inflammatory mediators causes airway narrowing after 3–4 hours and is maximal after 6–12 hours. This is much more difficult to reverse than the immediate reaction and there is an increase in level of airway hyperreactivity.

## Clinical features

Symptoms (breathlessness, chest tightness, cough, wheeze) classically show a diurnal variation often being worse at night. For example, nocturnal coughing is a common presenting symptom, especially in children.

Clinical features vary according to the severity of asthma (classified from mild to severe and either intermittent or persistent). Acute severe asthma in adults is diagnosed if:

- Patient cannot complete sentences in one breath
- Respiration rate ≥25 breaths/min
- Pulse ≥110 beats/min
- PEFR ≤50% of predicted or best.

**Fig. 7.17** Pathogenesis of asthma. (A) Preformed mediators; (B) newly generated mediators. IL5, interleukin 5; MBP, major basic protein; ECP, eosinophil cationic protein.

Life-threatening asthma is characterized by the following:

- PEFR < 33% of predicted or best
- Silent chest and cyanosis
- Bradycardia or hypotension
- Exhaustion, confusion or coma
- $P_aO_2 < 8kPa$.

## Investigations

Investigations include:

- Lung function tests—$FEV_1/FVC$ is reduced, RV may be increased; tests demonstrate an improvement in $FEV_1$ of more than 15% after bronchodilator administration
- Peak expiratory flow rate—morning and evening measurements. Useful in the long-term assessment of asthma; a characteristic morning dipping pattern is seen in poorly controlled asthma
- If PEFR < 50%, arterial blood gases should be tested
- Exercise laboratory tests
- Bronchial provocation tests—performed rarely in normal clinical practice, using histamine or methacholine to demonstrate bronchial hyperreactivity
- Chest radiography—no diagnostic features of asthma on chest radiograph; use to rule out a diagnosis of allergic bronchopulmonary aspergillosis
- Skin prick tests—allergen injections into the epidermis of the forearm, which are used to identify extrinsic causes. Look for weal development in sensitive patients.

## Treatment

Identify and avoid extrinsic factors. Follow the British Thoracic Society (BTS) guidelines with a stepwise approach to drug treatment:

- Occasional use of short-acting bronchodilators
- Regular inhaled anti-inflammatory agents
- High-dose inhaled steroids or low-dose plus long-acting inhaled bronchodilator
- High-dose inhaled steroids and regular bronchodilators
- Addition of regular steroid tablets.

Drugs used in treating asthma are discussed in Chapter 6.

# Bronchiectasis

Bronchiectasis is defined as an abnormal and permanent dilatation of the bronchi and is associated with chronic infection. Most cases arise in childhood.

## Aetiology

Bronchiectasis can either be acquired or, less commonly, congenital.

### Acquired bronchiectasis

Bronchiectasis is usually caused by a severe childhood infection (e.g. bronchopneumonia, measles or whooping cough). Inflammation can damage and weaken the bronchial wall, leading to dilatation. It may also be caused by bronchial obstruction (e.g. by a foreign body, tuberculous lymph nodes or tumour) followed by infection in the lung distal to the obstruction.

### Congenital bronchiectasis

Congenital abnormalities that interfere with ciliary function (e.g. primary ciliary dyskinesia, Kartagener's syndrome and Young's syndrome) impair the transport of mucus and cause recurrent infection. Kartegener's syndrome, which is a rare cause, is also associated with dextrocardia and sinusitis. The viscous mucus and recurrent infections of cystic fibrosis may also lead to bronchiectasis. Recurrent infections are also a feature of immunoglobulin deficiencies (e.g. IgA); therefore these are also associated with bronchiectasis.

## Pathology

Infection leads to obstruction, dilation of bronchi and often loss of cilia. Destruction of the alveolar walls and fibrosis of lung parenchyma occur and pulmonary haemodynamic changes can take place. The dependent portions of the lungs, usually the lower lobes, are affected most commonly.

## Symptoms

Cough is the most common symptom; this is often persistent and accompanied by sputum which may be mucopurulent or copious, purulent and foul-smelling. Systemic features of infection such as fever and malaise also occur.

Haemoptysis may be present and can be massive. Clubbing occurs and coarse inspiratory crackles are heard on auscultation.

## Complications

Complications of bronchiectasis include:

- Pneumonia
- Pneumothorax
- Empyema
- Meningitis
- Metastatic abscess (e.g. in brain)
- Amyloid formation (e.g. in kidney).

## Investigations

Bronchiectasis can be investigated through:

- Radiology—chest radiograph may be normal or show bronchial wall thickening. If disease is advanced, cystic spaces may be seen
- High-resolution CT—the investigation of choice to detect bronchial wall thickening
- Sputum tests—Gram stain, anaerobic and aerobic culture, and sensitivity testing are vital during an infective exacerbation. Major pathogens include *Staphylococcus aureus*, *Pseudomonas aeruginosa*, *Haemophilus influenzae* and anaerobes
- Tests for cystic fibrosis where appropriate (cystic fibrosis sweat test)
- Lung function spirometry (may show an obstructive pattern).

## Treatment

Aims of treatment are twofold:

- Control of infection
- Removal of secretions.

Infections should be eradicated with antibiotics if progression of the disease is to be halted. Treatment regimens depend on infecting organism (e.g. flucloxacillin 500 mg 6-hourly to treat *Staphylococcus aureus* infection). If there is no improvement with treatment, the patient is likely to be infected with *Pseudomonas aeruginosa*: treat with ceftazidime aerosol or parenterally. Secretions are removed by postural drainage for 10–20 minutes, three times a day. Patients are trained in the method by physiotherapists.

Bronchodilators are useful if demonstrable airflow limitation exists. Surgery is of limited value but may be indicated in a young patient with adequate lung function, if disease is localized to one lung or segment.

## Cystic fibrosis

Cystic fibrosis is a disorder characterized by the production of abnormally viscid secretions by exocrine glands and mucus-secreting glands, such as those in the pancreas and respiratory tract. Impaired mucociliary clearance in the airways leads to recurrent infections and bronchiectasis.

Cystic fibrosis is the commonest genetically transmitted disease in Caucasians. It is an autosomal recessive condition occurring in 1 : 2000 live births. The gene has been identified on the long arm of chromosome 7. Prevalence of heterozygous carriers is 4%.

### Aetiology

The commonest mutation is a specific gene deletion in the codon for phenylalanine at position 508 in the amino-acid sequence ($\Delta$F508). This results in a defect in a transmembrane regulator protein known as the cystic fibrosis transmembrane conductive regulator (CFTR). Mutation causes a failure of opening of the chloride channels in response to elevated cAMP in epithelial cells, leading to:

- Decreased excretion of chloride into the airway lumen
- Increased reabsorption of sodium into the epithelial cells
- Increased viscosity of secretions.

### Pathology

The thick secretions produced by the epithelial cells cause:

- Small airway obstruction, leading to recurrent infection and ultimately bronchiectasis
- Pancreatic duct obstruction, causing pancreatic fibrosis and ultimately pancreatic insufficiency.

### Clinical features

Presentation depends on age. Usually, the condition presents in infancy with gastrointestinal manifestations (Fig. 7.18).

| Cystic fibrosis | |
|---|---|
| **Respiratory manifestations** | **Gastrointestinal manifestations** |
| recurrent bronchopulmonary infection bronchiectasis | meconium ileus rectal prolapse diarrhoea failure to thrive malabsorption |

**Fig. 7.18** Manifestations of cystic fibrosis.

| Complications of cystic fibrosis | |
| --- | --- |
| **Respiratory complications** | **Other complications** |
| allergic aspergillosus | abdominal pain |
| bronchiectasis | biliary cirrhosis |
| cor pulmonale | delayed puberty |
| haemoptysis | diabetes mellitus |
| lobar collapse | gall stones |
| nasal polyps | growth failure |
| pneumothorax | male infertility |
| sinusitis | portal hypertension |
| wheezing | rectal prolapse |

**Fig. 7.19** Complications of cystic fibrosis.

| Summary of treatment | |
| --- | --- |
| **Respiratory** | **Gastrointestinal** |
| drain secretions, postural drainage | pancreatic enzyme supplements with all meals and snacks |
| prevent infection where possible | high-energy, high-protein diet |
| exercise encouraged | do not restrict fat in diet |
| regular sputum cultures | vitamin A, D, and E supplements |
| immunization against measles and influenza | |

**Fig. 7.20** Summary of treatment cystic fibrosis.

Stools are bulky, greasy, and offensive in smell. Respiratory signs are normal and symptoms are non-specific:

- Lungs are normal at birth
- Frequent infections with cough and wheeze as the child gets older
- Clubbing and dyspnoea occur.

Almost all men with cystic fibrosis are infertile; females may be subfertile.

## Investigations

Family history is sought (e.g. affected siblings). Genetic screening is available for couples with a family history.

Prenatal diagnosis is available by chorionic villous sampling or amniocentesis.

Tests include:

- Guthrie test
- Immunoreactive trypsin test (IRT)—positive test shows low levels
- Sweat test—raised levels of sodium and chloride in sweat.

The complications of cystic fibrosis are described in Fig. 7.19.

## Treatment

Treatment (Fig. 7.20) is based on:

- Physiotherapy
- Antibiotics (see below)
- DNase (see below)
- Anti-inflammatory drugs (steroids)
- Nutritional support.

IV antibiotics may be given at home (e.g. through implantable venous access devices) to reduce hospital admissions and improve patient independence.

Human DNase has been cloned, sequenced and expressed by recombinant techniques. This is:

- Capable of degrading DNA
- Shown to improve $FEV_1$
- Expensive.

Heart–lung and liver transplantations are possible in severely affected patients.

## Prognosis

Prognosis is improving: currently, mean survival is 29 years. Death is mainly caused by respiratory complications.

## Disorders of the pulmonary vessels

## Pulmonary congestion and oedema

Pulmonary oedema is defined as an abnormal increase in the amount of interstitial fluid in the lung. The two main causes are:

- Increased venous hydrostatic pressures
- Injury to alveolar capillary walls or vessels, leading to increased permeability.

Less common causes are blockage of lymphatic drainage and lowered plasma oncotic pressure.

## High-pressure pulmonary oedema

High-pressure or haemodynamic pulmonary oedema is cardiogenic; it may occur acutely as a result of a myocardial infarction or chronically in aortic and mitral valve disease.

Fluid movement between intravascular and extravascular compartments is governed by Starling forces (see Fig. 5.11, p. 80). Net fluid flow through a capillary wall (out of the blood) is governed by:

- Hydrostatic pressure (arterial blood pressure) at the arteriole end of the capillary bed
- Capillary permeability
- Opposing oncotic pressure exerted by serum proteins (mainly albumin); interstitial oncotic pressure may also contribute to the outflow.

Reabsorption of interstitial fluid is governed by:
- Plasma oncotic pressure (pulling pressure)
- Hydrostatic pressure in the interstitial space (tissue pressure)
- Fall in hydrostatic pressure at venous end of capillary.

Imbalances in Starling forces and a reduced plasma oncotic pressure will cause expansion of the interstitial spaces.

No pathological conditions cause a local reduction of plasma protein concentration within the lung capillaries. However, many conditions (e.g. left ventricular failure) cause an elevation of hydrostatic pressure. If left arterial pressure rises, so do pulmonary venous and capillary pressures, thereby raising hydrostatic pressure and causing oedema formation. Pulmonary oedema occurs only after the lymphatic drainage capacity has been exceeded. Lymphatic drainage can increase 10-fold without oedema formation. However, if lymphatic drainage is blocked (e.g. in cancer), oedema occurs more readily.

Oedema due to haemodynamic causes has a low protein content.

## Oedema caused by microvascular injury

This is the non-cardiogenic form of pulmonary oedema.

Capillary blood is separated from alveolar air by three anatomical layers:
- Capillary endothelium
- Narrow interstitial layer
- Alveolar epithelium.

## Damage to capillary endothelium

Normal alveolar capillary endothelial cells are joined by tight junctions containing narrow constrictions. Many conditions can damage the pulmonary capillary endothelium, resulting in movement of fluid and a transcapillary leak of proteins. Interstitial oncotic pressure rises; thus, a natural defence against oedema formation is disabled.

After damage, fibrinogen enters and coagulates within the interstitium. Interstitial fibrosis subsequently occurs, leading to impaired lymphatic drainage. Oedema caused by microvascular damage characteristically has a high protein content.

## Progression of pulmonary oedema

Fluid first accumulates in loose connective tissue around the bronchi and large vessels. Fluid then distends the thick, collagen-containing portions of the alveolar wall. The final stage of pulmonary oedema is accumulation of fluid within the alveolar spaces. If pulmonary oedema is chronic, recurrent alveolar haemorrhages lead to the accumulation of haemosiderin-laden macrophages along with interstitial fibrosis.

## Clinical features

Clinical features of oedema are as follows:
- Acute breathlessness
- Wheezing
- Anxiety
- Tachypnoea
- Profuse perspiration
- Production of pink sputum while coughing
- Peripheral circulatory shutdown
- Tachycardia
- Basal crackles and wheezes heard on auscultation
- Respiratory impairment with hypoxaemia
- Overloaded lungs predispose to secondary infection.

## Treatment

The patient should be placed in a sitting position and 60% $O_2$ administered. Intravenous diuretics give an immediate and delayed response. Morphine sedates the patient and causes systemic vasodilatation: if systemic arterial pressure falls below 90mmHg do not use morphine. Aminophylline can be infused over 10 minutes, but should be used only when bronchospasm is present.

# Adult respiratory distress syndrome (ARDS)

Adult respiratory distress syndrome (ARDS) is non-cardiogenic pulmonary oedema defined as diffuse pulmonary infiltrates, refractory hypoxaemia, stiff lungs and respiratory distress (Fig. 7.21). ARDS forms part of a systemic inflammatory reaction.

## Aetiology

Causes are as follows:

- Gram-negative septicaemia
- Trauma or shock
- Infection (e.g. pneumonia)
- Pancreatitis
- Gastric aspiration
- Perforated viscus
- Narcotic abuse
- Disseminated intravascular coagulation
- Oxygen toxicity
- Gas inhalation
- Ionizing radiation.

The underlying insult is damage to the alveolar capillary wall, leading to diffuse alveolar damage.

## Precipitating mechanisms of ARDS

Mechanisms include pulmonary capillary hypoxaemia, microembolism and loss of surfactant caused by pulmonary epithelium damage.

## Pathology

As noted above, the key feature of ARDS is non-cardiogenic pulmonary oedema. Pulmonary venous and capillary engorgement occurs, leading to interstitial oedema. Pulmonary epithelium damage also occurs.

Pulmonary hypertension is common; hypoxic vasoconstriction redirects blood to better areas of oxygenation.

A protein-rich intra-alveolar haemorrhagic exudate promotes formation of hyaline membranes that line alveolar ducts and alveoli.

In long-standing cases, pulmonary fibrosis ensues and the alveolar walls become lined by metaplastic cuboidal epithelium (Fig. 7.21).

### Resolution

Resolution occurs as follows:

- Resorption of oedema
- Ingestion of red cells and hyaline membranes by alveolar macrophages
- Regeneration of type II pneumocytes.

**Fig. 7.21** Cell types in adult respiratory distress syndrome. (A) Normal alveolar wall; (B) acute phase of ARDS; (C) organization phase of ARDS.

## Clinical features

Features change during the progression of ARDS. Patients with ARDS present with:

- Tachypnoea, often unexplained
- Dyspnoea
- Pulmonary oedema—fine crackles throughout both lung fields

- Arterial hypoxaemia, refractory to oxygen therapy.

Chest radiography shows bilateral diffuse shadowing.

## Management
- Treat underlying condition and provide supportive measures
- Treat as for pulmonary oedema: the aim is to achieve a negative fluid balance
- Provide cardiovascular support and mechanical ventilation (e.g. positive end expiratory pressure).

## Prognosis
Prognosis is dependent upon cause, but mortality is generally greater than 50%. With septic shock, mortality is 90%. With fat embolism, mortality is 10%.

Prognosis is poor in the elderly.

Death is caused by cardiac arrhythmias with sepsis, usually from Gram-negative organisms.

## Embolism, haemorrhage and infarction
Vascular disease of the lungs can be caused by:
- Vessel obstruction
- Vessel wall damage
- Intravascular pressure variations.

### Obstruction: pulmonary embolism
An embolus is an abnormal mass of material that is transported in the bloodstream from one part of the circulation to another and which impacts finally in the lumen of a vessel which has a calibre too small to allow passage. The end result of an embolus derived from venous thrombus is impaction in the pulmonary arterial tree. Most thrombi originate in the deep veins of the calf or pelvis.

This is a common condition: incidence of pulmonary emboli at autopsy has been reported to be 12%.

Pulmonary emboli rarely have a cardiac cause and are very rare in children.

### Predisposing factors
Predisposing factors are:
- Immobilization (e.g. prolonged bed rest)
- In women, the oral contraceptive pill—minor risk factor, increased by cigarette smoking
- Malignancy, especially of pancreas, uterus, breast and stomach

- Cardiac failure
- Chronic pulmonary disease
- Postoperative recovery
- Fractures of the pelvis or lower limb
- Hypercoagulable states (e.g. pregnancy).

When a patient presents postoperatively with sudden-onset chest pain, pulmonary embolism should be at the top of the list of differential diagnoses.

### Clinical features
Common symptoms are:
- Dyspnoea
- Tachypnoea
- Pleuritic pain
- Apprehension
- Tachycardia
- Cough
- Haemoptysis
- Leg pain/clinical DVT.

Symptoms are related to the size of the embolus and the corresponding volume of lung tissue deprived of blood in addition to the presence or absence of congestion in the pulmonary circulation at the time of impaction.

Pulmonary embolism can be classified as massive, moderate or small.

### Massive pulmonary embolism
A massive pulmonary embolism is a clinical emergency. The embolus is typically derived from a thrombus that occludes a long venous segment in the lower limb. The calibre of the main pulmonary arteries is greater than the iliac and femoral veins; therefore, thrombi must loosely bundle together to block the pulmonary arteries (as seen in a saddle embolus, which occurs at the bifurcation of the left and right pulmonary arteries).

Within normal human lung, occlusion of more than 50% of the pulmonary vascular bed is necessary for a massive pulmonary embolism to prove fatal.

## Clinical features

This is a clinical emergency presenting as sudden-onset severe chest pain and dyspnoea. Often onset occurs when straining during defaecation. Classically, a massive pulmonary embolism occurs a week or more after operation.

There are signs of shock: tachycardia, low blood pressure.

Right ventricular heave, gallop rhythm and a prominent a-wave in the jugular venous pulse may also be noted.

Sudden death can occur.

## Small or medium-sized pulmonary embolism

Moderate pulmonary embolism is caused by occlusion of a lobar or segmental artery. Perfusion of a segment may be reduced producing an area of localized necrosis.

An area of necrosis secondary to ischaemia is known as an infarct.

## Clinical features

Pulmonary infarction presents with sudden-onset pleuritic chest pain. Cough with haemoptysis and dyspnoea are other symptoms.

## Multiple microemboli

Multiple small emboli can occlude arterioles but this process is usually clinically silent. Gradual occlusion of the pulmonary arterial bed leads to pulmonary hypertension.

This is a rare condition characterized by exertional dyspnoea, tiredness and syncope. Basal crackles are heard on auscultation.

## Other forms of emboli
### Fat embolism

Fat embolism results from massive injury to subcutaneous fat or fracture of bones containing fatty marrow. Globules of lipid enter the torn vessels.

### Air embolism

Air embolism arises during childbirth or abortion or after chest wall injury. These microemboli can cause tiny infarcts in several organs.

### Tumour embolism

Tumour cells, like other particulate matter, become trapped in the pulmonary capillary bed. This is an important mechanism in the development of metastases.

### Amniotic fluid embolism

Amniotic fluid embolism can occur during childbirth or abortion, and may be fatal. Small fragments of trophoblast are commonly found in lungs of pregnant women at autopsy, but do not cause any symptoms.

## Investigations in suspected pulmonary emboli

Chest radiography is usually unremarkable, but valuable in excluding other causes. Electrocardiography may show signs of right ventricular strain (deep S waves in lead I, Q waves in lead III, and inverted T waves in lead III).

Arterial blood gases show arterial hypoxaemia and hypocapnia.

Radioisotope ventilation:perfusion scans demonstrate ventilated areas of lung and filling defects on the corresponding perfusion scans; these are assessed on the basis of probability of pulmonary embolism (see Chapter 10). In non-diagnostic scans, pulmonary angiography should be performed in the acutely ill patient or leg ultrasound if the patient is stable.

## Treatment

Treatment is based on:
- Supportive measures (analgesia, oxygen etc.)
- Anticoagulation
- Thrombolysis.

## Anticoagulation

Further emboli should be prevented (patients with a pulmonary embolism have a 30% chance of developing further emboli). Intravenous heparin is administered:
- Bolus: 10 000 IU
- Continuous infusion: 400–600 IU/kg daily.

Oral anticoagulants are given after 48 hours, and heparin is reduced. Oral anticoagulants are continued for between 6 weeks and 6 months.

## Thrombolysis

Thrombolysis is indicated in patients who are haemodynamically unstable (e.g. hypotensive). It is possible to break down thrombi by:
- Intravenous streptokinase 250 000 IU infusion over 30 minutes
- Intravenous streptokinase 100 000 IU hourly for up to 24 hours.

Surgery is performed only on massive pulmonary emboli in patients who fail to respond to thrombolysis.

## Prevention
This is by avoidance of deep vein thromboses:
- Early mobilization of patients after operation
- Use of tight elastic stockings
- Leg exercises
- Prophylactic anticoagulation.

## Pulmonary infarction
Less than 10% of pulmonary emboli cause infarction within the lung. Lung infarcts are more common in the lower lobes; infarction is less common in the lungs than in other organs because of the lungs' dual blood supply.

Pulmonary infarction is usually a consequence of a moderate pulmonary embolism. Pulmonary infarction is rare in young people.

### Predisposing factors
Predisposing factors for infarction include:
- Rise in pulmonary venous pressure
- Mitral stenosis or left ventricular failure
- Bronchial occlusion
- Pleural effusion
- Infection.

### Pathology
A wedge-shaped section of the lung downstream from the blockage becomes necrotic. The base of the wedge is situated toward the pleural aspect of the lung. Pleural inflammation over the infarcted area is common. Organization of pulmonary infarcts proceeds rapidly.

### Clinical features
Clinical features include sudden-onset pleuritic chest pain and dyspnoea.

### Investigations
Blood tests show increases in erythrocyte sedimentation rate and lactate dehydrogenase (LDH) levels. Polymorphonuclear leucocytosis is present.

Arterial blood gas measurement reveals hypoxaemia, but normal $PCO_2$.

Ventilation:perfusion scans show mismatching.

## Pulmonary hypertension and vascular sclerosis
Pulmonary hypertension occurs when blood pressure in the pulmonary circulation exceeds 30mmHg (Fig. 7.22).

| Pulmonary hypertension | |
|---|---|
| **Aetiology** | **Vascular lesion** |
| Cardiac disease | Precapillary (e.g. left-to-right shunt) |
| Hypoxia | Capillary (e.g. hypoxia) |
| Fibrosis | Postcapillary (e.g. left ventricular failure) |
| Miscellaneous | |
| Idiopathic (primary) | |

**Fig. 7.22** Classification of pulmonary hypertension. Note that pulmonary arterial changes depend on aetiology of the pulmonary hypertension.

Pulmonary hypertension can be caused by:
- Increased vascular resistance in the pulmonary circulation
- Increased pulmonary venous pressure
- Increased pulmonary blood flow.

The increase in vascular resistance is of most interest in respiratory medicine. This can occur due to:
- Chronic hypoxia
- Obstruction of pulmonary vessels
- Pulmonary fibrosis.

### Chronic hypoxia
Chronic airflow obstruction or living at high altitude can lead to chronic hypoxia. This is also seen in Pickwickian syndrome where pulmonary hypertension is caused by poor respiration associated with gross obesity. Because insignificant intimal fibrosis occurs, the condition is largely reversible.

### Obstruction of pulmonary vessels
This is seen in primary pulmonary hypertension, a rare condition of unknown aetiology, predominantly seen in women aged 20–30 years. The condition may be familial.

### Pulmonary fibrosis
Early changes of pulmonary vasculature are initially muscular in type and reversible. Obliterative fibrosis of pulmonary arteries and arterioles occurs later, with irreversible increases in pulmonary vascular resistance.

The other causes of pulmonary hypertension (those due to increased pulmonary venous pressure and increased pulmonary blood flow) are primarily cardiac and are not considered here.

### Pathology

Effects of pulmonary hypertension include:
- Enlarged proximal pulmonary arteries
- Right ventricular hypertrophy
- Right arterial dilatation
- Necrotizing arteritis.

### Clinical features

Clinical features are as follows:
- Symptoms of the underlying cause
- Chest pain and exertional dyspnoea
- Syncope and fatigue
- Prominent a-wave in jugular venous pulse
- Right ventricular heave
- Loud pulmonary component to second heart sound
- Midsystolic ejection murmur.

### Investigations

When investigating pulmonary hypertension, a possible cause should be sought.

A full blood count may show secondary polycythaemia. Chest radiography may reveal right ventricular enlargement, pulmonary artery dilatation, or oligaemic peripheral lung fields.

Electrocardiography may indicate right ventricular hypertrophy, right-axis deviation, a prominent R wave in V1, or inverted T waves in the right precordial leads.

Radioisotope lung scans and echocardiography may also be useful.

### Treatment

Treatment is dependent upon cause. Primary pulmonary hypertension is treated with anticoagulation therapy.

If the underlying cause of hypertension is untreatable, the patient will progress to cor pulmonale and death. Continuous oxygen therapy is beneficial in patients with cor pulmonale. Diuretics are used to treat fluid overload.

Heart–lung transplantation is recommended in young patients.

Prognosis is poor: 5-year survival rate is 40%.

### Cor pulmonale

Cor pulmonale is a major complication of pulmonary hypertension. It is defined as right heart failure secondary to lung disease and occurs as a result of any disorder that leads to pulmonary hypertension. Of

most interest here is its presence in lung disease. As noted above, lung disease that causes chronic hypoxia may lead to pulmonary hypertension and therefore cor pulmonale. The main respiratory diseases associated with cor pulmonale are:
- COPD
- Severe, chronic asthma
- Bronchiectasis
- Pulmonary emboli
- Pulmonary fibrosis.

The principal signs are those of the underlying disease in addition to oedema, raised JVP and atrial gallop rhythm. Arterial blood gases show hypoxaemia with or without hypercapnia.

## Disorders of the lung interstitium

This group of diseases can cause confusion because many different synonyms are used. The diseases themselves can be referred to as diffuse parenchymal lung diseases (DPLD), acknowledging that it is not just the interstitium that is affected. There are several synonyms for idiopathic fibrosing alveolitis (see below), pneumoconioses are also known as industrial dust diseases and extrinsic allergic alveolitis is the same as hypersensitivity alveolitis.

Remember that the interstitium is the space between the alveolar epithelium and capillary endothelium (see Fig. 3.12, p. 32).

### Pulmonary fibrosis

Pulmonary fibrosis is the end result of many respiratory diseases (Fig. 7.23) and is characterized by scar tissue in the lungs which decreases lung compliance, i.e. the lungs become stiffer.

The pathogenesis of pulmonary fibrosis is complex, involving many factors (Fig. 7.24). The main features are:

| Causes of pulmonary fibrosis | | | | | |
|---|---|---|---|---|---|
| Dusts | | Inhalants | Infection | Iatrogenic causes | Other causes |
| Mineral | Biological | | | | |
| coal | avian protein | oxygen | postpneumonic infection | cytotoxic drugs | sarcoidosis |
| silica | *Actinomyces* | sulphur dioxide | tuberculosis | non-cytotoxics | connective-tissue disease |
| asbestos | *Aspergillus* | nitrogen dioxide | — | radiation | chronic pulmonary oedema |

**Fig. 7.23** Causes of pulmonary fibrosis.

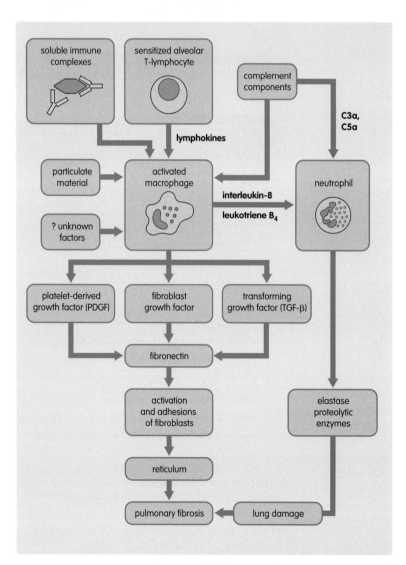

**Fig. 7.24** Pathogenesis of pulmonary fibrosis. Macrophages can be activated by several factors (e.g. soluble immune complexes and sensitized T-lymphocytes), resulting in the release of various cytokines leading to fibrosis. (From *Clinical Medicine* 3e, by P. Kumar and M. Clark. Baillière Tindall, 1994.)

- A lesion affecting the alveolar-capillary basement membrane
- Cellular infiltration and thickening by collagen of the interstitium of the alveolar wall
- Fibroblasts proliferate leading to further collagen deposition.

The end stage is characterized by a honeycomb lung, a non-specific condition in which cystic spaces develop in fibrotic lungs with compensatory dilatation of unaffected neighbouring bronchioles.

The end stage of chronic interstitial lung disease is termed honeycomb lung.

Note from Fig. 7.24 that the initial injury to the alveolar-capillary basement membrane may be caused by several different mechanisms. Some (e.g. dusts) are considered below.

## Clinical features

Patients become progressively breathless and develop a dry, non-productive cough. On examination, lung expansion is reduced and end-inspiratory crackles are heard.

## Investigations

Chest X-ray may show fine reticular, nodular or reticulonodular infiltration in the basal areas. High resolution CT (HRCT) or biopsy may be used to aid diagnosis. Lung function tests demonstrate a restrictive pattern along with a decreased transfer factor.

# The pneumoconioses

The pneumoconioses are a group of disorders caused by inhalation of mineral or biological dusts. The incidence is decreasing as working conditions continue to improve.

Four types of reaction occur:
- Inert (e.g. simple coal-worker's pneumoconiosis)
- Fibrous (e.g. asbestosis)
- Allergic (e.g. extrinsic allergic alveolitis)
- Neoplastic (e.g. mesothelioma).

Distribution of lung disease depends on the dust involved: particles measuring less than 2–3μm in diameter reach the distal alveoli. Dust particles that are phagocytosed by alveolar macrophages drain into peribronchial lymphatics and hilar lymph nodes.

Radiological appearances are related to the degree of associated fibrosis and atomic number of dust particles involved.

## Coal-worker's pneumoconiosis

The incidence of coal-worker's pneumoconiosis is related to total dust exposure: it is highest in men who work at the coal face. Two syndromes exist: simple pneumoconiosis and an advanced form, progressive massive fibrosis.

### Simple pneumoconiosis

Simple pneumoconiosis is the commonest type of pneumoconiosis, reflecting coal dust deposition within the lung. It is asymptomatic and diagnosis is made on the basis of chest X-rays. Opacities on chest radiographs are mainly in the upper zone and are graded as follows:
1. A few small, round opacities are present.
2. Numerous small, round opacities are present. Normal lung markings are visible.
3. Very numerous small, round opacities are present. Normal lung markings are partially or totally obscured.

Of patients with category 3 simple pneumoconiosis, 30% will develop progressive massive fibrosis.

### Progressive massive fibrosis

In progressive massive fibrosis, large, round fibrotic nodules measuring more than 10mm in diameter are seen, usually in the upper lobes. Scarring is present. Nodules may show central liquefaction and become infected by tuberculosis. The associated emphysema is always severe.

Symptoms include dyspnoea, cough and sputum production (which may be black as cavitating lesions rupture). Lung function tests show a mixed restrictive and obstructive pattern.

The disease may progress once exposure has ceased (unlike simple coal-worker's pneumoconiosis) and there is no specific treatment.

### Caplan's syndrome

Caplan's syndrome is the association of coal-worker's pneumoconiosis and rheumatoid arthritis.

Rounded lesions, measuring 0.5–5.0cm in diameter, are seen on X-ray.

## Asbestosis

Asbestosis is a diffuse fibrosis which is caused by the inhalation of asbestos. Asbestos is a mixture of silicates of iron, nickel, magnesium, aluminium and cadmium. It is mined in Southern Africa, the former Soviet Union and Canada. Several types of asbestos exist: amphiboles are the fibres that cause pulmonary disease in man, of which crocidolite (blue asbestos) is the most important.

Blue asbestos exists in straight fibres measuring 50μm in length and 1–2μm in width; they are resistant to macrophage and neutrophil enzyme destruction.

Asbestos fibres may become coated in acid mucopolysaccharide and encrusted with haemosiderin to form the drumstick-shaped asbestos bodies. Histology shows features of pulmonary fibrosis and honeycomb lung, affecting the lower lobes more commonly.

A considerable time lag exists between exposure and disease development. The first clinical symptoms are dyspnoea and a dry cough; signs include clubbing. Bilateral end inspiratory crackles indicate significant diffuse pulmonary fibrosis.

No treatment is available.

You might be forgiven for thinking that asbestosis is yet another synonym. But it does not simply mean exposure to asbestos (this in itself may not cause symptoms), nor is it a synonym for pleural plaques (you can have asbestosis with or without plaques) and mesothelioma is different again (see below).

## Sarcoidosis

Sarcoidosis is a multisystem granulomatous disorder of unknown aetiology. Sarcoidosis is a common cause of interstitial lung disease, with only lymph nodes involved more commonly than the lungs. Women are more likely to develop the condition, which has a peak incidence in patients aged 20–40 years. Prevalence in the UK is 19:100 000. A geographical distribution shows that it is common in the USA and rare in Japan. The course of the disease is more severe in American blacks.

## Clinical features

Sarcoidosis is asymptomatic in 30% of patients. The commonest presentation is with respiratory symptoms or radiographic abnormalities, notably bilateral hilar lymphadenopathy. Other symptoms include mild fever, malaise, arthralgia and erythema nodosum.

## Pulmonary infiltration

Pulmonary infiltration occurs as non-caseating granulomas distributed along the lymphatics and the walls of small airways and blood vessels. These granulomas usually heal with minimal fibrosis. In 10–20% the disease progresses and an interstitial fibrosis develops. If untreated, pulmonary fibrosis leads to progressive dyspnoea and cor pulmonale.

## Extrapulmonary manifestations

Extrapulmonary manifestations are as follows:
- Skin sarcoidosis (e.g. erythema nodosum)
- Eye manifestations (e.g. anterior uveitis)
- Metabolic manifestations (e.g. hypercalcaemia)
- Central nervous system involvement (e.g. cranial nerve palsies)
- Bone and joint involvement (e.g. arthralgia)
- Hepatosplenomegaly
- Cardiac involvement (e.g. cor pulmonale).

Sarcoidosis is diagnosed on histological evidence of widespread non-caseating epithelioid granulomas in more than one organ.

 History taking in these diseases should include a detailed evaluation of systemic features such as fever, rashes, eye signs etc.

## Investigations

Chest radiography can be useful:
- Bilateral hilar lymphadenopathy is a characteristic feature
- Reticular shadows typically appear in upper lobes after fibrosis starts.

Full blood count can show mild normochromic normocytic anaemia and raised erythrocyte sedimentation rate. Serum biochemistry can reveal hypercalcaemia. The tuberculin skin test is negative or depressed in most cases.

Lymph node transbronchial biopsy, which has superseded the Kveim test, gives positive results in 90% of cases of pulmonary sarcoidosis.

Serum ACE levels are two standard deviations above their normal mean value in 75% of patients. This test is non-specific, and is therefore of no diagnostic value, but can help to monitor response to treatment.

### Treatment

If the patient has hilar lymphadenopathy and no lung involvement, then no treatment is required.

If infiltration has occurred for more than 6 weeks treat with corticosteroids (20–40mg per day for 4–6 weeks then reduced dose for up to one year).

### Prognosis

Mortality is less than 5% in UK Caucasians and approximately 10% in Afro-Americans. If shadowing is present on chest radiographs for more than 2 years, the risk of fibrosis increases.

## Extrinsic allergic alveolitis

Hypersensitivity pneumonitis is also known as extrinsic allergic alveolitis. The condition is a widespread diffuse inflammatory reaction caused by a type III hypersensitivity reaction and results from the individual being already sensitized to the inhaled antigen. Antigens that can cause allergic lung disease include:

- Mouldy hay (e.g. farmer's lung)
- Bird faeces (e.g. in bird fancier's lung)
- Cotton fibres (e.g. byssinosis)
- Sugar cane fibres (e.g. bagassosis).

Clinical features are acute and severe if there is exposure to large doses of the antigen. Onset is more insidious in long-term exposure to small amounts.

### Farmer's lung

In farmer's lung, a fungus present in mouldy hay is inhaled and a type III immune complex reaction follows if the individual is already sensitized. Initial infiltration of small airways and alveolar walls with neutrophils occurs. Lymphocytes and macrophages then infiltrate, leading to the development of non-caseating granulomas, which may resolve or organize leading to pulmonary fibrosis.

Clinical features consist of fever, malaise, cough and dyspnoea developing several hours after initial exposure to the antigen. Coarse end-inspiratory crackles are heard on auscultation.

Investigations include polymorphonuclear leucocyte count, precipitating antibodies (evidence of exposure not disease), lung function tests and bronchoalveolar lavage.

Prevention is the aim of treatment. Corticosteroids help prevent onset of pulmonary fibrosis.

## Idiopathic pulmonary fibrosis

Also known as fibrosing alveolitis or cryptogenic fibrosing alveolitis, idiopathic pulmonary fibrosis is a rare, progressive chronic pulmonary fibrosis of unknown aetiology. It has a peak incidence in patients aged 45–65 years.

### Clinical features

Clinical features of idiopathic pulmonary fibrosis include, progressive breathlessness and a dry cough. Fatigue and considerable weight loss can occur. There is progression to cyanosis, respiratory failure, pulmonary hypertension and cor pulmonale over time.

Clubbing occurs in two-thirds of patients; chest expansion is reduced and bilateral, fine, end-inspiratory crackles are heard on auscultation.

> Interstitial lung diseases provide an opportunity for the examiner's favourite—questions about clubbing. Note that clubbing occurs in idiopathic fibrosing alveolitis and asbestosis but not in other interstitial diseases.

### Pathology

The alveoli walls are thickened because of fibrosis, predominantly in the subpleural regions of the lower lobes. An increased number of chronic inflammatory cells are in the alveoli and interstitium. This pattern is termed 'usual interstitial pneumonitis' and is a progressive condition.

Patterns of disease also include:

- Desquamative interstitial pneumonitis
- Bronchiolitis obliterans.

Idiopathic pulmonary fibrosis has been reported with a number of other conditions: connective-tissue disorders, coeliac disease, ulcerative colitis and renal tubular acidosis.

## Investigations
Several investigations are made:
- Transbronchial or open lung biopsy to confirm histological diagnosis
- CT scan
- Blood gases may show arterial hypoxaemia
- Full blood count may show raised erythrocyte sedimentation rate
- Lung function test shows a restrictive pattern
- Bronchoalveolar lavage shows increased numbers of neutrophils
- Autoantibody tests
- Antinuclear factor is positive in one-third of patients. Rheumatoid factor is positive in one-half of patients.

## Prognosis
Of patients with the condition, 50% die within 4–5 years.

## Treatment
About 50% of patients respond to immunosuppression. Combined therapy is recommended with:
- Prednisolone 0.5 mg/kg daily for one month and then tapered
- Azathioprine (2–3 mg/kg).

Cyclophosphamide may be substituted for azathioprine.

Single lung transplantation may be attempted where necessary.

Supportive treatment includes oxygen therapy.

## Diffuse pulmonary haemorrhage syndromes
### Goodpasture's syndrome
Goodpasture's syndrome is characterized by glomerulonephritis and respiratory symptoms. It usually begins with an upper respiratory tract infection. Goodpasture's syndrome is thought to be a type II hypersensitivity reaction.

### Clinical features
Clinical features include haemoptysis, haematuria and anaemia caused by massive bleeding.

Most patients have antiglomerular basement membrane antibody circulating in their blood, which causes glomerulonephritis and also acts on alveolar membranes, causing pulmonary haemorrhage. The course of the disease is variable: some patients resolve completely, others proceed to renal failure. There is an association with influenza virus $A_2$.

### Treatment
Treatment is by corticosteroids or plasmapheresis to remove antibodies.

## Idiopathic pulmonary haemosiderosis
Idiopathic pulmonary haemosiderosis is a rare condition, typically occurring in children aged under 7 years. An association with sensitivity to cow's milk has been suggested.

### Clinical features
Patients present with haemoptysis because of recurrent episodes of intra-alveolar haemorrhage, cough and dyspnoea.

### Pathology
The more acute form of idiopathic pulmonary haemosiderosis shows evidence of diffuse alveolar damage and type II pneumocyte hyperplasia. Haemosiderin-containing macrophages are found in the sputum.

### Treatment
Treatment is by corticosteroids and azathioprine. Prognosis is poor.

## Pulmonary eosinophilia
Pulmonary eosinophilia is a group of syndromes characterized by abnormally high levels of eosinophils in the blood, or in the case of acute eosinophilic pneumonia, in lung lavage fluid. The severity of these diseases can range from mild to fatal (Fig. 7.25).

## Bronchiolitis obliterans
In bronchiolitis obliterans, characteristic histological appearance shows:
- Polypoid masses of organizing inflammatory exudate
- Granulation tissue extending from alveoli to bronchioles.

| Pulmonary eosinophilia | | | | | | |
|---|---|---|---|---|---|---|
| Disease | Aetiology | Symptoms | Blood eosinophils (%) | Multisystem involvement | Duration | Outcome |
| simple | passage of parasitic larvae through lung | mild | 10 | none | <1 month | good |
| prolonged | unknown | mild/moderate | <20 | none | >1 month | good |
| asthmatic | often type 1 hypersensitivity to *Aspergillus* | moderate/severe | 5–20 | none | years | fair |
| tropical | hypersensitivity reaction to filarial infestation | moderate/severe | >20 | none | years | fair |
| hyper-eosinophilic syndrome | unknown | severe | >20 | always | months/years | poor |
| Churg–Strauss syndrome | possibly immune complex vasculitis | severe | >20 | always | months/years | poor/fair |

**Fig. 7.25** Table of causes of pulmonary eosinophilia.

Aetiology is unknown, although an association with a number of clinical conditions exists:
- Viral infections (e.g. respiratory syncitial virus)
- Aspiration
- Inhalation of toxic fumes
- Extrinsic allergic alveolitis
- Pulmonary fibrosis
- Collagen or vascular disorders.

Bronchiolitis obliterans is sensitive to corticosteroid treatment.

## Collagen disorders and vascular disorders
### Rheumatoid diseases
The respiratory system is affected in 10–15% of patients with rheumatoid disease; respiratory disease may occur before other systemic features. Patients characteristically have severe seropositive rheumatoid disease.

Diffuse pulmonary fibrosis can occur. Small-airway disease shows bronchiolitis obliterans or follicular bronchiolitis with lymphoid aggregates and germinal centres. Rheumatoid nodules are rare in the lung and when they do occur they usually cavitate. The pleura may show fibrosis and chronic unilateral pleural effusions are common.

### Systemic lupus erythematosus
In patients with systemic lupus erythematosus (SLE), pleurisy may develop, with or without an effusion. When present, effusions are small and bilateral.

Basal pneumonitis may be present and diffuse pulmonary fibrosis is rare.

## Desquamative interstitial pneumonitis
Desquamative interstitial pneumonitis is found in patients with fibrosing alveolitis. It is more diffuse than usual interstitial pneumonitis. A proliferation of macrophages in the alveolar airspaces occurs, along with interstitial thickening by mononuclear inflammatory cells. Lymphoid tissue and a small amount of collagen are sometimes present.

Desquamative interstitial pneumonitis has a distinctly uniform histological pattern. The alveolar walls show relatively little fibrosis.

Corticosteroids may be beneficial, and prognosis is good.

### Alveolar proteinosis
Alveolar proteinosis is a rare condition, also known as alveolar lipoproteinosis. The aetiology is unknown in the majority of cases and pathogenesis is uncertain. It has been hypothesized that there is increased destruction or decreased clearance of type II cells

and accumulation of eosinophilic material within the alveoli. Alveolar proteinosis is associated with a high incidence of concomitant fungal infections and may complicate other interstitial disease (e.g. desquamative interstitial pneumonitis.

The main symptoms of alveolar proteinosis are dyspnoea and cough. Chest pain and haemoptysis are rare.

The course of the disease is variable, but the majority of patients enjoy spontaneous remission.

## Neoplastic disease of the lung

### Bronchial carcinoma
Bronchial carcinoma accounts for 95% of all primary tumours of the lung and is the commonest malignant tumour in the Western world. Bronchogenic carcinoma affects men more than women (M:F ratio, 3.5:1) but incidence is rising in women and it is now the commonest cancer in both sexes. Typically patients are aged 40–70 years at presentation; only 2–3% occur in younger patients.

### Aetiology
Risk factors are summarized in Fig. 7.26. Cigarette smoking is the largest contributory factor:

- It is related to the amount smoked, duration and tar content
- The rise in incidence of lung cancer correlates closely to the increase in smoking over the past century

| Risk factors in lung cancer | |
| --- | --- |
| Factor | Relative risk |
| non-smoker | 1 |
| smoker, 1–2 packs/day | 42 |
| ex-smoker | 2 to 10 |
| passive smoke exposure | 1.5 to 2 |
| asbestos exposure | 5 |
| asbestos plus tobacco | 90 |

**Fig. 7.26** Risk factors in lung cancer. (Adapted from *Pulmonary Physiology* by G. Criner and G. D'Alonzo. Fence Creek Publishing, 1999, p. 303.)

- In non-smokers, the incidence is 3–5 cases per 100000. In the UK, there are 100 deaths per 100000 smokers per year
- The risk in those who give up smoking decreases with time
- Passive smoking also increases risk.

Environmental and occupational factors include:
- Radon released from granite rock
- Asbestos
- Air pollution (e.g. beryllium emissions).

### Histological types
There are four main histological types of bronchogenic carcinoma:
- Non-small-cell carcinomas (70%):
    Squamous cell carcinoma (52%).
    Adenocarcinoma (13%).
    Large-cell carcinoma (5%)
- Small-cell carcinomas (30%).

The different types of tumour are summarized in Fig. 7.27.

Tumours may occur as discrete or mixed histological patterns; the development from the initial malignant change to presentation is variable:
- Squamous cell carcinoma: 8 years
- Adenocarcinoma: 15 years
- Small-cell carcinoma: 3 years.

### Squamous cell carcinoma
Squamous cell carcinoma arises from squamous epithelium in the large bronchi. A strong association between cigarette smoking and squamous cell carcinoma exists. Males are affected most commonly, with a mean age at diagnosis of 57 years.

Squamous cell carcinomas are histologically well differentiated and are associated with keratinization. The cancer commonly produces a substance similar to parathyroid hormone (PTH) which leads to hypercalcaemia (see Fig. 7.29).

The major mass of the tumour may occur outside the bronchial cartilage and encircle the bronchial lumen, producing obstructive phenomena. The tumours are almost always hilar and are prone to massive necrosis and cavitation, with upper lobe lesions more likely to cavitate. Of squamous cell carcinomas, 13% show cavitation on chest radiographs. Peripheral lesions tend to be larger than those seen in adenocarcinomas.

**Fig. 7.27** Summary of tumour types.

| | Tumour types | | | |
|---|---|---|---|---|
| | Non-small-cell tumours | | | Small cell |
| | Squamous cell tumour | Adeno-carcinoma | Large cell | |
| incidence (%) | 52 | 13 | 5 | 30 |
| male/female incidence | M>F | F>M | M>F | M>F |
| location | hilar | peripheral | peripheral/central | hilar |
| histological stain | keratin | mucin | – | – |
| relationship to smoking | high | low | high | high |
| growth rate | slow | medium | rapid | very rapid |
| metastasis | late | intermediate | early | very early |
| treatment | surgery | | | chemotherapy |
| prognosis | 2-year survival = 50% | | | 3 months if untreated; 1 year if treated |

If squamous carcinoma occurs in the apical portion of the lung, it may produce Pancoast's syndrome (see below).

Squamous cell carcinoma is the least likely type to metastasize and untreated it has the longest patient survival of any of the bronchogenic carcinomas.

Adenocarcinoma of the lung is usually a peripheral tumour.

### Adenocarcinoma

Adenocarcinomas are most common in:
- Non-smoking elderly women
- The Far East.

Adenocarcinomas are associated with diffuse pulmonary fibrosis and honeycomb lung.

Bronchogenic tumours associated with occupational factors are mainly adenocarcinomas. Ninety per cent of adenocarcinomas occur between 40 and 69 years of age, with the mean age for diagnosis being 53.3 years. Two-thirds of adenocarcinomas are found peripherally. Usually, tumours measure more than 4 cm in diameter.

Adenocarcinoma arises from glandular cells such as mucus goblet cells, type II pneumocytes and clara cells. Histologically, they are differentiated from other bronchogenic tumours by their glandular configuration and mucin production. The gland structure may be acinar or papillary.

Clinically, two growth patterns are seen:
- Discrete nodule in the periphery with pleural tethering (most common)
- Multifocal and bilateral diffuse tumour (so-called bronchoalveolar cell carcinoma).

As the tumour is commonly in the periphery, obstructive symptoms are rare, so the tumour tends to be clinically silent. Symptoms include coughing, haemoptysis, chest pain and weight loss. A wide range of paraneoplastic syndromes are seen (see below). Malignant cells are detected in the sputum in 50% of patients, and the commonest radiological presentation is a solitary peripheral pulmonary nodule, close to the pleural surface.

Resection is possible in a small proportion of cases; 5-year survival rate is less than 10%. Invasion of the pleura and mediastinal lymph nodes is common, as too is metastasis to the brain and bones.

Metastasis in the gastrointestinal tract, pancreas or ovaries must be excluded after having made a diagnosis.

Large-cell anaplastic carcinomas lack features of differentiation.

## Large-cell anaplastic tumour

Large-cell anaplastic tumours are diagnosed by a process of elimination. No clear-cut pattern of clinical or radiological presentation distinguishes them from other malignant lung tumours.

Under light microscopy, findings include:
- Pleomorphic cells with a large, darkly staining nuclei
- Prominent nucleoli, abundant cytoplasm and well-defined cell borders
- Abundant mitoses.

Large-cell anaplastic tumours are variable in location, but are usually centrally located. Peripherally located lesions are larger than adenocarcinomas. The point of origin of the carcinoma influences symptomatic presentation of the disease: central lesions present earlier than peripheral lesions as they cause obstruction.

The tumour causes coughing, sputum production and haemoptysis. When a tumour occurs in a major airway, obstructive pneumonia can occur. Sputum cytology and bronchoscopy with bronchial biopsy make the diagnosis.

On electron microscopy, these tumours turn out to be poorly differentiated variants of squamous cell carcinoma and adenocarcinoma; they are extremely aggressive and destructive lesions. Early invasion of blood vessels and lymphatics occurs, and treatment is by surgical resection whenever possible.

Squamous cell carcinoma is the commonest cause of bronchogenic carcinoma.

## Small-cell carcinoma

Small-cell carcinomas arise from endocrine cells— Kulchitsky cells, members of the amine precursor uptake decarboxylase (APUD) system.

The incidence of this carcinoma is directly related to cigarette consumption and it is considered to be a systemic disease. Small-cell carcinomas are the most aggressive malignancy of all the bronchogenic tumours.

Most small-cell anaplastic tumours originate in the large bronchi and obstructive pneumonitis is frequently seen. Several histological subgroups of this carcinoma exist and all have:
- Cell size: 6–8μm
- High nucleus:cytoplasm ratio
- Hyperchromatism of the nuclei.

When almost no cytoplasm is present, and the cells are compressed into an ovoid form, the neoplasm is called an oat-cell carcinoma. On radiography, the oat-cell carcinoma does not cavitate.

There is a high occurrence of paraneoplastic syndromes associated with this type of tumour, so presentation may be varied. The most frequent presenting complaint is coughing. Spread is rapid, and metastatic lesions may be the presenting sign. Small-cell carcinomas metastasize through the lymphatic route.

Chest radiography may help in diagnosis, although the diagnosis must be confirmed by histological or cytological means.

Prognosis is very poor, with a mean survival time for untreated patients with small-cell carcinoma of 7 weeks after diagnosis. Death is generally caused by metastatic disease.

Small-cell carcinoma is the only bronchial carcinoma that responds to chemotherapy.

The majority of endocrine disturbances are caused by small-cell carcinomas.

## Mixed tumours

A number of mixed tumour types exist that are commonly seen in resection material at autopsy.

Many pathologists base their diagnosis on the prominent cell type present because the predominant cell type predicts prognosis of the condition.

## Clinical features

Features specific to the histological types have already been introduced above. There are no specific signs of bronchogenic carcinoma. Diagnosis always needs to be excluded in cigarette smokers who present with recurrent respiratory symptoms:

- Persistent cough—commonest presentation; may be productive if obstruction leads to infection
- Haemoptysis—occurs at some stage in disease in 50%
- Dyspnoea—rarely at presentation but occurs as disease progresses
- Chest pain—often pleuritic caused by obstructive changes
- Wheezing—monophonic, due to obstruction.

Unexplained weight loss is also a common presenting complaint. Other symptoms may be present due to complications decribed below.

In 10–30% of patients finger clubbing is present on examination.

## Complications
### Local complications

Symptoms may be caused by:

- Ulceration of bronchus; occurs in up to 50% of patients and produces haemoptysis in varying degrees
- Bronchial obstruction. The lumen of the bronchus becomes occluded; distal collapse and retention of secretions subsequently occur. This clinically causes dyspnoea, secondary infection and lung abscesses
- Central necrosis. Carcinomas can outgrow their blood supply leading to central necrosis. The main complication is then the development of a lung abscess.

Fig. 7.28 summarizes the effects of local spread.

### Pancoast's syndrome

Pancoast's syndrome can be caused by all types of bronchogenic carcinoma, although two-thirds

| Effects of local spread | |
| --- | --- |
| **Site of spread** | **Symptoms** |
| pleura/ribs | pain on respiration/pathological fractures |
| brachial plexus | shoulder pain and small muscle wasting of the hand |
| sympathetic ganglia | ipsilateral Horner's syndrome |
| recurrent laryngeal nerve | hoarse voice and bovine cough |
| superior vena cava | facial congestion; distended neck veins |

**Fig. 7.28** Effects and symptoms of local spread.

originate from squamous cells. As the tumour grows outward from the pulmonary parenchymal apex, it encroaches on anatomical structures, including:

- Chest wall
- Subpleural lymphatics
- Sympathetic chain.

As noted above, Pancoast's tumour can affect the sympathetic chain, resulting in loss of sympathetic tone and an ipsilateral Horner's syndrome. Intractable shoulder pain occurs when the upper rib is involved. The subclavian artery and vein may become compressed. Destruction of the inferior trunk of the brachial plexus leads to pain in the ulnar nerve distribution and may lead to small-muscle wasting of the hand.

Pancoast's tumour is diagnosed by percutaneous needle aspiration of the tumour.

### Metastatic complications

Local metastases to lymph nodes, bone, liver and adrenal glands occur.

Metastases to the brain present as:

- Change in personality
- Epilepsy
- Focal neurological lesion.

### Paraneoplastic syndromes

Paraneoplastic syndromes (Fig. 7.29) cannot be explained by direct invasion of the tumour. They are caused by production by tumour cells of polypeptides that mimic various hormones. Paraneoplastic syndromes are commonly associated with small-cell lung cancer.

| Paraneoplastic disorders associated with lung cancer | | | |
|---|---|---|---|
| | Mechanism | Clinical features | Lung cancer association |
| SIADH | excess scretion of ADH | headache, nausea, muscle weakness, drowsiness, confusion, eventually coma | small cell |
| ectopic ACTH | adrenal hyperplasia and secretion of large amounts of cortisol | Cushings: polyuria, oedema, hypokalaemia, hypertension, increased pigmentation | small cell or carcinoid |
| hypercalcaemia | ectopic PTH secretion | lethargy, nausea, polyuria, eventually coma | squamous cell (but may be due to bone metastases) |
| hypertrophic pulmonary osteoarthropathy | unknown | digital clubbing and periosteal inflammation | adenocarcinoma, squamous cell |
| gonadotrophins | ectopic secretion | gynaecomastia, testicular atrophy | large cell |

**Fig. 7.29** Paraneoplastic disorders associated with lung cancer.

## Investigations

Investigations are performed to confirm diagnosis and assess tumour histology and spread.

### Chest radiography

Good posteroanterior and lateral views are required. Seventy per cent of bronchial carcinomas arise centrally and chest radiography demonstrates over 90% carcinomas. The mass needs to be between 1–2cm in size to be recognized reliably. Lobar collapse and pleural effusions may be present.

### CT scan

CT scan gives good visualization of the mediastinum and is good at identifying small lesions. Valuable to assess extent of tumour and the operability of the mass. Lymph nodes >1.5cm are pathological.

Scan should include brain, liver and adrenals to identify distant metastases.

### Fibreoptic bronchoscopy

Confirms central lesion, assesses operability, and allows accurate cell type to be determined. Used to obtain cytological specimens. Mucus secretions plus sputum examined for presence of malignant cells.

If carcinoma involves the first 2cm of either main bronchus the tumour is inoperable.

### Transthoracic fine-needle aspiration biopsy

In transthoracic fine-needle aspiration biopsy, the needle is guided by X-ray or CT. Direct aspiration of peripheral lung lesion takes place through chest wall; 25% of patients suffer pneumothorax due to the procedure.

Implantation metastases do not occur.

## Staging

Small-cell and non-small-cell cancers are staged differently. Small-cell is staged as either limited or extensive whilst the TNM system (Fig. 7.30) is used for non-small-cell cancer.

## Treatment
### Surgery

The only treatment of any value in non-small-cell carcinoma is surgery; however, only 15% of cases are operable at diagnosis.

Surgery can only be performed after:
• Lung function tests show the patient has sufficient respiratory reserve
• CT scan shows no evidence of metastases.

### Radiation therapy

Treatment of choice if tumour is inoperable. Good for slowly growing squamous carcinoma.

Radiation pneumonitis develops in 10–15% and radiation fibrosis occurs to some degree in all cases.

| Staging in non-small-cell lung cancer | | |
|---|---|---|
| **Primary tumour** | | |
| T1 | <3 cm—no evidence of invasion proximal to a lobar brochus | |
| T2 | ≥3 cm or any site involving pleura or hilum; within a lobar bronchus or at least 2 cm distal to the carina | |
| T3 | any size extending into the chest wall, diaphragm, pericardium (not involving great vessels etc.) | |
| T4 | inoperable tumour of any size with invasion of the mediastium or involving heart great vessels, trachea, oesophagus, vertebral body or carina or malignant pleural effusion | |

| **Regional lymph nodes** | | **Distant metastases** | |
|---|---|---|---|
| N0 | no nodal involvement | M0 | no metastases |
| N1 | peribronchial and/or ipsilateral hilar nodes | M1 | distant metastases |
| N2 | ipsilateral mediastinal and sub-carinal lymph nodes | | |
| N3 | inoperable contralateral node involvement | | |

**Fig. 7.30** Staging in non-small-cell lung cancer.

### Chemotherapy

Only effective treatment for small-cell carcinoma, but is not undertaken with intent to cure. Platinum compounds can achieve good results.

### Terminal care

Endoscopic therapy and transbronchial stenting are used to provide symptomatic relief in patients with terminal disease. Daily prednisolone (maximum dose: 15mg) may improve appetite. Opioid analgesia is given to control pain and laxatives should be prescribed to counteract the opioid side effects. Candidiasis is a common treatable problem.

Both patient and relatives require counselling.

### Prognosis

Overall prognosis is poor; only 6–8% survive five years and mean survival is less than six months.

## Rarer types of lung tumours
### Malignant tumours
#### Bronchoalveolar cell carcinoma

A distinctive type of adenocarcinoma occurring in the distal portions of the pulmonary parenchyma accounting for 3% of all primary neoplasms of lung. The carcinoma affects males and females equally and the incidence is not related to cigarette consumption.

Unifocal point of origin within the lung with the major bulk of the tumour seen in the alveoli rather than the bronchi. The lesion grows very slowly and spreads by the bronchial route to implant on other portions of the respiratory epithelium. The lesion may be stable for 5–10 years.

Associated with profuse mucoid sputum production.

In the early stage, radiography may show a non-specific peripheral coin lesion. Diagnosis of the disease is based on histological examination of tissue obtained by transbronchial or open lung biopsy.

Surgical resection may be curative although surgical intervention is useless once dissemination has occurred.

### Bronchial carcinoid

Low-grade malignant tumour accounting for 1% of tumours found in the lungs. It affects males and females equally and presents <40 years.

Bronchial carcinoids are locally invasive, highly vascular tumours that cause recurrent haemoptysis. The tumour grows slowly, eventually blocking a bronchus.

Rarely gives rise to the carcinoid syndrome and the 5-year survival is >80%.

Malignant mesenchymal tumours (sarcomas) are extremely rare.

### Primary pulmonary lymphomas

Rare tumours composed of small B lymphocytes arising from the bronchus and bronchiole associated lymphoid tissue. Monotypic immunoglobulin may be secreted into the blood.

### Benign tumours
#### Adenomas

Arise from bronchial mucous glands. They present as polypoid or sessile lesions and symptoms are related to obstruction.

| Metastatic malignancy of lung and the resulting radiological appearance | | |
|---|---|---|
| Multinodular patterns | | Solitary nodule |
| Cannonball | Snowstorm | |
| salivary gland | breast | breast |
| kidney | kidney | kidney |
| bowel | bladder | bowel |
| uterus/ovarian | thyroid | |
| testis | prostate | |

**Fig. 7.31** Metastatic malignancy of lung and the resulting radiological appearance.

| Pulmonary manifestations of adverse drug reactions | |
|---|---|
| **Adverse reaction** | **Examples** |
| diffuse alveolar damage | bleomycin, methotrexate, amiodarone, radiotherapy |
| interstitial pneumonitis | methotrexate, busulphan, amiodarone, gold |
| eosinophilic pneumonia | bleomycin, naproxen, sulphasalazine |
| bronchiolitis obliterans | methotrexate, gold, mitomycin |
| pulmonary haemorrhage | amphotericin B, anticoagulants, hydralazine |
| pulmonary oedema | codeine, methadone, naloxone, salicylates |
| pleural effusions and fibrosis | amiodarone, hydralazine, bleomycin, bromocriptine |

**Fig. 7.32** Summary of pulmonary manifestations of adverse drug reactions.

## Benign mesenchymal tumours

Arise anywhere that mesenchyme occurs. The lesion is probably a hamartoma, it is a well circumscribed round lesion 1–2 cm composed of cartilage and found in the periphery of the lung. Rarely arises from a major bronchus and presents as an isolated coin lesion on radiographs.

## Metastatic malignancy to the lung

Metastases to the lung are a common clinical and radiological finding. Metastases are more likely to be multiple than solitary. Most haematogenous metastases are sharply circumscribed with smooth edges, and the appearance of multiple smoothly circumscribed nodules is highly suggestive of metastatic disease. Cavitation is unusual in metastatic lesions.

Solitary pulmonary metastases do occur as sarcomas of soft tissue or bone, carcinoma of the breast, colon and kidney.

Multinodular lung metastases may be of varying sizes (Fig. 7.31):
- Very large dimensions—cannonball pattern
- Many small nodules—snowstorm pattern.

## Diseases of iatrogenic origin

## Drug-induced lung disease

Pulmonary disease caused by medication is a growing problem. The mechanisms of drug-induced lung damage are either immunological or cytotoxic and the type of adverse reaction can be either:

- Predictable if caused by a dose-related effect
- Unpredictable if caused by the development of hypersensitivity reactions.

There are no specific clinical, functional or radiological findings in drug-induced pulmonary disease. The commonest symptoms include dyspnoea and cough (Fig. 7.32).

Examples of drug-induced lung diseases include:
- Bleomycin—the development of bleomycin-induced pulmonary disease is dose-dependent. Bleomycin causes oxygen-radical-induced lung damage. Incidence is approximately 3%, with a mortality rate of 1–2%
- Amiodarone—a class III antiarrhythmic drug, which can cause fatal interstitial pneumonitis. Lung damage has its onset several months after commencement of amiodarone treatment. Incidence of toxicity is 1–2%. The condition responds well to corticosteroid treatment
- β blockers—β blockers are contraindicated in patients with asthma as they also block airway β receptors, thus precipitating bronchoconstriction
- Aspirin—may induce asthma, either through decreased prostaglandin production or by increased leukotriene production. Recovery is usual on discontinuation of the drug.

| Lung transplantation | |
|---|---|
| **Indications** | **Diseases treated by transplantation** |
| age <60 years | pulmonary fibrosis |
| life expectancy <18 months without transplantation | primary pulmonary hypertension |
| no underlying cancer | bronchiectasis and cystic fibrosis |
| no serious systemic disease | emphysema including $\alpha_1$-antitrypsin deficiency |

**Fig. 7.33** Indications and diseases treated by lung transplantation.

## Complications of radiotherapy

The lungs are very sensitive to radiation. Clinical effects depend on the dose given, volume of lung irradiated, and length of treatment. Pulmonary response to radiation is characterized by:
- Acute phase of radiation pneumonitis
- Chronic phase of healing or fibrosis.

### Acute radiation pneumonitis

Acute radiation pneumonitis is defined as an acute infiltrate precisely confined to the radiation area and occurring within 3 months of radiotherapy. Acute radiation pneumonitis rarely produces symptoms within the first month after therapy. Symptoms have an insidious onset and include non-productive cough, shortness of breath on exertion, and low-grade fever.

Diffuse alveolar damage occurs, consisting of a proteinaceous exudate of material in the alveolar air spaces associated with hyaline membranes, especially in alveolar ducts. Endothelial damage, loss of normal respiratory epithelium, and hyperplasia of type II pneumocytes also occur.

Radiation pneumonitis results in a restrictive lung defect and corticosteroids should be given in the acute phase.

### Chronic fibrosis

Acute radiation pneumonitis can resolve spontaneously or progress to pulmonary fibrosis. The chronic fibrosing state is usually asymptomatic. Proliferation and fragmentation of elastic fibres occurs and bronchiolitis obliterans and bronchial fibrosis may be present.

Chronic fibrosis is not precisely confined to irradiated areas.

| Complications of lung transplantation | |
|---|---|
| **Complication** | **Time** |
| hyperacute rejection | seconds/minutes |
| pulmonary oedema | 12–72 hours |
| bacterial lower respiratory tract infection: donor-acquired recipient-acquired | hours/days days/years |
| acute rejection | day 5/years |
| airway complications | week 1/months |
| opportunistic infection | week 4/years |
| chronic rejection (e.g. bronchiolitis obliterans) | week 6/years |

**Fig. 7.34** Summary of the complications of lung transplantation.

## Lung transplantation

Single lung transplantation is preferred to double transplantation because of donor availability. Bilateral lung transplantation is required in infective conditions to prevent bacterial spill-over from a diseased lung to a single lung transplant.

Patients must have end-stage lung or pulmonary vascular disease with no other treatment options (Fig. 7.33).

### Complications

The complications of lung transplantation are described in Fig. 7.34.

### Strategies for avoiding rejection

Lung transplantation does not require any significant degree of matching based on tissue type. The main criteria are compatibility of blood group and size match between organ and recipient.

### Suppression of the immune system

All transplant patients require immunsuppression for life. This begins immediately before transplantation; drugs used include:
- Prednisolone
- Azathioprine
- Cyclosporin.

Large doses are given in the initial postoperative period. Lower maintenance doses are achieved after

| Pleural effusions | | | |
|---|---|---|---|
| **Transudate** | | **Exudate** | |
| protein | <30 g/L | protein | >30 g/L |
| lactate dehydrogenase | <200 IU/L | lactate dehydrogenase | >200 IU/L |
| usually bilateral | | unilateral in focal disease; bilateral in systemic disease | |

**Fig. 7.35** Classification of pleural effusions.

| Causes of transudates and exudates | |
|---|---|
| **Transudate** | **Exudate** |
| left heart failure | bacterial pneumonia |
| hypoproteinaemia | carcinoma bronchus |
| constrictive pericarditis | pulmonary infarction |
| hypothyroidism | tuberculosis |
| cirrhosis | connective-tissue disease |

**Fig. 7.36** Causes of transudates and exudates.

a few months. Rejection episodes are treated with high-dose intravenous corticosteroids.

## Prognosis
One-year survival rates are 60–70%.

# Diseases of the pleura

## Pleural effusions
A pleural effusion is the presence of fluid between the visceral and parietal pleura. Effusions can be categorized as transudative or exudative, depending on the protein concentration (Fig. 7.35). Transudative pleural effusions (<30g/L) occur as a result of an imbalance between hydrostatic and osmotic forces, for example in congestive cardiac failure (hydrothorax). Exudative pleural effusions (>30g/L) occur when local factors influencing pleural fluid formation and reabsorption are altered specifically through injury or inflammation. Causes of each type of effusion are shown in Fig. 7.36. Exudative effusions often occur as a complication of pneumonia; these are termed parapneumonic effusions.

### Gross appearance
On examination, the pleural fluid may be clear and straw-coloured, turbid (signifying infection) or haemorrhagic. If a haemorrhagic effusion exists, neoplastic infiltration, pulmonary infarction and TB need to be excluded. Leading malignancies that have associated pleural effusions are breast carcinoma, bronchial carcinoma and lymphomas/leukaemia.

### Clinical features
Pleural effusions are typically asymptomatic until >500mL of fluid is present. Pleuritic chest pain may develop in addition to dyspnoea, which is dependent on the size of effusion.

Signs on examination include stony dull percussion note; see Chapter 9.

### Investigations
Features on a chest radiograph include blunting of costophrenic angles. Ultrasound is used to detect small effusions not seen on CXR and for guiding aspiration which is performed for microbiological examination or therapeutically.

A pleural biopsy with Abrams' needle may be necessary if the aspiration is inconclusive.

### Treatment
Treat the underlying disease. If the patient is symptomatic drain the effusion. Drain fluid slowly. Malignant effusions—chemical pleurodesis can provide temporary relief. Use bleomycin/tetracycline.

Questions on the cause of exudative and transudative pleural effusions are common in clinical examinations.

## Empyema
Also known as a pyothorax, this is a collection of pus within the pleural cavity caused by:
- Complication of thoracic surgery
- Rupture of lung abscess into the pleural space

| Haemothorax | |
|---|---|
| **Degree** | **Management** |
| minimal (<350 mL) | blood usually reabsorbs spontaneously with conservative treatment |
| moderate (300–1500 mL) | thoracentesis and tube drainage with underwater seal drainage |
| massive (>1500 mL) | two drainage tubes inserted; immediate or early thoracotomy may be necessary to arrest bleeding |

**Fig. 7.37** Management of haemothorax.

- Perforation of oesophagus
- Mediastinitis
- Bacterial spread of pneumonia.

The empyema cavity can become infected by anaerobes. The patients are pyrexial and ill. The pus must be removed and appropriate antibiotic treatment should be initiated immediately.

## Haemothorax

Blood in the pleural cavity. Common in both penetrating and non-penetrating injuries of the chest and may cause hypovolaemic shock and reduce vital capacity through compression. Due to the defibrinating action that occurs with motions of respiration and the presence of an anticoagulant enzyme the clot may be defibrinated and leave fluid radiologically indistinguishable from effusions of another cause.

Blood may originate from lung, internal mammary artery, thoracicoacromial artery, lateral thoracic artery, mediastinal great vessels, heart, or abdominal structures via diaphragm. See Fig. 7.37 for the management of haemothorax.

## Chylothorax

Accumulation of lymph in the pleural space. Commonest causes are rupture or obstruction of the thoracic duct due to surgical trauma or neoplasm, e.g. lymphoma. A latent period between injury and onset of 2–10 days occurs. The pleural fluid is high in lipid content and is characteristically milky in appearance. The prognosis is generally good.

### Chylous effusion

Caused by the escape of chyle into the pleural space from obstruction or laceration of the thoracic duct.

### Chyliform effusion

Results from degeneration of malignant and other cells in pleural fluid.

## Pneumothorax

Pneumothorax is the accumulation of air in the pleural space. It may occur spontaneously or following trauma.

### Spontaneous

Results from rupture of a pleural bleb, the pleural bleb being a congenital defect of the alveolar wall connective tissue. Patients are typically tall, thin, young males. M:F ratio 6:1. Spontaneous pneumothoraces are usually apical affecting both lungs with equal frequency.

Secondary causes of spontaneous pneumothorax occur in patients with underlying disease such as, COPD, TB, pneumonia, bronchial carcinoma, sarcoidosis and cystic fibrosis.

Patients present with sudden onset of unilateral pleuritic pain and increasing breathlessness.

The main aim of treatment is to get the patient back to active life as soon as possible.

### Investigations

Chest radiography may show an area devoid of lung markings. May be more clearly seen on the expiratory film.

### Management

Small pneumothorax: no treatment, but review in 7–10 days. Moderate pneumothorax: admit for simple aspiration.

### Tension pneumothorax

Medical emergency.

Commonest causes:
- Positive pressure ventilation
- Stab wound or rib fracture.

Air escapes into pleural space and the rise above atmospheric pressure causes the lung to collapse. At each inspiration intrapleural pressure increases as the pleural tear acts as a ball valve that permits air to enter but not leave the pleural space. Venous return to the heart is impaired as pressure rises and patients experience dyspnoea and chest pain. They may also be cyanotic.

165

**Fig. 7.38** Radiograph of a tension pneumothorax. Tension pneumothorax displacing mediastinum and depressing left hemidiaphragm. Extensive consolidation and cavitation in both lungs is due to tuberculosis. A pleural adhesion (arrowheads) is visible. (Courtesy of Dr D. Sutton and Dr J.W.R. Young.)

Clinically:
- Mediastinum pushed over into contralateral hemithorax. Tracheal deviation
- Hyperresonance, absence of breath sounds
- Intercostal spaces widened on ipsilateral side.

On ECG there is a rightward shift in mean frontal QRS complex, diminution in QRS amplitude, and inversion of precordial T waves.

Diagnosed on needle insertion.

Treat with immediate thoracostomy with underwater seal drainage, before requesting chest radiographs. See Fig. 7.38 for a radiograph of a tension pneumothorax. Fig. 7.39 gives a summary of non-inflammatory pleural effusions.

A tension pneumothorax should never be diagnosed by chest radiography. It is a clinical diagnosis which requires treatment before requesting a chest radiograph.

| Noninflammatory pleural effusions | | |
|---|---|---|
| **Disorder** | **Collection** | **Cause** |
| haemothorax | blood | chest trauma; rupture of aortic aneurysm |
| hydrothorax | proteinaceous fluid | congestive cardiac failure |
| chylothorax | lymph | neoplastic infiltration; trauma |
| pneumothorax | air | spontaneous; traumatic |

**Fig. 7.39** Summary of non-inflammatory pleural effusions.

## Neoplasms of the pleura

### Malignant mesothelioma

Malignant mesothelioma is a tumour of mesothelial cells most commonly affecting the visceral or parietal pleura. The incidence of mesothelioma is rising rapidly. In 90% of cases it is associated with occupational exposure to asbestos, especially fibres which are <0.25 µm diameter, e.g. crocidolite and amiosite. The latent period between exposure and death is long, ranging from 15 to 67 years.

Two histological varieties exist—50% of mesotheliomas have elements of both:
- Epithelial: tubular structure
- Fibrous: solid structure with spindle-shaped cells.

The tumour begins as nodules in the pleura and goes on to obliterate the pleural cavity.

### Clinical features:
- Initial symptoms are very vague
- Pain is the main complaint, often affecting sleep and results from infiltration of the tumour into the chest wall with involvement of intercostal nerves and ribs.

Other features include:
- Dyspnoea
- Weight loss
- Finger clubbing.

### Investigations
Features of chest radiograph are:
- Pleural effusions
- Unilateral pleural thickening
- Nodular appearance.

Open lung biopsy may be needed to confirm diagnosis.

## Prognosis

No treatment is available and the condition is universally fatal. Pain responds poorly to therapy.

Metastases are common to hilar and abdominal lymph nodes with secondary deposits arising in lung, liver, thyroid, adrenals, bone, skeletal muscle and brain. The patient's symptoms become worse until death occurs, usually within 2 years of diagnosis; the cause of death is usually infection, vascular compromise or pulmonary embolus.

Patients eligible for industrial injuries benefit include those with mesothelioma, asbestosis, asbestos related carcinoma of bronchus, and coal-worker's pneumoconiosis.

## Pleural fibroma

Rare neoplasm of the pleura not related to asbestos exposure which consists of:

- Fibrous connective tissue
- Mesothelial cells.

A solitary mass can grow to be very large and hypertrophic pulmonary osteoarthropathy is a frequent association. Affects females most commonly with the mean age at presentation 50 years.

Aetiology unknown. Most patients are asymptomatic.

**Fig. 7.40** Mesothelioma of the right pleura. The patient had a long history of asbestos exposure and has now developed a large pleural mass. (Courtesy of Professor C.D. Forbes and Dr W.F. Jackson.)

Tumours grow slowly and behave generally in a benign fashion although malignant tumours do exist.

Surgical excision usually results in complete cure.

Up to 80% of localized fibrous tumours arise in relation to the visceral pleura.

Figure 7.40 is a radiograph showing pleural thickening.

- Describe the two main ways in which atelectasis can occur.
- Classify and give examples of the causes of atelectasis.
- List the causes of pulmonary oedema.
- List the multifactoral aetiology of adult respiratory distress syndrome.
- List the investigations required to diagnose pulmonary embolism.
- Describe the consequences of pulmonary hypertension.
- What are the definitions of chronic bronchitis and emphysema?
- Describe the management of patients with COPD.
- Describe the management of a patient with bronchial asthma.
- What is the pathology of bronchiectasis?
- List the complications of cystic fibrosis.
- Describe the management of a patient with pneumonia.
- What is the pathogenesis of tuberculosis?
- List the common causes of pneumonia in the immunocompromised patient.
- What is the pathogenesis of pulmonary fibrosis.
- Describe the different forms of pneumoconioses.
- What is the relationship between cigarette smoking and bronchogenic carcinomas?
- Describe the differences between small-cell and non-small-cell carcinomas.
- Describe the endocrine manifestations of bronchogenic carcinomas.
- Describe the relationship between asbestos and pleural disease.

# CLINICAL ASSESSMENT

# 8. Presentations of Respiratory Disease

## Common presentations

The principal symptoms of respiratory disease (breathlessness, cough, sputum, haemoptysis, wheeze and chest pain) are common to many different conditions. Clinical findings often overlap considerably and this can make diagnosis seem difficult. However, a good history focusing on the time course and progression of the illness will often reveal recognizable patterns of symptoms and enable you to narrow down the differential diagnoses. Chapter 9 gives a framework for history taking; the main symptoms of respiratory disease and the key details that you should establish are described below.

It is important to remember that extreme lung disease does not necessarily produce clinical signs (e.g. a silent chest is an ominous sign in severe asthma).

## Breathlessness

Breathlessness or dyspnoea is a difficulty or distress in breathing and is a symptom of many different diseases (Fig. 8.1). Breathlessness is a very common reason for referral to a respiratory clinic.

The patient may describe the symptom in a variety of ways. Common terms used are 'puffed', 'can't get enough air' and 'feeling suffocated'. A number of physiological factors (Fig. 8.2) underlay this sensation and sometimes several mechanisms co-exist to cause breathlessness. However, understanding the physiological basis of dyspnoea is of limited help clinically; it is a good history that is vital in diagnosing the underlying disease. Key points to establish include the speed of onset of breathlessness (Figs 8.3–8.5), its progression and variability, exacerbating and relieving factors and response to any treatment. Ask specifically about breathlessness on lying flat (orthopnoea), which can occur in severe airflow obstruction or cardiac failure.

The severity of the symptom should be assessed by questioning the patient on how it affects their daily life (Fig. 8.6).

Although dyspnoea is a subjective sensation you may be able to see objective evidence of respiratory distress e.g. use of accessory muscles of inspiration, or obvious tachypnoea. See Chapter 9 for more key signs.

## Cough

A cough is the commonest manifestation of lower respiratory tract disease. The cough reflex is a complex centrally mediated defence reflex, resulting from the appropriate chemical or mechanical stimulation of the larynx and the more proximal portion of the tracheobronchial tree. The basic pattern of a cough can be divided into four components:

- Rapid deep inspiration
- Expiration against a closed glottis
- Sudden glottal opening
- Relaxation of expiratory muscles.

A cough may be voluntary but is usually an involuntary response to an irritant such as:

- Infection (URTI/LRTI)
- Cigarette smoke
- Dusts
- Danders (e.g. from cats).

Common respiratory diseases causing cough are shown in Fig. 8.7. Remember that gastro-oesophageal reflux or ACE inhibitor therapy can cause a patient to cough. Cough can also be due to paralysis of the vocal cords; this 'bovine' cough is low-pitched and occurs when the recurrent laryngeal nerve is compressed, for example by a tumour.

Enquire about the timing of the cough (morning or evening), its chronicity and nature (i.e. productive or unproductive). Answers to these questions should allow you to differentiate between two common causes of cough: asthma and chronic bronchitis (Fig. 8.8).

**Causes of breathlessness**

| | |
|---|---|
| physiological | exercise |
| | high altitude |
| pathological | respiratory disorders |
| | cardiac disorders |
| | obesity |
| | anaemia |
| psychological | anxiety (hyperventilation) |
| pharmacological | drug-induced respiratory disorders |
| | drug-induced cardiac disorders |

**Fig. 8.1** Causes of breathlessness. (Adapted from *Macleod's Clinical Examination* 10e, edited by J.F. Munro and I.W. Campbell. Churchill Livingstone, 2000.)

**Physiology of dyospnoea**

| Mechanism causing dyspnoea | Responds to: |
|---|---|
| chemoreceptors | hypercapnia and to lesser extent hypoxaemia |
| lung receptors (stretch and J receptors) | lung pathology (congestion etc.) |
| chest wall receptors | awareness by receptors of increased work |
| sense of effort | awareness by skeletal muscles of increased effort |
| afferent mismatch | relationship between force generated and lung volume produced; mismatch may lead to dyspnoea |

**Fig. 8.2** Physiology of dyspnoea.

**Conditions associated with breathlessness, grouped according to onset**

| Sudden onset | Onset occurring over hours | Onset occurring over weeks |
|---|---|---|
| Pulmonary embolism | Pneumonia | Chronic obstructive pulmonary disease (COPD) |
| Spontaneous pneumothorax | Exacerbation of asthma | Pleural effusion |
| Acute pulmonary oedema | Pulmonary oedema | Bronchial carcinoma |
| Inhalation of foreign body | | Pulmonary fibrosis |
| Acute asthma | | Anaemia |

**Fig. 8.3** Onset of breathlessness.

# Sputum

Everybody produces airway secretions. In a healthy non-smoker, approximately 100–150mL of mucus is produced every day. Normally, this mucus is transported up the airway's ciliary mucus escalator and swallowed. This process is not normally perceived. However, expectorating sputum is always abnormal, and is a sign that excess mucus has been generated. This can result from irritation of the respiratory tract (commonly caused by cigarette smoking or the common cold) or from infection.

Sputum may be classified as:
- Mucoid: clear, grey or white
- Serous: watery or frothy
- Mucopurulent: a yellowish tinge
- Purulent: dark green/yellow.

Always try to inspect the sputum and note its volume, colour, consistency and odour. These details can provide clues as to the underlying pathology (Fig. 8.9). A yellow/green colour usually means infection and is due to myeloperoxidase produced by eosinophils or neutrophils. However, note that sputum in asthma contains high numbers of eosinophils and is often yellow or green without underlying infection.

Most bronchogenic carcinomas do not produce sputum. The exception is alveolar cell carcinoma, which produces copious amounts of mucoid sputum.

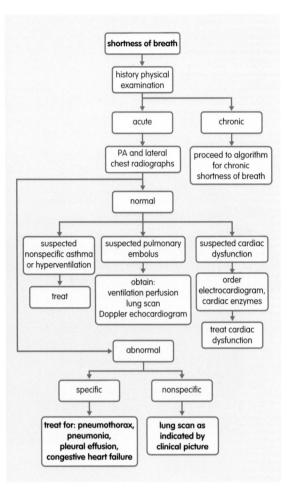

**Fig. 8.4** Diagnostic algorithm of breathlessness. (Adapted with permission from *Clinical Medicine*, 2e by H.L. Greene *et al*. Mosby Year Book, 1996.)

**Fig. 8.5** Diagnostic algorithm of chronic breathlessness. (Adapted with permission from *Clinical Medicine*, 2e by H.L. Greene *et al*. Mosby Year Book, 1996.)

| Key questions in assessing breathlessness |
| --- |
| How far can you walk upstairs/uphill without stopping? <br> How far can you walk on the flat without stopping? <br> Do you feel breathless when washing or dressing? <br> Do you feel breathless at rest? |

**Fig. 8.6** Assessing the severity of breathlessness.

| Common respiratory causes of cough | |
| --- | --- |
| Cause | Nature |
| asthma | worse at night; dry or productive |
| COPD | worse in morning; often productive |
| bronchiectasis | related to posture |
| post-nasal drip | persistent |
| tracheitis | painful |
| croup | harsh |
| interstitial fibrosis | dry |

**Fig. 8.7** Common respiratory causes of cough.

173

| Patterns of cough in asthma and chronic bronchitis | | |
|---|---|---|
| | **Asthma** | **Chronic bronchitis** |
| **timing** | worse at night | worse in the morning |
| **chronicity** | dry (may be green sputum) | productive |
| **nature** | intermittent | persistent |
| **response to treatment** | associated wheeze is reversible | associated wheeze is irreversible |

**Fig. 8.8** Patterns of cough in asthma and chronic bronchitis.

| Types of sputum | |
|---|---|
| **Character** | **Cause** |
| pink/frothy | pulmonary oedema |
| yellow/green | infections/eosinophils in asthma |
| rusty | pneumococcal pneumonia |
| foul-tasting | anaerobic infection |
| viscous, difficult to cough up | asthma/infections |
| large volumes | bronchiectasis |
| black | cavitating lesions in coal miners |
| blood-stained | see Figs 8.10 and 8.11 |

Detailed questioning about cough is needed in patients with chronic bronchitis. Useful questions include: Do you cough up sputum/spit/phlegm from your chest on most mornings? Would you say you cough up sputum on most days for as much as three months a year? Do you often need antibiotics from your GP in winter?

**Fig. 8.9** Types of sputum.

You may have to prompt the patient when investigating the volume of sputum. Do they cough up enough to fill a teaspoon/tablespoon/eggcup/sputum pot?

Chronic bronchitis is a particularly important cause of sputum production. This is defined as a cough productive of sputum for most days during at least three consecutive months, for more than two successive years.

## Haemoptysis

Haemoptysis is coughing up blood; this needs to be differentiated from other sources of bleeding within the oral cavity and haematemesis (vomiting blood). This distinction is usually obvious from the history. Haemoptysis is not usually a solitary event and so if possible the sputum sample should be inspected.

Haemoptysis is a serious and often alarming symptom that requires immediate investigation (Fig. 8.10). A chest radiograph is mandatory in a patient with haemoptysis, and the symptom should be treated as bronchogenic carcinoma until proved otherwise. Despite appropriate investigations, often no obvious cause can be found and the episode is attributed to a simple bronchial infection.

Important respiratory causes of haemoptysis are:
- Bronchial carcinoma
- Pulmonary infarction

**Fig. 8.10** Diagnostic algorithm of haemoptysis. (Adapted with permission from *Decision Making in Medicine* by H.L. Greene, W.P. Johnson and M.J. Maricic. Mosby Year Book, 1993.)

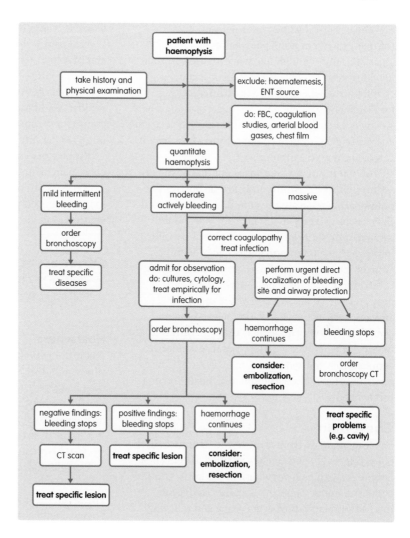

- T.B
- Pneumonia (particularly pneumococcal)
- Bronchiectasis
- Acute/chronic bronchitis.

In investigating the cause of haemoptysis, ask about any preceding events, such as respiratory infection or deep vein thrombosis (DVT) and establish the frequency, volume and whether it is fresh or altered blood. Figure 8.11 gives some characteristic patterns of haemoptysis and possible diagnoses.

| Patterns of haemoptysis | |
|---|---|
| **Pattern** | **Possible diagnosis** |
| recurrent blood-streaked sputum | bronchial carcinoma |
| frank, becoming progressively darker over 24/48 h | infarction |
| recurrent over years, with purulent sputum | bronchiectasis |

**Fig. 8.11** Patterns of haemoptysis.

## Wheeze

Wheezing is a common complaint, complicating many different disease processes. Establish exactly what a patient means by 'wheeze'; used correctly the term describes musical notes heard mainly on expiration and caused by narrowed airways.

Wheezes are classified as either polyphonic (of many different notes) or monophonic (just one note). Poylphonic wheezes are common in widespread airflow obstruction; it is the characteristic wheeze heard in asthmatics. A localized monophonic wheeze suggests that a single airway is partially obstructed; this can also occur in asthma (e.g. by a mucus plug) but may be a sign of narrowing due to a tumour.

The symptom of wheezing is not diagnostic of asthma, although asthma and chronic obstructive pulmonary disease are the commonest causes and they can be difficult to distinguish. You should establish whether the patient wheezes first thing in the morning (common in chronic bronchitis), at night (common in asthma) or on exercising.

Stridor is an audible *inspiratory* noise and indicates partial obstruction of the upper, larger airways, such as the larynx, trachea and main bronchus. It is very important that you differentiate between a wheeze and stridor because stridor is a serious sign requiring urgent investigation. Causes of obstruction include tumour and inhalation of a foreign body.

## Chest pain

Pain can originate from most of the structures in the chest (Fig. 8.12) and can be classified as central or lateral. As with pain anywhere in the body, enquire about site, mode of onset, character, radiation, intensity, precipitating, aggravating and relieving factors and response to any analgesics taken. Make sure you ask specifically about the pain's relationship to breathing, coughing or movement; if it is made worse by these it is likely to be pleural in origin. Pleural pain is sharp and stabbing in character and may be referred to the shoulder tip if the diaphragmatic pleura is involved. It can be very severe and often leads to shallow breathing, avoidance of movement and cough suppression. The commonest causes of pleural pain are pulmonary infarction or infection.

Respiratory causes of central, or retrosternal, chest pain include bronchitis and acute tracheitis. This pain is often made worse by coughing and may be relieved when the patient coughs up sputum.

## Other associated symptoms

In addition to the principal presentations, there are several other symptoms that you should note.

### Hoarseness

Ask if the patient's voice has changed at all in recent times, and if so, was there anything that preceded the change, e.g. overuse of the voice, thyroidectomy etc. There may be a simple, benign cause of hoarseness such as:

- Cigarette smoking
- Acute laryngitis as part of an acute URTI
- Use of inhaled steroids.

However, there may be a more sinister cause: like the bovine cough noted above, hoarseness may be a sign that a lung tumour is compressing the recurrent laryngeal nerve.

### Weight loss

Unintentional weight loss is always an important sign, raising suspicion of carcinoma. Establish how much weight the patient has lost, over what period, and whether there is any loss of appetite. Note, however, that it is common for patients with severe emphysema to lose weight.

### Ankle swelling

A patient with chronic obstructive pulmonary disease (COPD) may comment that their ankles swell during acute exacerbations. Ask about this and check for oedema as part of your examination (see p. 199); it is an important sign of cor pulmonale.

| Causes of chest pain | |
| --- | --- |
| Structure | Possible cause of pain |
| pleura | pneumothorax, pulmonary infarction |
| muscle | strain (e.g. from coughing) |
| bone | rib fracture or tumour |
| costochondral junctions | Tietze's syndrome |
| nerves | herpes zoster, Pancoast's syndrome |
| heart and great vessels | cardiac ischaemia/infarction aortic dissection/aneurysm |
| oesophagus | spasm, reflux |

**Fig. 8.12** Causes of chest pain.

# Acute presentations

## Respiratory failure

Respiratory failure is not a presentation seen in isolation but a possible outcome of many different respiratory diseases.

In the initial stages of lung disease, the body may be able to maintain normal blood gases by adapting to increased ventilatory demand. However, if the underlying disease progresses, the ventilatory workload may become excessive. The result is a failure to oxygenate the blood or failure to remove carbon dioxide by ventilation. The patient is said to be in respiratory failure, a state which can be diagnosed on the clinical picture and by blood gas analysis. The patient will usually have signs of underlying disease in addition to the clinical features of respiratory failure, which are principally those of hypoxia (Fig. 8.13).

Respiratory failure can be classified into two types, depending on the presence or absence of hypercapnia. It is important to distinguish the two types because this impacts on the therapy given.

### Type I respiratory failure

This is the most common type of respiratory failure. The features are:
- Acute hypoxaemia: $P_aO_2$ low (<8kPa)
- $P_aCO_2$ normal or low.

The patient is hypoxic (and becomes cyanotic, confused and restless) but is normo- or hypocapnic. This can be explained by the patient's response to an initial rise in $P_aCO_2$. Alveolar ventilation is stimulated and the excess carbon dioxide (and sometimes more than the excess) is excreted.

Almost all acute lung diseases can cause type I respiratory failure. The underlying mechanism for the failure of gas exchange is frequently ventilation:perfusion mismatch. Some common examples are:
- Severe acute asthma
- Pneumonia
- Pulmonary embolism
- Pulmonary oedema.

### Type II respiratory failure

The features of type II respiratory failure are:
- $P_aO_2$ low (<8kPa)
- $P_aCO_2$ high (>6.5kPa).

The patient is hypoxic and hypercapnic. As the $P_aCO_2$ rises, the patient will develop additional symptoms and signs including headache, warm peripheries and bounding pulse; with severe hypercapnia a flapping tremor may develop.

Type II respiratory failure is also known as ventilatory failure; the rise in $P_aCO_2$ is no longer matched by an increase in alveolar ventilation. This can be because:
- Ventilatory drive is insufficient
- The work of breathing is excessive
- The lungs are unable to pump air in and out efficiently.

Type II respiratory failure can therefore occur in neuromuscular disorders, CNS depression or when a lung collapses, for example after tension pneumothorax. However, the commonest cause is an acute exacerbation of COPD. Patients with COPD are often hypoxaemic for many years with morning headache being the only sign that $P_aCO_2$ is slightly raised. An acute exacerbation (e.g. due to respiratory infection) then increases the work of breathing still further, leading to 'acute-on-chronic' respiratory failure.

 If the respiratory failure develops quickly, increased $P_aCO_2$ leads to a rise in pH: respiratory acidosis. If it develops more slowly, there is time for renal compensation and pH may be normal or near-normal. Always look at bicarbonate levels to see if they have risen in compensation.

Management of respiratory failure is discussed in detail in Chapter 6. However, it is important to note here that you should be cautious in giving oxygen to patients with type II respiratory failure. Respiratory drive in these patients has become relatively insensitive to hypercapnia; hypoxaemia plays a more important role in stimulating ventilation. Giving high concentrations of oxygen will therefore suppress ventilatory drive and $P_aCO_2$ may rise rather than fall.

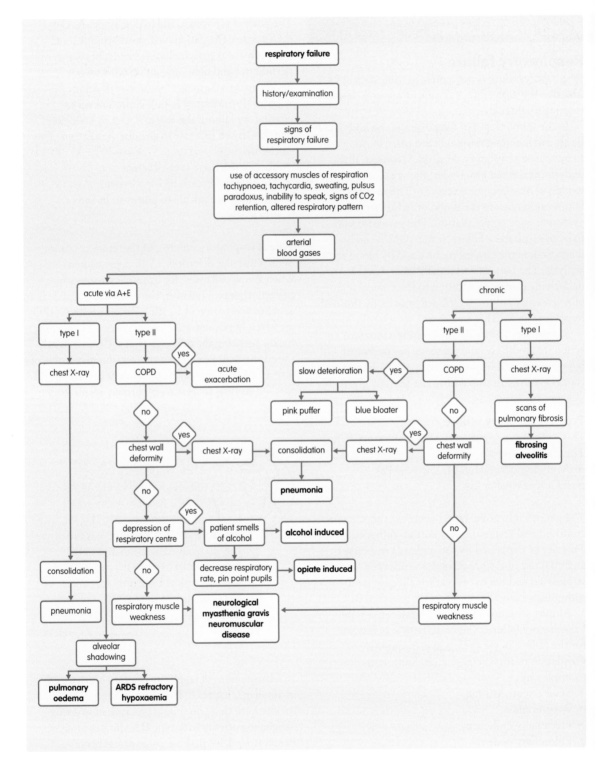

**Fig. 8.13** Diagnostic algorithm of respiratory failure. ARDS: adult respiratory distress syndrome. (Adapted with permission from *Clinical Medicine*, 2e by H.L. Greene *et al.* Mosby Year Book, 1996.)

- What are the key differences in presentation between a patient with COPD and one with asthma?
- What important facts do you need to establish if a patient complains of coughing up blood?
- Explain the difference between type I and II respiratory failure, in terms of blood gases and symptoms.
- What are the three basic mechanisms that contribute to type II respiratory failure?
- Why do you need to exercise caution in administering oxygen to a patient with COPD who is in respiratory failure?

179

# 9. History and Examination

## Taking a history

In respiratory medicine your skills in history taking will be tested by both:

- Acute presentations—diagnosis must be quick but may be hindered by the patient's condition
- Chronic presentations—documenting the key features in an illness that may span many years.

Each situation has its specific challenges and in each a good history should tell you the diagnosis.

> This section outlines a generic approach to history taking. In practice, you should tailor your history to the possible diagnoses. In a female patient with a suspected deep vein thrombosis (DVT) you will need to ask about pregnancy, oral contraceptive pill, recent travel or surgery and family history of DVT or PE. Obviously, you will need a different set of questions to establish a diagnosis of asthma.

## Initial observations

Before you begin take a few minutes to introduce yourself and to put the patient at ease.

Simple observation at the bedside can often give a good clue to the likely diagnosis:
- Inhalers and oxygen bottles
- Sputum pots
- Walking sticks or frames.

How does the patient appear during the interview? Agitated, or distressed? Is there a visible tremor? Are they too breathless to speak in full sentences? Is their voice rough or hoarse? Simple observations now will save time later.

## Structure of the history
### Presenting complaint (PC)
The presenting complaint is a concise statement of the symptoms felt by the patient. Use the patient's own words—this is not a diagnosis. For example, for shortness of breath the patient might use 'out of puff' or 'can't get any air in'.

### History of presenting complaint (HPC)
Build up a picture of the presenting complaint, investigating each symptom as described in Chapter 8. You should establish the following details:
- Onset: acute or gradual
- Pattern: intermittent or continuous
- Frequency: daily, weekly or monthly
- Duration: minutes or hours
- Progression: better or worse than in the past
- Severity: mild, moderate or severe
- Character: e.g. is the pain sharp, dull or aching?
- Precipitating and relieving factors: e.g. are any medications used?
- Associated symptoms: e.g. cough, wheeze, haemoptysis, dyspnoea, chest pain, orthopnoea
- Systemic symptoms: e.g. fever, malaise, anorexia, weight loss?

Has the patient had the problem before? If so, what was the diagnosis, treatment and outcome?

Ask the patient how disabling the problem is and how it affects daily life. In patients with chronic illness, you should establish their exercise tolerance and whether this has declined.

### Past medical history (PMH)
Present the PMH in chronological order, listing any hospital admissions, surgical operations and major illnesses.

Take a careful note of anything that might contribute to the presenting complaint; for example:
- Pneumonia—complications include pleural effusion, bronchiectasis
- 'Wheezy bronchitis' as a child—possibly asthma
- Severe measles or whooping cough in childhood—may lead to bronchiectasis

- Previous pulmonary embolism (PE) or deep vein thrombosis (DVT)
- Pregnancy—risk of PE
- Recent surgery—PE, hospital acquired or aspiration pneumonia
- Eczema or hayfever—evidence of atopy.

Has the patient received BCG immunization or experienced tuberculosis contact in the past? Has he or she ever had a chest radiograph: it may be useful for comparison.

Note any other factors that might have contributed, for example:

- Recent travel—DVT, legionella
- Recent life events (e.g. moving house)—stress, house dust.

## Drug history (DH)

When taking the drug history, list the patient's current intake of both prescribed and over-the-counter (OTC) drugs, recording dosage, frequency and duration of treatment. Ask the patient what each tablet is for and when it is taken; this gives an indication of the patient's understanding of his or her problems and compliance. Remember that some drugs (e.g. beta-blockers or NSAIDs) can make asthma worse. The oral contraceptive pill is a risk factor for pulmonary embolism. ACE inhibitors prescribed for hypertension can cause cough.

## Drug allergies

Ask about any allergies; if the patient mentions an allergy, ask what exactly happened, and how long ago it happened.

## Family history (FH)

When noting a family history, it may be easier to draw a pedigree chart. Do any members of the family suffer from a respiratory disorder? A family history of premature emphysema or liver cirrhosis may indicate $\alpha_1$ antitrypsin deficiency. Is there a family history of pulmonary embolism or deep vein thrombosis. Ask about atopy, asthma, eczema and hayfever. Does anybody in the family smoke?

## Social history (SH)

Social history is hugely important in the respiratory system; many respiratory diseases can be caused, or worsened, by social factors such as housing, occupation, hobbies or pets.

## Home and social situation

Ask who lives with the patient at home and are they fit and well? Do they have any additional help around the home?

Ask about accommodation:

- Type: house, flat (which floor?) or bedsit
- Heating: coal fire, gas fire or central heating
- Conditions: damp or dry
- Number of people living in the accommodation
- Area of town: gives an indication of socioeconomic class
- Pets: dogs, cats or birds.

Asking about pets is important in a respiratory history. For example, cat dander may precipitate an asthma attack or allergic rhinitis and pet birds are a rare cause of pneumonia.

Ask about the patient's financial situation: is he or she entitled to any state benefits (e.g. social support)? Enquire about diet and exercise.

## Smoking and alcohol

A detailed smoking history is essential. You should record:

- Age started
- Age stopped (if applicable)
- Whether cigarettes, cigars or pipe
- Average smoked per day.

It may help to convert this information into 'pack years' (where one pack year is 20 cigarettes smoked each day for a year).

The smoking history gives clues to correct diagnosis. Most patients with COPD have a 20 or more pack year history. A patient with a diagnosis of COPD and a 10 pack year history may be a misdiagnosed asthmatic.

| Occupational causes of lung disease | |
|---|---|
| **Disease** | **Area of work** |
| asbestosis | vehicle body workers, ship building, demolition |
| malignant mesothelioma | as above |
| byssinosis | textile workers |
| stannosis | tin mining |
| farmer's lung | farming (exposure to mouldy hay) |
| coal worker's pneumoconiosis | coal mining |
| silicosis | mining, quarrying, foundry work etc. |
| occupational asthma | see Fig. 7.15 |
| beryllosis | electronic industries |

**Fig. 9.1** Occupational causes of lung disease.

Ask if the patient drinks alcohol. If yes, convert the weekly intake into units if possible. One glass of wine or one-half pint of beer is equivalent to 1 unit. Remember that some forms of pneumonia (*S. aureus* and *Klebsiella*) occur in alcoholics.

### Occupation
Present the patient's jobs in chronological order starting from the time the patient left school. Some respiratory conditions have a long latent period between time of exposure and presentation.

Enquire about occupational related disorders (e.g. asbestos exposure and mesothelioma). The length of each job and the job description need to be recorded. Figure 9.1 lists some lung diseases associated with specific occupations. Hobbies may also be relevant.

Once you have finished, check that you have not missed anything and then summarize the key points to add clarity and ease presentation.

## Communication skills

The sections above outline the information you need to elicit from the patient. Being able to gather all this information in a pleasant but efficient manner is dependent on the rapport you generate with the patient and your ability to communicate. Communication skills are now an important part of the curriculum at most medical schools and form part of structured clinical exams (OSCEs). These skills can take time to develop, but with practice you can pick up a lot of extra marks. Rehearse some communication scenarios with friends and practise on the wards if you can. Watching 'good' and 'bad' communicators in action can also be helpful. Some of the basic techniques are discussed below.

Asthma is a favourite with OSCE examiners. Practise explaining to an imaginary patient:
- The pathological basis of the illness (without using jargon).
- How it should be managed.
- The difference between preventers and relievers.
- How to use an inhaler/peak flow meter.

## Verbal skills
How we say things is as important as what we say. Be aware that the tone, pitch and speed of your speech will have an effect on the consultation. Tailor your language to the patient's understanding and avoid jargon.

### Open questions
Effective consultations often begin with an open question, i.e. one that encourages the patient to give a spontaneous account. Allow the patient to speak for a minute or two without interruption before picking up on aspects of their narrative. Open questions can also help to gather information when a new subject is introduced. Examples include:
- What made you come to the surgery/hospital today?
- Tell me how your breathing has been
- Tell me more about the chest pain.

### Closed questions
These ask for specific information and can fill in any gaps in the history. Questions such as 'Does the pain

catch when you breathe in?' focus the narrative and speed it up. Closed questions can be a useful prompt when patients are reluctant to give specific facts, for example on how much they are smoking. Supplying an answer of 'About 40 a day?' may elicit a gasp followed by a reasonably truthful answer.

## Responses

Your response to the narrative can encourage the patient and confirm your understanding. The appropriate response may:

- Demonstrate empathy and build trust: 'That must have been very frightening'
- Show you are actively listening: 'Yes, go on...'
- Pick up on cues from the patient: 'You mentioned that your breathing was worse at night...'
- Clarify: 'What did you mean by...?'

## Non-verbal skills

A large proportion of our communication is non-verbal. Be aware of your own posture, facial expressions and gestures and be alert to those of the patient—they may give you clues as to their concerns. You should also ensure that you:

- Position yourself so that you face the patient and there is a comfortable distance between you. Sit beside the desk rather than across it.
- Maintain good eye contact, even if the patient doesn't
- Use non-verbal cues to demonstrate you are listening (smiling, nodding etc.)
- Try to minimize any irritating habits you may have—other people may be able to point these out to you!

## Obstacles to communication

Many factors can provide a barrier to effective communication. The following may help to minimize them.

- If possible find a quiet room or cubicle with reasonable privacy
- If the patient is in pain, determine whether they need analgesia before the history
- Be patient and persistent if the history is hindered by a patient's symptoms (e.g. breathlessness)
- Try to minimize language and cultural barriers by having an interpreter or family member present.

## Framework for the consultation

A mental checklist can be useful, particularly in pressurized situations such as exams. Examiners will be looking for a 'patient-centred' approach; you should explore the patient's ideas, concerns and expectations and demonstrate an intention to involve them in decisions about their treatment. One such framework is:

- Introduce yourself and explain what you would like to do
- Find out why the patient has presented to you
- Establish how much the patient knows about their problem
- What do they expect from the consultation?
- Explore the problem through history and examination
- Explain your diagnosis clearly
- Check that the patient understands
- Ask the patient if they have any questions
- Literature—provide leaflets or written notes to take away
- Follow-up. Clarify what the next step is, e.g. appointment for bronchoscopy.

These last four points can be remembered as CALF. Gain some extra marks at an OSCE station by running through these at the end.

## Examination

### Overview

As with any examination, it is important that you:

- Introduce yourself if you have not already done so
- Wash your hands before you begin and when you finish the examination
- Explain to the patient what you propose to do and ask if this is acceptable.

The structure of the examination is inspection, palpation, percussion and auscultation. For a respiratory examination, patients should be fully exposed to the waist, comfortable, and sitting at 45°, with their hands by their sides.

In clinical examinations, purposefully walk to the end of the bed to observe the patient; this emphasizes that you are observing the patient and also gives you thinking time. Give a running commentary of what you are doing, this needs practice as you will be nervous.

## General inspection

The initial observation is vital. If you have not already done so as part of the history, stand at the end of the bed and look at the locker for sputum pots, inhalers and charts. Note any drip stands that are present, venous cannulae, or bandages.

Stand back and note the patient's general appearance. Are they:
- Obviously unwell or distressed?
- Alert or confused?
- Thin or overweight?

There are some signs (e.g. use of accessory muscles of inspiration or pallor) that you may notice immediately. Does the patient have a cough and, if so, does it sound productive? Is there any abnormality (e.g. hoarseness) in the voice?

Then run through a systematic general inspection. You should look generally at muscle bulk, noting any cachexia (Fig. 9.2) and then inspect the skin in detail

(Fig. 9.3). You may want to inspect the thorax at this point too; these aspects are discussed below.

It is essential that you look closely at how the patient is breathing. In addition to respiratory rate (Fig. 9.4), which is easier to test with the pulse, you should note:

| Inspection of skin | | |
|---|---|---|
| Test performed | Signs observed | Diagnostic inference |
| observe the general state of the skin | steroidal skin: shiny excessive bruising thin | prolonged use of corticosteroids: chronic obstructive pulmonary disease asthma fibrosing alveolitis systemic disease (e.g. Crohn's disease) |
| | generalized dryness and scaling of skin | ichthyosis vulgaris acquired ichthyosis hypothyroidism sarcoidosis |
| | thin skin | ageing Cushing's syndrome topical or systemic steroid use |
| observe the colour of the skin | pale skin | pallor anaemia leukaemia shock |
| | light brown coloured spots on skin | café-au-lait spots neurofibromatosis tuberous sclerosis |

**Fig. 9.3** Tests, signs and diagnostic inferences found when inspecting the skin.

| Cachexia | | |
|---|---|---|
| Test performed | Signs observed | Diagnostic inference |
| observe muscle bulk and general condition of the skin | generalized muscle wasting and lack of nutrition; pallor; dry and wrinkled skin | malignant disease bronchial carcinoma chronic disease renal disease hepatic disease cardiac failure tuberculosis other anorexia nervoso malnutrition emotional disturbance |

**Fig. 9.2** Tests, signs and diagnostic inferences found in cachexia.

| Abnormal ventilation rate | | |
|---|---|---|
| Test performed | Signs observed | Diagnostic inference |
| discretely count the respiratory rate while feeling the patient's pulse | 12–20 breaths per minute | normal |
| | >12 breaths per minute (tachypnoea) | anxiety pain infection pneumothorax pulmonary embolism |
| | <12 breaths per minute (bradypnoea) | hypothyroidism increased intracranial pressure |

**Fig. 9.4** Tests, signs and diagnostic inferences found when checking the breathing rate.

- Signs of dyspnoea (e.g. use of accessory muscles of inspiration such as the sternomastoids, patient 'fixing' upper body by leaning forward, mouth breathing, nasal flaring)
- Unusual patterns of breathing (Fig. 9.5)
- Any noises you can hear unaided (e.g. wheeze or stridor).

## Hands and limbs
### Examination of the hands
The hands can reveal key signs of respiratory disease. Take both the patient's hands and note their temperature. Abnormally warm and cyanosed hands are a sign of $CO_2$ retention. Check the fingers for nicotine staining. One important sign of respiratory disease is finger clubbing (Figs 9.6 and 9.7). This is a painless, bulbous enlargement of the distal fingers; it is accompanied by softening of the nail bed and loss of nail bed angle. Also assess for:

- Muscle wasting (Fig. 9.8)
- Rheumatoid hands (Fig. 9.9)
- Hypertrophic pulmonary osteoarthropathy (HPOA) (Fig. 9.10)
- Hand tremor (Fig. 9.11).

| Abnormal patterns of breathing | |
| --- | --- |
| **Signs observed** | **Diagnostic inference** |
| hyperventilation with deep sighing respirations (Kussmaul's respiration) | diabetic ketoacidosis aspirin overdose acute massive pulmonary embolism |
| increased rate and volume of respiration followed by periods of apnoea (Cheyne–Stokes respiration) | terminal disease increased intracranial pressure |
| prolongation of expiration | airflow limitation |
| pursed lip breathing | air trapping |

**Fig. 9.5** Unusual patterns of breathing.

Know the causes of clubbing before any clinical examination. Note that chronic bronchitis does not cause clubbing.

### Examination of the pulse
A normal resting pulse in an adult is between 60–100 b.p.m. Bradycardia is defined as a pulse rate of less than 60 b.p.m. and tachycardia of greater than 100. Palpate the radial pulse, wait for a moment and then count for 15 seconds. You can then multiply by four to give a rate per minute. Is the pulse regular and if not how is it irregular? (Fig. 9.12).

| Clubbing | | |
| --- | --- | --- |
| **Test performed** | **Sign observed** | **Diagnostic inference** |
| view the nail from the side at eye level; rock the nail from side to side on the nail-bed; look at the nail-bed and nail angle. place nails back to back; a diamond-shaped area is evident between them if clubbing does not exist. | increase in the soft tissues of the nail-bed and fingertip, with increased sponginess of the nail-bed loss of angle between nail and nail-bed transverse curvature of nail increases in final stages, whole tip of the finger becomes clubbed clubbing may also affect the toes bones are normal | pulmonary causes: tumour (bronchial carcinoma, mesothelioma) chronic pulmonary sepsis (empyema, lung abscess, bronchiectasis, cystic fibrosis) fibrosing alveolitis asbestosis hypertrophic pulmonary osteoarthropathy cardiac causes: congenital bacterial endocarditis other causes: idiopathic causes cirrhosis inflammatory bowel disease |

**Fig. 9.6** Tests, signs and diagnostic inferences found in clubbing.

**Fig. 9.7** One method of inspecting for clubbing. Normal fingers: note diamond-shaped area.

In addition to testing pulse volume and character, which are better assessed from the carotid pulse, you should also check for the presence of pulsus paradoxus. In normal individuals the pulse decreases slightly in volume on inspiration and systolic blood pressure falls by 3–5mmHg. In severe obstructive diseases (e.g. severe asthma) the contractile force of respiratory muscles is so great that there is a marked fall in systolic pressure on inspiration. A fall of greater than 10mmHg is pathological. Figure 9.13 shows how to test for this sign.

| Muscle wasting | | |
| --- | --- | --- |
| **Test performed** | **Sign observed** | **Diagnostic inference** |
| look at the dorsal aspect of the hand for any reduction in muscle bulk<br><br>always compare both hands together | muscle wasting: note the distribution and if it is unilateral or bilateral | localized:<br>unilateral<br>– Pancoast's tumour<br>bilateral<br>– disuse atrophy;<br>rheumatoid arthritis<br>generalized:<br>diabetes<br>thyrotoxicosis<br>anorexia nervosa |

**Fig. 9.8** Tests, signs and diagnostic inferences found in muscle wasting.

| Rheumatoid hands | | |
| --- | --- | --- |
| **Test performed** | **Sign observed** | **Diagnostic inference** |
| look at the hands for signs of rheumatoid disease | ulnar deviation of fingers swan-neck or boutonniere deformity Z-deformity of thumb subluxation of proximal phalanx wasting of small muscles | rheumatoid disease, which may affect the lung:<br>pulmonary nodules<br>pleural effusion |

**Fig. 9.9** Tests, signs and diagnostic inferences found in rheumatoid hands.

| Hypertrophic pulmonary osteoarthropathy | | |
| --- | --- | --- |
| **Test performed** | **Sign observed** | **Diagnostic inference** |
| apply pressure to the wrist | tenderness on palpation of the wrist; the pain is over the shafts of the long bones adjacent to the joint<br><br>arthralgia and joint swelling | hypertrophic pulmonary osteoarthropathy, a nonmetastatic complication of malignancy – subperiosteal new-bone formation in the long bones of the lower limbs and forearms; clubbing is also present – 90% of cases are associated with bronchogenic carcinoma, especially squamous cell carcinoma<br><br>other causes:<br>rheumatoid arthritis<br>systemic sclerosis |

**Fig. 9.10** Tests, signs and diagnostic inferences found in hypertrophic pulmonary osteoarthropathy.

**Fig. 9.11** Tests, signs and diagnostic inferences found in hand tremor.

| Hand tremor | | |
|---|---|---|
| **Test performed** | **Sign observed** | **Diagnostic inference** |
| ask patient to hold fingers outstretched and spread in front; place a piece of paper on the dorsal aspect of the hands; observe hands at eye level from the side | very fine finger tremor on outstretched fingers; finger tremor is made more obvious by placing a piece of paper on top of the hands | • stimulation of β-receptors by bronchodilator drugs especially nebulized drugs.<br>• thyrotoxicosis |
| ask patient to hold arm outstretched in front; fully extend the wrists; apply pressure to hands; leave patient like this for 30 seconds | flapping tremor (asterixis) against your hands, which is coarse and irregular in nature; maximum activity at wrist and metacarpophalangeal joints | $CO_2$ retention hepatic failure encephalopathy metabolic diseases subdural haematoma |

| Abnormal radial pulse | |
|---|---|
| **Sign observed** | **Diagnostic inference** |
| rate <100 beats per minute | normal |
| rate >100 beats per minute (tachycardia) | pain shock infection thyrotoxicosis sarcoidosis pulmonary embolism drugs e.g. salbutamol iatrogenic causes |
| full, exaggerated arterial pulsation (bounding pulse) | $CO_2$ retention thyrotoxicosis fever anaemia hyperkinetic states |

**Fig. 9.12** Tests, signs and diagnostic inferences found when testing the radial pulse.

You will gain marks if your examination looks fluent and professional. It is easy to move smoothly from introducing yourself and shaking the patient's hand to examination of the hands to testing the radial pulse. Then you can discreetly test for respiratory rate without the patient realising and altering their breathing.

## Examination of the limbs

Examine the axillary lymph nodes as shown in Fig. 9.14. Check the patient's ankles for oedema by applying pressure with fingers and thumb for a few seconds. If there is subcutaneous fluid you may see pitting persisting. Bilateral pitting oedema is seen in many conditions including congestive cardiac failure, liver failure and, important to your respiratory enquiry, cor pulmonale.

# Head and neck
## Examination of the face

First, observe the face generally. You may notice:
• Signs of superior vena cava obstruction (Fig. 9.15)
• Cushingoid features (Fig. 9.15).

Look at the mouth for signs of:
• Candida infection—white coating on tongue often seen after steroids or antibiotics
• Central cyanosis (Fig. 9.16).

Then examine the eyes (Figs 9.17 and 9.18) and test for anaemia (Fig. 9.19).

Remember that an anaemic patient may be dangerously desaturated without appearing cyanosed.

**Fig. 9.13** Tests, signs and diagnostic inferences found in pulsus paradoxus.

| Pulsus paradoxus | | |
|---|---|---|
| **Test performed** | **Sign observed** | **Diagnostic inference** |
| measure blood pressure using a sphygmomanometer: cuff pressure is reduced and systolic sound is heard; this initially occurs only in expiration; with further reduction of cuff pressure you can hear systole in inspiration as well; the pressure difference between the initial systolic sound in expiration and when it is present throughout the breathing cycle is what is measured | pulse volume decreases with inspiration, the reverse of normal<br><br>large fall in systolic blood pressure during inspiration | severe asthma<br>other causes:<br>  cardiac tamponade<br>  massive pulmonary embolism<br><br>fall is exaggerated when venous return to the right heart is impaired |

| Enlarged axillary lymph nodes | | |
|---|---|---|
| **Test performed** | **Sign observed** | **Diagnostic inference** |
| Method 1: face the patient; place the patient's right arm on your right arm; patient's arm must be relaxed; palpate axilla with left hand; place the patient's left arm on your left arm; palpate left axilla | enlarged lymph node (axillary lymphadenopathy) | localized spread of viral or bacterial infection tuberculosis human immunodeficiency virus (HIV) infection actinomycosis cytomegalovirus (CMV) infection measles |
| Method 2: ask the patient to place hands behind head; palpate axilla by placing your fingers high up in axilla; press tips of fingers against chest wall; move fingers down over ribs | | axial lymphadenopathy is often present in breast carcinoma |

**Fig. 9.14** Tests, signs and diagnostic inferences found when examining the axillary lymph nodes.

| Observation of the face | | |
|---|---|---|
| **Test performed** | **Sign observed** | **Diagnostic inference** |
| observe the patient's face | oedema cyanosis puffy eyes fixed, engorged neck veins | superior vena cava obstruction:<br>  bronchial carcinoma<br>  lymphoma<br>  mediastinal goitre<br>  fibrosis |
| | features associated with Cushing's syndrome:<br>  moon face<br>  plethora<br>  acne<br>  hirsute<br>  oral candidiasis | long-term administration of steroids<br>  ACTH secretion by small-cell bronchial carcinoma |

**Fig. 9.15** Tests, signs and diagnostic inferences found when observing the face.

## Examination of the neck

Examine tracheal position and measure the crico-sternal distance (Figs 9.20 and 9.21). Then make sure the patient is at 45° and test the jugular venous pulse (Figs 9.22 and 9.23). Finally, test for cervical lymphadenopathy from behind (Figs 9.24 and 9.25).

Develop a set system of palpating the lymph nodes of the neck (as mentioned above). Sit the patient up and examine from behind with both hands.

| Central cyanosis | | |
|---|---|---|
| **Test performed** | **Sign observed** | **Diagnostic inference** |
| good natural light is needed<br><br>ask the patient to stick tongue out<br><br>look at the mucous membranes of the lips and tongue | blue discoloration to skin and mucous membrane<br><br>central cyanosis cannot be accurately identified in black and Asian patients | level of deoxygenated haemoglobin >5 g/dL<br>diseases caused by marked ventilation–perfusion mismatch will cause central cyanosis:<br>  severe pulmonary fibrosis<br>  chronic bronchitis<br>  right–left heart shunts<br>  pneumonia<br>  respiratory failure<br>  bronchiectasis<br>  chronic obstructive<br>  pulmonary disease |

**Fig. 9.16** Tests, signs and diagnostic inferences found in central cyanosis.

| Examination of the eyes | | |
|---|---|---|
| **Test performed** | **Sign observed** | **Diagnostic inference** |
| Look at the eyes, noting the position of the eyelid and pupil size; always compare with the other side.<br><br>If an abnormality is present, check that the pupils are reactive to light | Dropping of upper eyelids so that upper part of iris and pupil are covered (ptosis) | Third nerve palsy (with dilated pupil).<br>Horner's syndrome (with small reactive pupil): involvement of the sympathetic chain on the posterior chest wall by an apical bronchial carcinoma; T1 wasting and sensoryloss also occur.<br>Idiopathic (usually in young females).<br>Myasthenia gravis (with bilateral ptosis)<br>Dystrophia.<br>Mitochondrial disease (rare) |
|  | Small pupil | Old age.<br>Horner's syndrome.<br>Argyll Robertson's pupil: miotic and responsive to accommodation effort, but not to light.<br>Disease in pons.<br>Cerebrovascular accident.<br>Drugs (e.g. opiates). |

**Fig. 9.17** Tests, signs and diagnostic inferences found when examining the eyes.

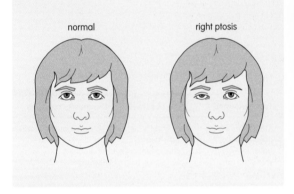

normal       right ptosis

**Fig. 9.18** Typical appearance of a patient with ptosis.

| Anaemia | | |
|---|---|---|
| **Test performed** | **Sign observed** | **Diagnostic inference** |
| ask patient to look up, then evert lower lid of eye<br><br>note the colour of mucous membrane | pale mucous membrane | indication of anaemia; however, anaemia can only be conclusively diagnosed by measuring haemoglobin levels |

**Fig. 9.19** Tests, signs and diagnostic inferences found in anaemia.

Before a clinical examination, learn the lymph nodes of the neck and into which set of nodes different structures drain.

## The thorax
### Observation of the thorax

As already noted, it is often easier to inspect the thorax as part of your general inspection. In addition to observing chest wall movement, you should note any lesions, thoracic scars (Fig. 9.26) or radiotherapy tatoos (small green or blue dots used as guidance for radiotherapy). Then observe the shape of the thorax

| Tracheal position and crico-sternal distance | | |
|---|---|---|
| **Test performed** | **Sign observed** | **Diagnostic inference** |
| stand at the front of the patient; pressing gently, place one finger on the trachea | deviation of the trachea away from the midline | pulled to side of collapse |
| judge if the finger slides to one side (tracheal deviation gives an indication of the position of the upper mediastinum; however, the only conclusive method of judging the position is chest radiography) | | pushed away from mass or fluid contralateral side to tension pneumothorax |
| measure the distance (in finger breadths) between the sternal notch and cricoid cartilage during a full inspiration | three or four finger breaths | normal |
| | reduced distance | air flow limitation |

**Fig. 9.20** Tests, signs and diagnostic inferences found when checking the trachea.

from the front, side and back and look at the curvature of the spine. Chest deformities may be asymptomatic or they may restrict the ventilatory capacity of the lungs. Common chest abnormalities and their clinical significance are shown in Figs 9.27 and 9.28.

Scoliosis and kyphosis can lead to respiratory failure caused by compressional effects.

## Palpation

You should palpate any lumps or depressions you noticed on inspection and test for the symmetry and extent of chest expansion (Fig. 9.29). Testing chest expansion from the posterior is illustrated in Fig. 9.30.

Test for the position of the apex beat by moving your hand inwards from the lateral chest until you feel the pulsation. The apex beat should be in the fifth intercostal space at the midclavicular line. The

clinical significance of deviations are shown in Fig. 9.31.

Test for tactile vocal fremitus as shown in Fig. 9.32.

## Percussion

The percussion note tells us the consistency of the matter underlying the chest wall, i.e. if it is air, fluid or solid. The correct method of percussion is shown in Fig. 9.33. Percuss in a logical order, comparing one side with other and remember to include the axilla (Fig. 9.34). A normal percussion note is described as resonant. In lung pathology (Fig. 9.35) the percussion note may be:
- Hyperresonant
- Dull
- Stony dull.

Map out any abnormality you find but don't confuse the cardiac borders or liver edge with lung pathology; they will sound dull normally. The note also sounds muffled in a very muscular or obese patient.

When percussing, remember that the upper lobe predominates anteriorly and the lower lobe predominates posteriorly.

## Auscultation

Normal breath sounds are described as vesicular and have a rustling quality heard in inspiration and the first part of expiration. Listen to the patient's chest:
- Using the bell of the stethoscope
- In a logical order comparing the two sides (as for percussion)
- With the patient taking fairly quick breaths through an open mouth.

You should listen for:
- Diminished vesicular breaths (Fig. 9.36)
- Bronchial breathing (Fig. 9.36)
- Added sounds, such as wheezes or stridor (Fig. 9.37), crackles (Fig. 9.38) or pleural rub (Fig. 9.39).

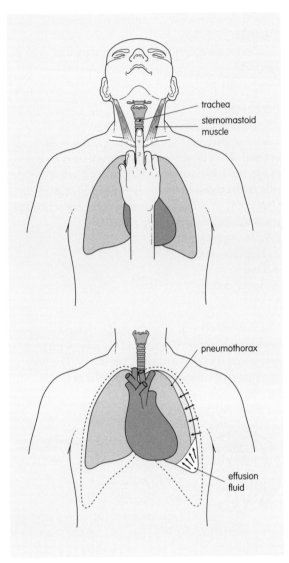

trachea

sternomastoid
muscle

pneumothorax

effusion
fluid

**Fig. 9.21** Palpation to determine tracheal position.

With auscultation always
think **BAR** [**B**—**B**reath
sounds; **A**—**A**dded sounds;
**R**—vocal **R**esonance].
Added sounds that disappear
when the patient coughs are not
significant.

### Vocal resonance

The tests for vocal resonance and whispering
petoriloquy are shown in Figs 9.40 and 9.41.

### Summary

Once you have finished your examination, sum up
the positive findings in a clear and concise manner.
Figure 9.42 shows some possible findings on
examination for a patient with COPD. Figure 9.43 is
a summary of the signs found on examination of the
respiratory system as a whole.

| Jugular venous pressure | | |
|---|---|---|
| **Test performed** | **Sign observed** | **Diagnostic inference** |
| patient must be at 45° looking straight ahead; good light is needed; ask patient to rest head comfortably against a pillow, neck slightly flexed; the patient's neck must be relaxed, as it is impossible to assess jugular venous pressure if the sternomastoid muscles are tensed | elevated jugular venous pressure | resting pressure in thorax is raised:<br>• tension pneumothorax<br>• severe hyperinflation in asthma |
| a normal jugular pulse becomes visible just above the clavicle between the two heads of sternocleidomastoid; jugular venous pressure is difficult to assess and needs much practice; if the jugular pulse is not seen, try the hepatojugular reflex: apply pressure to the liver, increasing venous return to the heart, and so increasing the jugular venous pressure | elevated nonpulsatile jugular venous pressure | superior vena cava obstruction, usually caused by malignant enlargement of the right bronchus |
| | elevated pulsatile jugular venous pressure | paratracheal lymph nodes<br>cor pulmonale |
| time against the contralateral pulse and measure the height of the pulse above the heart (giving a measure of pressure); the normal height of the pulse above the atrium is <4 cm | depressed jugular venous pressure | shock<br>dehydration<br>severe infection |

**Fig. 9.22** Tests, signs and diagnostic inferences found when checking the jugular venous pulse.

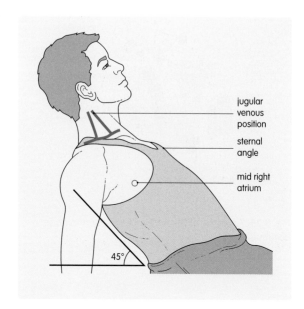

**Fig. 9.23** Measurement of the height of the jugular venous pulse.

| Cervical lymphadenopathy | | |
|---|---|---|
| **Test performed** | **Sign observed** | **Diagnostic inference** |
| examine the cervical chain of lymph nodes from behind the patient; it helps if the neck is slightly flexed; most patients extend neck to try and help you<br><br>know the nodes which you are feeling<br><br>using both hands, start at the mandibular ramus, palpate the submandibular nodes then anterior chain nodes, supraclavicular nodes, and posterior chain nodes in a Z-fashion | cervical lymphadenopathy<br><br>note number of palpable nodes<br><br>describe as for any lump | infection<br>carcinoma<br>tuberculosis<br>sarcoidosis<br>hard node: calcified<br>soft, matted node: tuberculous |

**Fig. 9.24** Tests, signs and diagnostic inferences found in cervical lymphadenopathy.

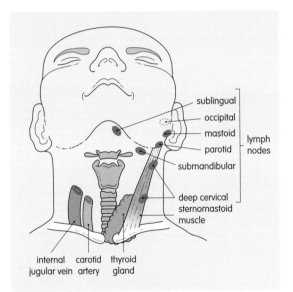

**Fig. 9.25** Anatomy of the neck including lymph node distribution.

| Thoracic scars | | |
|---|---|---|
| **Test performed** | **Sign observed** | **Diagnostic inference** |
| look at the thorax for any obvious scars, remembering to look at the front and back of the chest, axilla, and under the breasts | scars present from previous operations | median sternotomy (most open-heart surgery; cardiopulmonary bypass)<br><br>posteriolateral thoracotomy (ligation of posterior descending artery; lung and oesophageal resections)<br><br>lateral thoracotomy (pneumothorax)<br><br>left thoracotomy (closed mitral valvotomy) |

**Fig. 9.26** Tests, signs and diagnostic inferences found in thoracic scars.

### Assessing the chest wall and spine

| Test performed | Sign observed | Diagnostic inference |
|---|---|---|
| look at the sternum and its relationship to the ribs | depressed in pectus excavatum (funnel chest) | benign condition requiring no treatment. On chest radiograph, the heart may be displaced and appear enlarged |
| | prominent in pectus carinatum (pigeon chest) | may be secondary to severe childhood asthma |
| observe the patient from the side; ask patient to fold arms and take a deep inspiration | anteroposterior diameter of chest > lateral diameter (barrel chest) | hyperinflation asthma |
| ask the patient to stand; stand directly behind the patient and look at the curvature of the spine | increased lateral curvature of the spine (scoliosis) | structural abnormality developmental abnormality vertebral disc prolapse |
| next, stand at the side of the patient and again look at the curvature of the spine | increased forward curvature of the spine (kyphosis) | osteoporosis ankylosing spondylitis |

**Fig. 9.27** Tests, signs and diagnostic inferences found in chest wall abnormalities.

**Fig. 9.28** Features of scoliosis and kyphosis.

### Chest expansion

| Test performed | Sign observed | Diagnostic inference |
|---|---|---|
| place the flat of both hands on the pectoral region of the chest; ask the patient to take a deep breath, and note any asymmetry | symmetrical rise of hands as chest expands | normal |
| | asymmetrical rise | unilateral pathology on the depressed side |
| put fingers of both hands as far around the chest as possible; bring thumbs together in the midline; keep thumbs off chest wall; ask patient to take a deep breath in; note distance between thumbs; examine both front and back | – | – |
| place a tape measure around the internipple line and measure the difference between inspiration and expiration | >4 cm expansion | normal |
| | <4 cm expansion | reduced expansion |

**Fig. 9.29** Tests, signs and diagnostic inferences found in chest expansion.

expiration

inspiration

**Fig. 9.30** Examining chest expansion from the back. (Adapted from *Respiratory Care: A Guide to Clinical Practice* 4e, by G.C. Burton, J.E. Hodgkin and J.J. Ward. Lippincott-Raven, 1977, p. 171.)

| Apex beat | |
|---|---|
| **Sign observed** | **Diagnostic inference** |
| pulsation in fifth intercostal space midclavicular line | normal |
| deviated pulsation; lower mediastinum displacement | left deviation: cardiomegaly pulmonary fibrosis scoliosis pectus excavatum bronchiectasis right deviation: pneumothorax pleural effusion dextracardia |

**Fig. 9.31** Signs and diagnostic inferences found in examination of the apex beat.

| Tactile vocal fremitus | | |
|---|---|---|
| **Test performed** | **Sign observed** | **Diagnostic inference** |
| place either the ulnar edge or the flat of your hand on the chest wall; ask the patient to repeatedly say '99' or '1, 2, 3'; repeat for front and back, comparing opposite zones | increased resonance | solid areas of lung with open airways consolidation pneumonia tuberculosis extensive fibrosis |
| | decreased resonance | feeble voice pleural thickening blocked bronchus |
| the vibrations produced by the manoeuvre are transmitted through the lung substance and felt by the hand; alterations in disease are the same as for vocal resonance | | |

**Fig. 9.32** Tests, signs and diagnostic inferences found in tactile vocal fremitus.

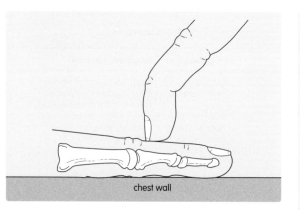

**Fig. 9.33** Correct method of percussion (see text for explanation).

**Fig. 9.34** Sites for percussion. (From *Macleod's Clinical Examination* 10e. Edited by J.F. Munro, I. W. Campbell Churchill Livingstone, 2000, p. 135.)

| Percussion | | |
|---|---|---|
| **Test performed** | **Sign observed** | **Diagnostic inference** |
| place your nondominant hand on the chest wall, palm downwards, with fingers slightly separated; the second phalanx of the middle finger should be in an intercostal space directly over the area to be percussed; strike this finger with the terminal phalanx of the middle finger of the other hand | increased resonance (resonance depends on the thickness of the chest wall and the amount of air in the structures underlying it) | increased air in lung:<br>• emphysema<br>• large bullae<br>• pneumothoracies<br>• asthma |
| to achieve a good percussion note, the striking finger should be partially flexed and striked at right angles to the other finger; the striking movement must be a flick of the wrist<br><br>on percussion you will hear a percussion note and feel vibrations<br><br>percuss from top to bottom including axilla; to check for disease in the lung apices, percuss directly onto the clavicles; do not percuss more heavily than you need and always compare both sides, front and back | dullness (solid lung tissue does not reflect sound as readily as aerated lung); if a dull area exists, map out its limits by percussing from the resonant to the dull area | consolidation:<br>• fibrosis<br>• collapse<br>• pleural thickening<br>• tuberculosis<br>• extensive carcinoma |
| dullness occurs as you percuss over the liver; note that the right diaphragm is higher than the left diaphragm | stony dullness | fluid present:<br>• pleural effusion |

**Fig. 9.35** Tests, signs and diagnostic inferences found when doing percussion of the thorax.

| Auscultation of the thorax | |
|---|---|
| **Sign observed** | **Diagnostic inference** |
| vesicular breath sounds | breath sounds are produced in the larger airways where flow is turbulent; sounds are transmitted through smaller airways to the chest wall; vesicular breath sounds are normal |
| | if vesicular breath sounds are reduced or absent:<br>• airway obstruction<br>• asthma<br>• chronic obstructive pulmonary disease<br>• tumour |
| bronchial breath sounds (described in relation to timing; a gap exists between inspiration and expiration, which are of equal duration; harsh clear breath sounds) | normal, if heard at the tip of the scapula; otherwise caused by:<br>• consolidation<br>• pneumonia<br>• lung abscess |
| | if inaudible:<br>• severe emphysema<br>• bullae<br>• pneumothorax<br>• pleural effusion |

**Fig. 9.36** Tests, signs and diagnostic inferences found in auscultation of the thorax.

| Wheeze and stridor | |
|---|---|
| **Sign observed** | **Diagnostic inference** |
| prolonged musical sound | none: the amount of wheeze is not a good indicator of the degree of airway obstruction |
| polyphonic sound (many musical notes), mainly in expiration | small airway obstruction: narrowing caused by combination of smooth muscle contraction; inflammation within airways; increased bronchial secretions |
| monophonic sound | large airway obstruction: a worrying finding, suggesting a single narrowing (e.g. tumour) |
| loud inspiratory sound | large airway narrowing (larynx, trachea, main bronchi):<br>• laryngotracheobronchitis<br>• epiglotitis<br>• laryngitis |

**Fig. 9.37** Signs and diagnostic inferences found in stridor and wheeze.

| Crackles | | |
|---|---|---|
| **Test performed** | **Sign observed** | **Diagnostic inference** |
| listen to the patient breathing<br><br>crackles may be mimicked by rolling hair on your temple between two fingers; timing during the respiratory cycle is of huge significance | nonmusical, short, uninterrupted sounds heard during inspiration | crackles represent equalization of intraluminal pressure as collapsed small airways open during inspiration |
| | early inspiratory crackles | diffuse airflow limitation<br>chronic obstructive pulmonary disease<br>pulmonary oedema |
| | late inspiratory crackles | conditions that largely involve alveoli:<br>• fibrosis<br>• fibrosing alveolitis<br>• bronchiectasis |

**Fig. 9.38** Tests, signs and diagnostic inferences found in crackles.

| Pleural rub | | |
|---|---|---|
| **Test performed** | **Sign observed** | **Diagnostic inference** |
| listen to the patient breathing | leathery creaking sound associated with each breath<br><br>inspiratory and expiratory sound that is not shifted by cough; reoccurs at the same time in each respiratory cycle | caused by inflamed surfaces of pleura rubbing together:<br>• pneumonia<br>• pulmonary embolism<br>• emphysema<br>• pleurisy |

**Fig. 9.39** Tests, signs and diagnostic inferences found in pleural rub.

| Vocal resonance | | |
|---|---|---|
| **Test performed** | **Sign observed** | **Diagnostic inference** |
| auscultatory equivalent to vocal fremitus; place the stethoscope on to the chest and ask the patient to repeatedly say '99' or '1, 2, 3' | normal lung attenuates high-frequency notes; normally, booming low-pitched sounds are heard | as for vocal fremitus |

**Fig. 9.40** Tests, signs and diagnostic inferences found in vocal resonance.

| Whispering pectoriloquy | | |
|---|---|---|
| **Test performed** | **Sign observed** | **Diagnostic inference** |
| place the stethoscope on to the chest and ask the patient to repeatedly whisper '99' or '1, 2, 3' | words are clear and seem to be spoken right into the listener's ears (whispering pectoriloquy) | whispered speech cannot usually be heard over healthy lung; solid lung tissue conducts sound better than normally aerated lung, indicating consolidation, cavitation, tuberculosis, or pneumonia |

**Fig. 9.41** Tests, signs and diagnostic inferences found in whispering pectoriloquy.

| Signs of COPD | |
|---|---|
| on inspection | central cyanosis |
| | barrel chest |
| | use of accessory muscles |
| | intercostal indrawing |
| | pursed-lip breathing |
| | flapping tremor |
| | tachypnoea |
| on palpation | tachycardia |
| | tracheal tug |
| | reduced expansion |
| on percussion | hyperresonant lung fields |
| on auscultation | wheeze |
| | prolongation of expiration |

**Fig. 9.42** Signs found on examination of a patient with COPD.

| Signs found on examination of the respiratory system | | | | | |
|---|---|---|---|---|---|
| | **Consolidation** | **Pneumothorax** | **Pleural effusion** | **Lobar collapse** | **Pleural thickening** |
| **Chest radiograph** |  | | | | |
| **Mediastinal shift** | none | none (simple), away (tension) | none or away | towards | none |
| **Chest wall excursion** | normal or decreased | normal or decreased | decreased | decreased | decreased |
| **Percussion note** | normal or decreased | increased | decreased (stony) | decreased | decreased |
| **Breath sounds** | increased (bronchial) | decreased | decreased | decreased | decreased |
| **Added sounds** | crackles | click (occasional) | rub (occasional) | none | none |
| **Tactile vocal fremitus or vocal resonance** | increased | decreased | decreased | decreased | decreased |

**Fig. 9.43** Summary table of signs found on examination of the respiratory system.

- Why is the social history so important in respiratory medicine?
- What features of a patient's past medical history might be relevant?
- Give an example of an open and a closed question; how is each type used?
- Give a brief framework for a consultation.
- Why is the initial observation of the patient important?
- Describe the visible effects of long-term steroid use.
- List the causes of tachypnoea.
- List the different patterns of breathing and their significance.
- Describe the common causes of clubbing and how to look for clubbing.
- Describe the significance of unilateral muscle wasting of the hand.
- Describe the relevance of tracheal position in tension pneumothorax.
- Name the common scars seen on the thorax and the possible operations that the patient may have undergone.
- List the surface markings of the lungs for percussion.
- Describe the relationship between added sounds and disease.
- How does lung disease alter examination findings?

# 10. Investigations and Imaging

## Introduction

There are a large number of investigations in respiratory medicine, ranging from basic bedside tests to more invasive procedures such as bronchoscopy. As you read this chapter, you should bear in mind that some of the investigations below are performed only rarely in specialized pulmonary laboratories whilst others are performed by patients at home every day. The investigations that are most commonly performed, and which you should have a thorough knowledge of, include:

- Arterial blood gas analysis
- Sputum examination
- Basic tests of pulmonary function
- Bronchoscopy
- Chest X-rays.

## Routine investigations

### Haematology

In the associated figures, you will find some of the commonly performed haematological tests:

- Full blood count (Fig. 10.1)
- Differential white blood cell count (Fig. 10.2)
- Other haematological tests (Fig. 10.3).

### Clinical chemistry

The commonly performed biochemical tests are shown in Fig. 10.4.

If malignancy is suspected, you should also perform liver function tests and test alkaline phosphatase as an indicator of metastases. In addition, endocrine tests should be performed for paraneoplastic manifestations.

### Tests of blood gases
#### Arterial blood gas analysis

Blood gas analysis of an arterial blood sample is mandatory in all acute pulmonary conditions. The analysis should always be repeated soon after starting oxygen therapy to assess response to treatment.

A heparinized sample of arterial blood is tested using a standard automated machine, which measures:

- $P_aO_2$
- $P_aCO_2$
- Oxygen saturation. Blood pH, standard bicarbonate and base excess are either given on the standard readout or can be calculated.

The patient's results are compared with the normal ranges (Fig. 10.5) and assessed in two parts:
- Degree of arterial oxygenation—is the patient hypoxic?
- Acid–base balance disturbances.

Before accurate interpretation of the results, a detailed history of the patient including a detailed drug history is needed.

### Pulse oximetry

This is a simple, non-invasive method of monitoring the percentage of haemoglobin that is saturated with oxygen. The patient wears a probe on their finger or ear lobe and this is linked to a unit which displays the readings. The unit can be set to sound an alarm when saturation drops below a certain level (usually 90%). The pulse oximeter works by calculating the absorption of light by haemoglobin, which alters depending on whether it is saturated or desaturated with oxygen. A number of factors may lead to inaccurate oximeter readings. These include:

- Poor peripheral perfusion
- Carbon monoxide poisoning
- Skin pigmentation
- Nail varnish
- Dirty hands.

### Microbiology

Microbiological examination is possible with samples of sputum, bronchial aspirate, pleural aspirate, throat swabs and blood. The aim of examination is to identify bacteria, viruses or fungi.

Tests to request are microscopy, culture and drug sensitivity. The microbiological findings should be interpreted in view of the whole clinical picture.

| Full blood count | | | |
|---|---|---|---|
| | | **diagnostic inference** | |
| **test** | **normal values** | **increased values** | **decreased values** |
| haemoglobin (g/dL) | male: 13–18<br>female: 11.5–16.5 | decreased in anaemia<br>(look at MCV for further information);<br>a normal MCV (i.e. normocytic<br>anaemia) is common in chronic<br>disease | |
| mean cell volume (fl) | 76–98 | macrocytosis. (B12 or folate<br>deficiency etc.) | microcytosis (common in<br>iron deficiency anaemia and<br>thalassaemias) |
| red blood cells ($\times10^9$) | male: 4.5–6.5<br>female: 3.8–5.8 | polycaethemia; may be secondary<br>to chronic lung disease, smoking,<br>altitude | |

**Fig. 10.1** Tests performed and diagnostic inference for full blood count.

| Differential white blood cell count | | | |
|---|---|---|---|
| | | **Diagnostic inference** | |
| **Cell type** | **Normal values** | **Increased values** | **Decreased values** |
| white blood cell | $4–11 \times 10^9$/L | bacterial infections<br>malignancy<br>pregnancy | viral infections<br>drugs<br>systemic lupus erythematosus<br>overwhelming bacterial infection |
| neutrophil | $2.5–7.5 \times 10^9$/L 60–70% | bacterial infections<br>malignancy<br>pregnancy | viral infections<br>drugs<br>systemic lupus erythematosus<br>overwhelming bacterial infection |
| eosinophil | $0.04–0.44 \times 10^9$/L 1–4% | allergic reactions<br>asthma<br>sarcoidosis<br>pneumonia<br>eosinophilic granulomatosus | steroid therapy |
| monocyte | $0.2–0.8 \times 10^9$/L 5–10% | tuberculosis | chronic infection |
| lymphocyte | $1.5–4.0 \times 10^9$/L 25–30% | infection<br>cytomegalovirus infection<br>toxoplasmosis<br>tuberculosis | tuberculosis |

**Fig. 10.2** Tests performed and diagnostic inference for differential white blood cell count.

# Bacteriology
## Sputum
Testing of sputum for the presence of bacteria is the most common microbiological test performed in respiratory medicine. Obtain the sample, preferably of induced sputum, before antibiotic treatment is started. Collect into a sterile container, inspect the sample, and send to the laboratory.

| Other haematological tests | | | |
|---|---|---|---|
| | | Diagnostic inference | |
| Test performed | Normal values | Increased values | Decreased values |
| C-reactive protein (CRP) | Normal < 4 mg/L Changes more rapidly than erythrocyte sedimentation rate | Acute infection; inflammation; same as erythrocyte sedimentation rate | Levels often normal in malignancy |
| Anti-streptolysin O (ASO) titre | Normal < 200 IU/mL | Confirms recent streptococcal infection | |

Fig. 10.3 Other haematological tests and their diagnostic inference.

| Biochemical blood tests | | | |
|---|---|---|---|
| | | Diagnostic inference | |
| Test performed | Normal values | Increased values | Decreased values |
| potassium | 3.5–5.0 mmol/L | | adrenocorticotropic hormone (ACTH) secreting tumour β-agonists |
| angiotensin converting enzyme (ACE) | 10–70 U/L | sarcoidosis | |
| calcium | 2.12–2.65 mmol/L | malignancy sarcoidosis squamous cell carcinoma of the lung | |
| glucose | 3.5–5.5 mmol/L | adrenocorticotropic hormone (ACTH) secreting tumour long-term steroid use pancreatic dysfunction | |

Fig. 10.4 Biochemical tests and their diagnostic inference.

Request Gram stain, Ziehl–Neelson stain, and anaerobic cultures. Culture on Lowenstein–Jensen medium to detect tuberculosis. A sputum sample is valuable in diagnosing suspected pneumonia, tuberculosis and aspergillosis, or if the patient presents with an unusual clinical picture.

Failure to isolate an organism from the sputum is not uncommon.

Resistance to commonly used antibiotics is often found in bacteria responsible for respiratory tract infections; therefore, antibiotic sensitivity testing is vital.

## Blood culture

A blood culture should always be performed in patients with fever and lower respiratory tract infection. Collect a large volume of blood and divide it equally into two bottles of nutrient media, 20mL of blood per culture bottle. Collect two or three cultures over 24 hours.

| Arterial blood gases | | | |
| --- | --- | --- | --- |
| | | Diagnostic inference | |
| Test performed | Normal values | Increased values | Decreased values |
| pH | 7.35–7.45 | alkalosis<br>hyperventilation | acidosis<br>$CO_2$ retention |
| $P_aO_2$ | >10.6 kPa | | hypoxic |
| $P_aCO_2$ | 4.7–6.0 kPa | respiratory acidosis (if pH decreased) | respiratory alkalosis (if pH increased) |
| base excess | ±2 mmol/L | metabolic alkalosis | metabolic acidosis |
| standardized bicarbonate | 22–25 mmol/L | metabolic alkalosis | metabolic acidosis |

**Fig. 10.5** Tests performed and diagnostic inference for arterial blood gases.

Blood cultures identify systemic bacterial and fungal infections. Results may be positive while sputum culture is negative.

### Upper respiratory specimens
Microscopy is generally unhelpful because of the abundant commensals of the upper respiratory tract, which contaminate samples.

Throat specimens can be collected using Dacron or calcium alginate swab. The tonsils, posterior pharynx and any ulcerated areas are sampled. Avoid contact with tongue and saliva, as this can inhibit identification of group A streptococci.

A sinus specimen is collected with a needle and syringe. The specimen is cultured for aerobic and anaerobic bacteria. Common pathogens of sinuses are *Streptococcus pneumoniae*, *Haemophilus influenzae*, *Mycoplasma catarrhalis*, *Staphylococcus aureus* and anaerobes.

*Coxiella bunetti*, *Mycoplasma pneumoniae* and *Legionella* are difficult to culture; therefore, results of serology must be used.

### Lower respiratory specimens
Techniques used to collect samples include expectoration, cough induction with saline, bronchoscopy, bronchial alveolar lavage, transtracheal aspiration and direct aspiration through the chest wall. Some these techniques are considered below under the more invasive procedures.

### Viral testing
Because of the small size of viral particles, light microscopy provides little information: it is able to visualize viral inclusions and cytopathic effects of viral infection.

### Viral serology
Viral serology is the most important group of tests in virology. Serological diagnoses are obtained when viruses are difficult to isolate and grow in cell culture.

Specimens should be collected early in the acute phase because viral shedding for respiratory viruses lasts 3–7 days; however, symptoms commonly persist for longer. A repeated sample should be collected 10 days later.

Specimens should be tested serologically only after the second sample has been received. The laboratory measures antibody type and titre in response to the viral infection: a four-fold increase in titre (rising titre) taken over 10 days is significant.

Viral serology also identifies the virus and its strain or serotype, and is able to evaluate the course of infection.

### Cell culture
Specimens for cell cultures are obtained from nasal washings, throat swabs, nasal swabs and sputum. Viruses cannot be cultured without living cells.

### Fungal testing
Fungal infections may be serious, especially in the immunocompromised patient, where they can cause systemic infection; invasive fungal infections require blood culture. Repeated specimens from the site need to be taken to rule out contaminants in cultures.

Common fungal infections are *Candida* and *Aspergillus*. Microscopic identification may be difficult for *Aspergillus* because it is common in the environment. Culture is rarely helpful in identifying *Aspergillus*; the *Aspergillus precipitans* test is of more use.

## More invasive procedures

### Bronchoscopy

Bronchoscopy allows the visualization of the trachea and larger bronchi and can be used to sample tissues via brushings, lavage or biopsy. Two types of bronchoscope are used:
- Flexible fibreoptic bronchoscope
- Rigid bronchoscope (under general anaesthetic).

In practice, the flexible bronchoscope is used in most instances. Patients may be lightly sedated to reduce anxiety and suppress the cough mechanism. Topical lidocaine is used to anaesthetize the pharynx and vocal cords.

The main indications for bronchoscopy are:
- Diagnosis of lung cancer (e.g. after an abnormal chest X-ray or haemoptysis)
- Staging of lung cancer
- Diagnosis of diffuse lung disease
- Diagnosis of infections (especially in immunocompromised hosts).

### Bronchoalveolar lavage (BAL)

Sterile saline is infused down the flexible bronchoscope and then aspirated. This technique is commonly used to look for evidence of neoplasms or opportunistic infections in immunocompromised patients.

### Transbronchial biopsy

Transbronchial biopsy provides samples from outside the airways, e.g. of alveolar tissue. The technique is performed using biopsy forceps attached to a flexible bronchoscope. The bronchoscopist cannot directly visualize the biopsy site and may be assisted by fluoroscopic imaging. Complications include pneumothorax or haemorrhage.

### Percutaneous fine needle aspiration

This technique is used to sample peripheral lesions under the guidance of radiography.

### Open and thorascopic lung biopsy

In some cases of diffuse lung disease, or where a lesion cannot easily be reached, more extensive lung biopsy is required for diagnosis. Open lung biopsy is performed through a thoracotomy with the patient under general anaesthesia. However, video-assisted thorascopic techniques are increasingly used as a less invasive alternative.

## Histopathology

Histopathology is the investigation and diagnosis of disease from the examination of tissues.

### Histopathological examination of biopsy material

The histopathological examination is a vital test in cases of suspected malignancy, allowing a definitive diagnosis to be made. Biopsy material is obtained from the techniques described above, in addition to:
- Pleural biopsy
- Lymph node biopsy.

Histological features of malignant neoplasms are:
- Loss of cellular differentiation
- Abundant cells undergoing mitosis, many of which are abnormal
- High nuclear:cytoplasm ratio
- Cells or nuclei varying in shape and size.

Other uses of histopathology include diagnosing interstitial lung diseases such as cryptogenic fibrosing alveolitis.

### Cytological examination of sputum

Cytological examination is useful in diagnosing bronchial carcinoma and has the advantage of being a non-invasive, quick test; however, it is dependent upon adequate sputum production. Sputum is obtained by:
- Induction–inhalation of nebulized hypertonic saline
- Transtracheal aspiration
- Bronchoscopy
- Bronchial washings.

Exfoliated cells (in the sputum, pleural fluid, bronchial brushings/washings, or fine-needle aspirate of lymph nodes and lesions) are examined, primarily for signs of malignancy.

# Investigations of pulmonary function

Tests of pulmonary function are used in:
- Diagnosis of lung disease
- Monitoring disease progression
- Assessing patient response to treatment.

 Pulmonary function tests can seem confusing but there are just three basic questions that most tests aim to answer:
1. Are the airways narrowed? (PEFR, $FEV_1$, $FEV_1$:FVC, flow volume loops).
2. Are the lungs a normal size? (TLC, RV and FRC).
3. Is gas uptake normal? ($T_LCO$ and $KCO$).

So, as a minimum, make sure you have a good understanding of peak flow monitoring and spirometry and know how you would measure RV, FRC and gas transfer.

## Tests of ventilation

Ventilation can be impaired in two basic ways:
- The airways become narrowed (obstructive disorders)
- Expansion of the lungs is reduced (restrictive disorders).

These two types of disorder have characteristic patterns of lung function (see Chapter 4) which can be measured using the tests below.

### Forced expiration

Peak expiratory flow rate (PEFR) is a simple and cheap test that uses a peak flow meter (Fig. 10.6) to measure the maximum expiratory rate in the first 10ms of expiration. Peak flow meters can be issued on prescription and used at home by patients to monitor their lung function.

Before measuring PEFR (Fig. 10.7), the practitioner should instruct the patient to:
- Take a full inspiration to maximum lung capacity

**Fig. 10.6** Peak flow meter.

**Fig. 10.7** Patient performing peak expiratory flow rate test.

- Seal the lips tightly around the mouthpiece
- Blow out forcefully into the peak flow meter, which is held horizontally.

The best of three measurements is recorded and plotted on the appropriate graph. At least two recordings per day are required to obtain an accurate pattern. Normal PEFR is 400–650L/min in healthy adults.

PEFR is reduced in conditions that cause airway obstruction:
- Asthma, where there is wide diurnal variation in PEFR known as 'morning dipping' (Fig. 10.8)

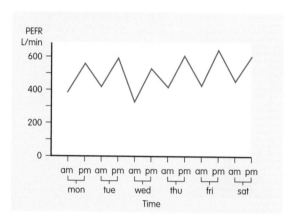

**Fig. 10.8** Typical peak expiratory flow rate graph for an asthmatic patient.

- Chronic obstructive pulmonary disease
- Upper airway tumours.

Other causes of reduced PEFR include expiratory muscle weakness, inadequate effort and poor technique. PEFR is not a good measure of air flow limitation because it measures only initial expiration; it is best used to monitor progression of disease and response to treatment.

Visit an asthma nurse and ask for a demonstration of PEFR tests.

## Forced expiratory volume and forced vital capacity

The forced expiratory volume in one second ($FEV_1$) and the forced vital capacity (FVC) are measured using a spirometer. The spirometer works by converting volumes of inspiration and expiration into a single line trace. The subject is connected by a mouthpiece to a sealed chamber (Fig. 10.9). Each time the subject breathes, the volume inspired or expired is converted into the vertical position of a float. The position of the float is recorded on a rotating drum by means of a pen attachment. Electronic devices are becoming increasingly available.

## $FEV_1$ and FVC

$FEV_1$ and FVC are related to height, age and sex of the patient.

$FEV_1$ is the volume of air expelled in the first second of a forced expiration, starting from full inspiration. FVC is a measure of total lung volume exhaled; the patient is asked to exhale with maximal effort after a full inspiration.

### $FEV_1$:FVC ratio

The $FEV_1$:FVC ratio is a more useful measurement than $FEV_1$ or FVC alone. $FEV_1$ is 80% of FVC in normal subjects. The $FEV_1$:FVC ratio is an excellent measure of airway limitation and allows us to differentiate obstructive from restrictive lung disease.

In restrictive disease:
- Both $FEV_1$ and FVC are reduced, often in proportion to each other
- $FEV_1$:FVC ratio is normal or increased (>80%).

Whereas, in obstructive diseases:
- High intrathoracic pressures generated by forced expiration cause premature closure of the airways with trapping of air in the chest
- $FEV_1$ is reduced much more than FVC
- $FEV_1$:FVC ratio is reduced (<80%).

Patterns of lung function are often tested in exams. Chapter 4 (p. 46) contains more details on patterns of obstructive and restrictive diseases.

### Flow–volume loops

Flow–volume loops are graphs constructed from maximal expiratory and inspiratory manoeuvres performed on a spirometer. The loop shape can identify the type and distribution of airway obstruction. After a small amount of gas has been exhaled, flow is limited by:
- Elastic recoil force of the lung
- Resistance of airways upstream of collapse.

Flow–volume loops are useful in diagnosing upper airway obstruction (Fig. 10.10). In restrictive diseases:
- Maximum flow rate is reduced
- Total volume exhaled is reduced
- Flow rate is high during latter part of expiration because of increased lung recoil.

**Fig. 10.9** Spirometry. The measurement of lung volume by displacement of a float within a sealed chamber is recorded on a paper roll by a pen.

pulley

sealed chamber (containing air)

spirometer trace

water

paper

pen holder and counter balance

pen

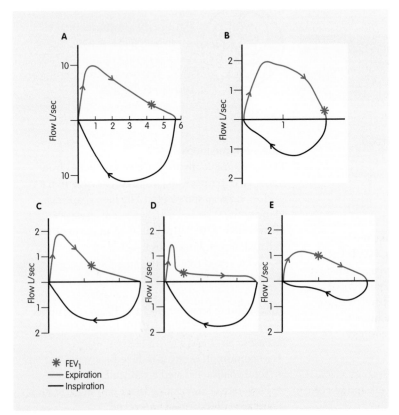

**Fig. 10.10** Typical flow–volume loops. (A) Normal. (B) Restrictive defect (phrenic palsy). (C) Volume-dependent obstruction (e.g. asthma). (D) Pressure-dependent obstruction (e.g. severe emphysema). (E) Rigid obstruction (e.g. tracheal stenosis).

✳ FEV₁
— Expiration
— Inspiration

In obstructive diseases:

- Flow rate is low in relation to lung volume
- Expiration ends prematurely because of early airway closure
- Scooped out appearance is often seen after point of maximum flow.

## Tests of lung volumes

The amount of gas in the lungs can be thought of as being split into subdivisions (Fig. 4.3, p. 45), with disease processes altering these volumes in specific ways. In measuring tidal volume and vital capacity, we use spirometry; alternative techniques are needed for the other volumes.

### Residual volume (RV) and functional residual capacity (FRC)

One important lung volume, residual volume (RV), is not measured in simple spirometry, because gas remains in the lungs at the end of each breath (otherwise the lungs would collapse). Without a measure for RV, we cannot calculate functional residual capacity (FRC) or total lung capacity (TLC).

> Remember that FRC is the volume of gas remaining in the lung at the end of a quiet expiration. RV is the volume remaining at the end of a maximal expiration. Look back at the subdivisions of lung volumes on p. 45 (Fig. 4.3) if you are unsure as to how FRC, RV and TLC relate to each other.

RV is a useful measure in assessing obstructive disease. In a healthy subject, residual volume is approximately 30% of total lung capacity. In obstructive diseases, the lungs are hyperinflated with 'air trapping' so that RV is greatly increased and the ratio of RV:TLC is also increased. There are three methods of measuring RV: helium dilution, plethysmography and nitrogen washout.

### Helium dilution

The patient is connected to a spirometer containing a mixture of 10% helium in air. Helium is used because it is an insoluble, inert gas that does not cross the alveolar–capillary membrane. At the end of an expiration, the patient begins to breathe from the closed spirometer; after several breaths, the helium concentration in the spirometer and lung becomes equal.

The helium concentration is known at the start of the test and is measured when equilibrium has occurred. The dilution of helium is related to total lung capacity. Residual volume can be calculated by subtracting vital capacity from total lung capacity.

The helium dilution method measures only gas that is in communication with the airways.

### Body plethysmography

Plethysmography determines changes in lung volume by recording changes in pressure. The patient sits in a large air-tight box and breathes through a mouthpiece (Fig. 10.11). At the end of a normal expiration, a shutter closes the mouthpiece and the patient is asked to make respiratory efforts. As the patient tries to inhale, box pressure increases. Using Boyle's law, lung volume can be calculated.

This method measures all intrathoracic gas including cysts, bullae and pneumothoraces. In contrast to the helium dilution method, body

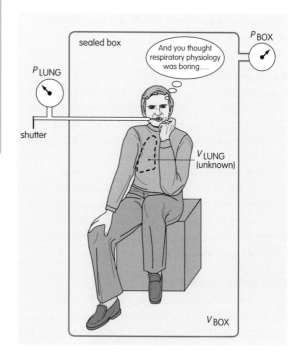

**Fig. 10.11** Plethysmography. This assumes pressure at the mouth is the pressure within the lung.

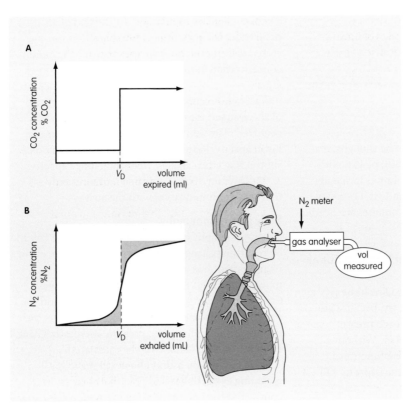

**Fig. 10.12** Measurement of anatomical dead space. (A) Using Fowler's method it would be expected that the gas expired from those areas not undergoing gaseous exchange (anatomical dead space) would contain no nitrogen and thus a stepwise change would occur to the nitrogen concentration of expired gas; the volume at which this occurs would be equal to the anatomical dead space volume. (B) On a graph showing the real-world results, a dotted line has been drawn to approximate the step change in nitrogen concentration.

plethysmography defines the extent of non-communicating airspace within the lung; this is important in subjects with chronic obstructive pulmonary disease (e.g. emphysema).

### Nitrogen washout

Following a normal expiration, the patient breathes 100% oxygen. This 'washes out' the nitrogen in the lungs. The gas exhaled subsequently is collected and its total volume and the concentration of nitrogen are measured. The concentration of nitrogen in the lung before washout is 80%. The concentration of nitrogen left in the lung can be measured by a nitrogen meter at the lips measuring end expiration gas. Assuming no net change in the amount of nitrogen (it does not participate in gas exchange) it is possible to estimate the FRC.

### Anatomical dead space

The volume of anatomical dead space (i.e. areas of the airway not involved in gaseous exchange) is usually about 150mL, or 2mL/kg of bodyweight. In a healthy person, the physiological and anatomical deadspaces are nearly equal; however, in patients with alveolar disease and nonfunctioning alveoli (e.g.

in emphysema), physiological deadspace may be up to 10 times that of the anatomical deadspace.

### Fowler's dead space

Fowler's dead space method uses the single-breath nitrogen test to measure anatomical dead space.

The patient makes a single inhalation of 100% $O_2$. On expiration, the nitrogen concentration rises as the deadspace gas (100% $O_2$) is washed out by alveolar gas (a mixture of nitrogen and oxygen). If there were no mixing of alveolar and dead space gas during expiration there would be a stepwise increase in nitrogen concentration when alveolar gas is exhaled (Fig. 10.12A). In reality, mixing does occur which means that the nitrogen concentration increases slowly, then rises sharply. As pure alveolar gas is expired, nitrogen concentration reaches a plateau (the alveolar plateau). Nitrogen concentration is plotted against expired volume; deadspace is the volume at which the two areas under the plot are equal (Fig. 10.12B).

## Tests of diffusion

Oxygen and carbon dioxide pass by diffusion between the alveoli and pulmonary capillary blood.

The diffusing capacity of carbon monoxide (CO) measures the ability of gas to diffuse from inspired air to capillary blood, and also reflects the uptake of oxygen from the alveolus into the red blood cells. Carbon monoxide is used because:
- It is highly soluble
- It combines rapidly with haemoglobin.

The single-breath test is the test most commonly used to determine diffusing capacity.

## Single-breath test
The patient takes a single breath from residual volume to total lung capacity. The inhaled gas contains 0.28% carbon monoxide and 13.5% helium. The patient is instructed to hold his or her breath for 10 seconds before expiring. The concentration of helium and carbon monoxide in the final part of the expired gas mixture is measured and the diffusing capacity of carbon monoxide is calculated. You need to know the haemoglobin level before the test.

In practice, the transfer factor is used in preference to the diffusing capacity. In the normal lung, the transfer factor accurately measures the diffusing capacity of the lungs whereas, in diseased lung, diffusing capacity also depends on:
- Area and thickness of alveolar membrane
- Ventilation:perfusion relationship.

## Transfer factor
Transfer factor ($T_L$CO) is defined as the amount of carbon monoxide transferred per minute, corrected for the concentration gradient of carbon monoxide across the alveolar capillary membrane (Fig. 10.13).

The transfer factor is reduced in conditions where there are:

- Fewer alveolar capillaries
- Ventilation:perfusion mismatches
- Reduced accessible lung volumes.

Gas transfer is a relatively sensitive but nonspecific test, useful at detecting early disease in lung parenchyma; transfer coefficient is a better test. The transfer coefficient ($KCO$) is corrected for lung volumes and is useful in distinguishing causes of low $T_L$CO due to loss of lung volume:
- $T_L$CO and $KCO$ are low in emphysema and fibrosing alveolitis
- $T_L$CO is low, but $KCO$ is normal in pleural effusions and consolidation.

It might help to think of the difference between $T_L$CO and $KCO$ in terms of a patient who has had a lung removed. Clearly, lung volumes are reduced and therefore so is $T_L$CO. But $KCO$ corrects for the lost volume, and if the remaining lung is normal, $KCO$ is also completely normal.

## Tests of blood flow
Pulmonary blood flow can be measured by two methods: the Fick method and the indicator dilution technique.

### Fick method
The amount of oxygen taken up by the blood passing through the lungs is related to the difference in

|  | Decreased transfer factor | Increased transfer factor |
|---|---|---|
| **Conditions that affect the transfer factor** | | |
| Pulmonary causes | emphysema; loss of lung tissue; diffuse infiltration | pulmonary haemorrhage |
| Cardiovascular causes | low cardiac output; pulmonary oedema | thyrotoxicosis |
| Other causes | anaemia | polycythaemia |

**Fig. 10.13** Conditions that affect the transfer factor.

oxygen content between arterial and mixed venous blood. Oxygen consumption is measured by collecting expired gas in a large spirometer and measuring its oxygen concentration.

### Indicator dilution technique
Dye is injected into the venous circulation; the concentration and time of appearance of the dye in the arterial blood are recorded.

## Testing patterns of ventilation
### Ventilation:perfusion relationships
Ventilation:perfusion relationships are measured by means of isotope scans; these are described in the section on imaging below.

### Inequality of ventilation
In diseases such as asthma or COPD the lungs may be unevenly ventilated. Inequality of ventilation is measured using the single-breath nitrogen test, similar to the method for measuring anatomic dead space described above.

Four phases are recognized in the single-breath nitrogen test, according to the composition of exhaled breath:
1. Pure deadspace.
2. Mixture of deadspace and alveolar gas.
3. Pure alveolar gas.
4. Towards the end of expiration, an abrupt increase in nitrogen concentration is seen.

The third phase, the alveolar plateau, is almost flat in healthy subjects. In patients with lung disease, alveolar nitrogen concentration continues to rise during expiration because of:
- Uneven dilution of the alveolar nitrogen by inspired oxygen
- The poorly ventilated alveoli (i.e. those containing more nitrogen) emptying last.

The change in nitrogen percentage concentration occurring between 750mL and 1250mL of expired volume is used as an index of uneven ventilation.

## Testing lung mechanics
### Lung compliance
Compliance is a measure of distensibility. It is defined as the volume change per unit of pressure across the lung. Lung compliance increases in emphysema, as the lung architecture is destroyed. In

| Causes of altered lung compliance | |
|---|---|
| **Reduced compliance** | **Increased compliance** |
| pulmonary venous pressure increased | old age |
| alveolar oedema | emphysema |
| fibrosis | bronchoalveolar drugs |
| airway closure | |

**Fig. 10.14** Causes of altered lung compliance.

contrast, pulmonary fibrosis stiffens alveolar walls and decreases compliance (Fig. 10.14).

Lung compliance is measured by introducing a balloon into the oesophagus to estimate intrapleural pressure. A lung of high compliance expands to a greater extent than one of low compliance when both are exposed to the same transpulmonary pressure.

To measure compliance:
- The patient breathes out from total lung capacity into a spirometer in steps
- Oesophageal pressure is measured simultaneously
- The lung is given time to stabilize for a few seconds after each step, so that equalization of pressure is achieved at a number of lung volumes throughout inspiration and expiration
- A pressure–volume curve is obtained, which displays the elastic behaviour of the lung.

### Airway resistance
A large proportion of the resistance to air flow is offered by the upper respiratory tract. Airway resistance is defined as the pressure difference between the alveolus and mouth required to produce airflow of 1 L/s.

A number of disease states increase airway resistance including:
- Asthma
- COPD
- Endobronchial obstruction (e.g. tumour or foreign body).

Airway resistance can be measured by plethysmography. The patient is seated in a constant pressure within the body plethysmograph and instructed to pant. The pressure within the plethysmograph changes: during inspiration the volume increases whereas during expiration it decreases. The greater the airway resistance, the greater are the pressure swings in the chest and plethysmograph.

In practice, estimates of airway resistance are much more commonly used than plethysmography. PEFR and $FEV_1$ are both useful estimates of resistance, based on the relationship between resistance and airflow.

## Closing volume

As lung volumes decrease on expiration there is a point at which smaller airways begin to close; this is known as the closing volume of the lungs (Fig. 10.15). Closing volume is usually expressed as a percentage of vital capacity. In young subjects, closing volume is approximately 10% of vital capacity and increases with age, being approximately 40% of vital capacity at 65 years of age.

In diseases such as asthma or COPD the smaller airways close earlier, i.e. at a higher lung volume. An increase in closing volume against predicted values is a sensitive measure of early lung disease and may even show changes caused by cigarette smoking before the patient is symptomatic.

The test uses the single-breath nitrogen method, as described above, but in this case it is phase 4 that is of most interest. The start of phase 4 indicates the lung volume above residual volume at which closure of lung airways first occurs. Phase 4 is caused by preferential emptying of the apex of the lung after the lower zone airways have closed.

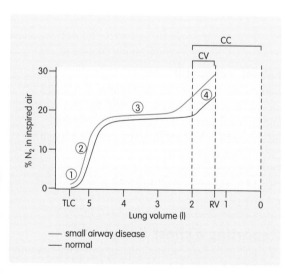

**Fig. 10.15** Closing volume. Airways in lower lung zones close at low lung volumes and only those alveoli at the top of the lungs continue to empty. Because concentration of nitrogen in alveoli of upper zones is higher, the slope of the curve abruptly increases (phase 4). Phase 4 begins at larger lung volumes in individuals with even minor degrees of airway obstruction, increasing closing volume. CV = closing volume; CC = closing capacity; TLC = total lung capacity. (Courtesy of The Ciba Collection of Medical Illustrations, illustrated by Frank H. Netter, 1979.)

## Exercise testing

Exercise testing is primarily used to:
- Diagnose unexplained breathlessness which is minimal at rest
- Assess the extent of lung disease, by stressing the system
- Determine the level of impairment in disability testing
- Assist in differential diagnosis (e.g. when it is not known whether a patient is limited by cardiac or lung disease)
- Test the effects of therapy on exercise capacity
- Prescribe a safe and effective exercise regime.

There are a number of established tests, including the shuttle test and a progressive exercise test, which is commonly performed on a cycle ergometer.

### Shuttle test

This is a standardized test in which the patient walks up and down a 10 metre course, marked by cones. The test is divided into levels by signals played from a tape recorder. The test is stopped if the patient becomes too breathless or if they cannot reach the cone in the time allowed.

### Cycle ergometer progressive exercise test

This is performed in a laboratory and stresses the patient to a predetermined level based on heart rate. A number of tests are made as the patient exercises, including:
- ECG
- Volume of gas exhaled

- Concentration of oxygen and carbon dioxide in exhaled gas.

The volume of gas exhaled per minute ($V_E$ L/min), oxygen consumption ($VO_2$ L/min) and carbon dioxide output ($VCO_2$ L/min) are then calculated. The test indicates whether exercise tolerance is limited by the cardiovascular or respiratory system and assesses increases in heart rate and ventilation against a known oxygen uptake.

## Imaging of the respiratory system

### Ultrasound

Ultrasound uses high frequency sound waves to image internal structures. In respiratory medicine the technique is primarily used in the investigation of pleural effusions and empyemas. Ultrasound can detect an effusion that is not seen on chest X-ray, or localize an effusion before it is drained by thoracentesis.

A variation on this technique, Doppler ultrasound, is a non-invasive method for detecting deep vein thrombosis. It is used in investigating patients with suspected pulmonary thromboembolism. The technique examines blood flow and can detect thrombus in the veins above the popliteal fossa.

### Plain radiography

The plain film radiograph is of paramount importance in the evaluation of pulmonary disease. The standard radiographic examinations of the chest are described below.

#### Posteroanterior erect radiograph (PA chest)

In the PA erect radiograph, X-rays travel from the posterior of the patient to the film, which is held against the front of the patient (Fig. 10.16). The scapula can be rotated out of the way, and accurate assessment of cardiac size is possible. The radiograph is performed in the erect position because:

- Gas passes upwards, making the detection of pneumothorax easier
- Fluid passes downwards, making pleural effusions easier to diagnose
- Blood vessels in mediastinum and lung are represented accurately.

**Fig. 10.16** Normal posteroanterior chest radiograph. The lungs are equally transradiant, the pulmonary vascular pattern is symmetrical. AA = aortic arch; SVC = superior vena cava; PA = pulmonary artery; LAA = left atrial appendage; RA = right atrium; LV = left ventricle; IVC = inferior vena cava. (Courtesy of Dr D. Sutton and Dr J.W.R. Young.)

### Lateral radiograph

Lateral views help to localize lesions seen in PA views; they also give good views of the mediastinum and thoracic vertebrae (Fig. 10.17). Valuable information can be obtained by comparison with older films, if available.

In women of reproductive age, radiography should be performed within 28 days of last menstruation.

### Reporting a chest X-ray

Always view chest radiographs on a viewing box and follow a set routine for reporting plain films. If possible, compare with the patient's previous films.

Follow a set pattern for reading chest X-rays—that way you will not miss anything.

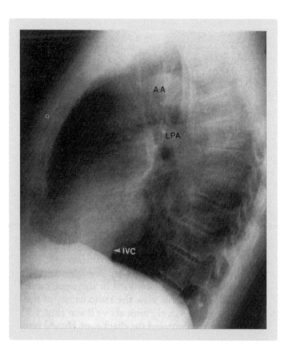

**Fig. 10.17** Normal lateral chest radiograph. AA = aortic arch; LPA = left pulmonary artery; IVC = inferior vena cava. (Courtesy of Dr D. Sutton and Dr J.W.R. Young.)

## Clinical data

Take down the following details:
- Patient's name
- Age and sex
- Clinical problem
- Date of radiography.

## Technical qualities

Note that radiographs contain right- or left-side markers.

With good penetration of X-rays, you should just be able to see the vertebral bodies through the cardiac shadow. In overpenetration, the lung fields appear too black. Conversely, in underpenetration, the lung fields appear too white.

Note the projection (AP, PA or lateral; erect or supine). To deduce whether the patient was straight or rotated, compare the sternal ends of both clavicles.

With adequate inspiration, you should be able to count six ribs anterior to the diaphragm. Make sure that the whole lung field is included.

## Heart and mediastinum

When examining the cardiac shadow, observe the position, size and shape of the heart. Are the cardiac borders clearly visible?

Note whether the trachea is central or deviated to either side. Identify blood vessels and each hilum.

## Other

Note the following points:
- Diaphragm—visible behind the heart. Costophrenic angles acute and sharp
- Lungs—divide the lungs into zones (upper, middle and lower); compare like with like
- Bones—ribs, clavicles, sternum, thoracic vertebra
- Finally, recheck the apices, behind the heart, and hilar and retrodiaphragmatic regions.

## Lateral radiograph

On a lateral radiograph, note the following:
- Diaphragm—right hemidiaphragm seen passing through heart border
- Lungs—divide lungs into area in front, behind and above the heart
- Retrosternal space—an anterior mass will cause this space to be white
- Fissures—horizontal fissure (faint white line that passes from midpoint of hilum to anterior chest wall); oblique fissure (passes from T4/5 through hilum to the anterior third of the diaphragm)
- Hilum
- Bones—check vertebral bodies for shape, size and density; check sternum.

# Interpreting abnormalities

Once you have completed your overall review of the film, return to any areas of abnormal lucency or opacity and assess them according to:
- Number—single or multiple
- Position and distribution (lobar etc.)
- Size, shape and contour
- Texture (homogenous, calcified etc.).

The radiological features of common lung conditions are described below.

## Collapse

Atelectasis (collapse) is loss of volume of a lung, lobe or segment for any cause. The most important mechanism is obstruction of a major bronchus by tumour, foreign body or bronchial plug.

Fig. 10.18 The silhouette sign.

| The silhouette sign | |
| --- | --- |
| **Nonaerated area of lung** | **Border that is obscured** |
| Right upper lobe | Right border of ascending aorta |
| Right middle lobe | Right heart border |
| Right lower lobe | Right diaphragm |
| Left upper lobe | Aortic knuckle and upper left cardiac border |
| Lingula of left lung | Left heart border |
| Left lower lobe | Left diaphragm |

PA and lateral radiographs are required. Compare with old films where available. The silhouette sign can help localize the lesion (Fig. 10.18).

> The lateral borders of the mediastinum are silhouetted against the air-filled lung that lies underneath. This silhouette is lost if there is consolidation in the underlying lung.

### Signs of lobar collapse

Signs of lobar collapse are:
- Decreased lung volume
- Displacement of pulmonary fissures
- Compensatory hyperinflation of remaining part of the ipsilateral lung
- Elevation of hemidiaphragm on ipsilateral side
- Mediastinal and hilar displacement. Trachea pulled to side of collapse
- Radiopacity (white lung)
- Absence of air bronchogram.

Some signs are specific to lobe involvement.

In upper lobe collapse of the right lung, a PA film is most valuable in making the diagnoses; the collapsed lobe lies adjacent to mediastinum (Fig. 10.19A).

In the left lung, a lateral film is most valuable in making diagnoses; the lobe collapses superiomedially and anteriorly (Fig. 10.19B).

Lower lobe collapse causes rotation and visualization of the oblique fissure on PA film.

A lateral film is most valuable in diagnosing middle lobe collapse. Thin, wedge-shaped opacity between horizontal and oblique fissures is seen.

### Consolidation

Consolidation is seen as an area of white lung and represents fluid or cellular matter where there would normally be air (Figs 10.20 and 10.21). There are many causes of consolidation including:
- Pneumonia
- Pulmonary oedema.

In contrast to collapse:
- The shadowing is typically heterogeneous (i.e. not uniform)
- The border is ill-defined
- Fissures retain their normal position.

There are two patterns of distribution:
- Segmental or lobar distribution
- Bat's-wing distribution.

Peripheral lung fields may be spared (e.g. in pulmonary oedema). Air bronchograms may be seen, because they are delineated by surrounding consolidated lung.

>  The presence of air bronchograms can be a useful pointer to the correct diagnosis. They are mostly seen in infection, when consolidated alveoli are lying adjacent to air-filled small and medium bronchioles.

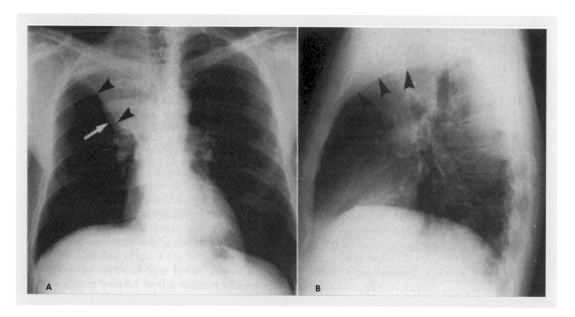

**Fig. 10.19** (A and B) Right upper lobe collapse. The horizontal and oblique fissures (black arrowheads) are displaced. There is a mass (white arrow) at the right hilum. (Courtesy of Dr D. Sutton and Dr J.W.R. Young.)

| Radiological distribution of alveolar processes | | |
|---|---|---|
| | **Bat-wing pattern** | |
| **Segmental pattern** | **Acute** | **Chronic** |
| pneumonia | pulmonary oedema | atypical pneumonia |
| pulmonary infarct | pneumonia | lymphoma |
| segmental collapse | pulmonary haemorrhage | sarcoidosis |
| alveolar cell carcinoma | | pulmonary alveolar proteinosis |
| | | alveolar cell carcinoma |

**Fig. 10.20** Radiological distribution of alveolar processes.

## Interstitial patterns

Three types of interstitial pattern exist (linear, nodular and honeycomb), and overlap may occur.

### Linear pattern

A linear pattern is seen as a network of fine lines running throughout the lungs. These lines represent thickened connective tissue and are termed Kerley A and B lines:

A Upper lobes—long, thin lines.
B Lower lobes—short, thin horizontal lines 1–2 cm in length.

Kerley B lines can help to limit the possible diagnoses. They are caused by increased fluid between alveoli, in the interlobular septa. They are seen in pulmonary oedema and malignant lymphatic infiltration.

Fig. 10.21 Consolidation of the right upper lobe. (Courtesy of Professor C.D. Forbes and Dr W.F. Jackson.)

Fig. 10.22 Tuberculosis in a Greek immigrant to the UK. This film shows multiple areas of shadowing, especially in the upper lobes, and several lesions have started to cavitate. (Courtesy of Professor C.D. Forbes and Dr W.F. Jackson.)

### Nodular pattern

This pattern is seen as numerous well-defined small nodules (1–5mm) evenly distributed throughout the lung. Causes include miliary tuberculosis and chickenpox pneumonia.

### Honeycomb pattern

A honeycomb pattern indicates extensive destruction of lung tissue, with lung parenchyma replaced by thin-walled cysts. Pneumothorax may be present. Normal pulmonary vasculature is absent. Pulmonary fibrosis leads to a honeycomb pattern.

## Pulmonary nodules

### Solitary nodules

The finding of a solitary pulmonary nodule on a plain chest radiograph is not an uncommon event. The nodule, which is commonly referred to as a coin lesion, is usually well circumscribed, less than 6cm in diameter, lying within the lung. The rest of the lung appears normal and the patient is often asymptomatic.

A solitary nodule on a chest X-ray may be an artefact or it may be due to:

- Malignant tumour—bronchial carcinoma or secondary deposits
- Infection—tuberculosis (Fig. 10.22) or pneumonia
- Benign tumour—hamartoma.

If the patient is older than 35 years of age, then malignancy should be at the top of the list of possible differential diagnoses. If the lesion is static for a long period of time, as determined by reviewing previous radiographs, then it is likely to be a benign lesion. However, a slow-growing nodule in an elderly patient is likely to be malignant.

It is important to take into account clinical history and compare with a past chest radiograph if available. You should be able to distinguish carcinoma from other causes:

- Size of lesion—if lesions is >4cm diameter, be suspicious of malignancy
- Margin—an ill-defined margin suggests malignancy
- Cavitation indicates infection or malignancy
- Calcification—unlikely to be malignancy
- Presence of air bronchogram—sign of consolidation, not malignancy.

### Multiple nodules

Metastases are usually seen as well-defined nodules varying in size, which are more common at the periphery of lower lobes (Fig. 10.23); cavitation may be present. Abscesses are cavitated with thick and irregular wall. Cysts are often large.

Other nodules include:

- Rheumatoid nodules
- Wegener's granulomatosis
- Multiple arteriovenous malformations.

## Hilar masses

Normal hilar complex includes:

- Proximal pulmonary arteries and bifurcations
- Bronchus
- Pulmonary veins
- Lymph nodes, not seen unless enlarged.

**Fig. 10.23** Snowstorm mottling in both lung fields. In this case, the underlying diagnosis was testicular seminoma, with disseminated haematogenous metastases. (Courtesy of Professor C.D. Forbes and Dr W.F. Jackson.)

Hilar size varies from person to person, so enlargement is difficult to diagnose (Fig. 10.24). Radiological features of the hilum are:

- Concave lateral margin
- Equal radiopacity
- Left hilum lies higher than right.

PA films are most valuable in assessing hilar shadow, but you must always consult the lateral film. Technical qualities of the film need to be adequately assessed before conclusions can be made because patient rotation commonly mimics hilar enlargement.

Sarcoidosis commonly presents as bilateral lymphadenopathy.

## Mediastinal masses

A mediastinal mass typically has a sharp, concave margin, visible due to the silhouette sign. Lateral films may be particularly useful. Mediastinal masses are frequently asymptomatic and are grouped according to their anatomical position (Fig. 10.25). Computerized tomography (CT) is advised where there is a doubt as to the nature of the lesion.

| Causes of hilar enlargement | | |
|---|---|---|
| | **Bilateral enlargement** | |
| **Unilateral enlargement** | **Enlarged lymph nodes** | **Enlarged vessels** |
| bronchial carcinoma | lymphomas | left-to-right cardiac shunts |
| metastatic malignancy | sarcoidosis | pulmonary arterial hypertension |
| lymphomas | cystic fibrosis | chronic obstructive pulmonary disease |
| primary tuberculosis | infectious mononucleosis | left heart failure |
| sarcoidosis | leukaemia | pulmonary embolism |
| pulmonary embolus | | |
| pulmonary valve stenosis | | |

**Fig. 10.24** Unilateral and bilateral causes of hilar enlargement.

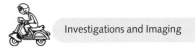
**Fig. 10.25** Mediastinal masses.

| Mediastinal masses | | |
| --- | --- | --- |
| **Anterior masses** | **Middle masses** | **Posterior masses** |
| retrosternal thyroid | bronchial carcinoma | neurogenic tumour |
| thymic mass | lymphoma | paravertebral abscess |
| dermoid cyst | sarcoidosis | oesophageal lesions |
| lymphomas | primary tuberculosis | aortic aneurysm |
| aortic aneurysm | bronchogenic cyst | |

## Anterior mediastinal masses

Characteristics of anterior mediastinal masses are:

- Hilar structures still visible
- Mass merges with the cardiac border
- A mass passing into the neck is not seen above the clavicles
- Small anterior mediastinal masses are difficult to see on PA films.

## Middle mediastinal masses

- A middle mediastinal mass merges with hila and cardiac border
- The majority are caused by enlarged lymph nodes.

## Posterior mediastinal masses

In posterior mediastinal masses the cardiac border and hila are seen but the posterior aorta is obscured. Vertebral changes may be present.

## Pleural lesions

### Pneumothorax

Pneumothorax is usually obvious on normal inspiratory PA films. Look carefully at upper zones, because air accumulates first here; you will see an area devoid of lung markings (black lung), with the lung edge outlined by air in the pleural space. Small pneumothoraces can be identified on the expiratory film and may be missed in the supine film.

### Tension pneumothorax

Tension pneumothorax is seen as a displacement of the mediastinum and trachea to the contralateral side, depressed ipsilateral diaphragm, and increased space between the ribs.

Tension pneumothorax is a medical emergency. Review an expiratory film if possible and bear in mind the patient's clinical state. If breathlessness is progressive and you suspect a tension pneumothorax, start treatment without waiting for a chest X-ray.

### Pleural effusions

PA erect radiography is performed. Classically, there is a radiopaque mass at the base of the lung and blunting of the costophrenic angle, with the pleural meniscus higher laterally than medially. Large effusions can displace the mediastinum contralaterally.

A horizontal upper border implies that a pneumothorax is also present. An effusion has a more homogeneous texture than consolidation and air bronchograms are absent.

### Mesothelioma

Mesothelioma is a malignant tumour of the pleura, which may present as discrete pleural deposits or as a localized lesion.

Thickened pleura is observed with irregular medial margin on radiography; in 50% of cases, pleural plaques are elsewhere. Pleural effusions are common, usually containing blood (Fig. 10.26). Rib destruction is uncommon.

**Fig. 10.26** Small pleural effusions. Both costophrenic angles are blunted. (Courtesy of Dr D. Sutton and Dr J.W.R. Young.)

## Vascular patterns
### Normal vascular pattern
Lung markings are vascular in nature. Arteries branch vertically to upper and lower lobes. On erect films, upper lobe vessels are smaller than the lower lobe vessels. It is difficult to see vessels in the peripheral one-third of lung fields.

### Pulmonary venous hypertension
On erect films, upper lobe vessels are larger than the lower lobe vessels. Pulmonary venous hypertension is associated with oedema and pleural effusions.

### Pulmonary arterial hypertension
Pulmonary arterial hypertension is seen as bilateral hilar enlargement associated with long-standing pulmonary disease.

## Ventilation:perfusion scans
Ventilation:perfusion scans are primarily used to detect pulmonary emboli. The principle is that a pulmonary embolus produces a defect on the perfusion scan (a 'filling defect') which is not matched by a defect on the ventilation scan i.e. there is an area of the lung that is ventilated but not perfused.

## Ventilation scans
Ventilation is detected by inhalation of a gas or aerosol labelled with the radioisotope, $Xe^{133}$. The patient breathes and rebreathes the gas until it comes into equilibrium with other gases in the lung.

## Perfusion scans
Radioactive particles larger than the diameter of the pulmonary capillaries are injected intravenously, where they remain for several hours. $Tc^{99m}$-labelled macro-aggregated albumin (MAA) is used. A gamma camera is then used to detect the position of the MAAs. The pattern indicates the distribution of pulmonary blood flow.

## Diagnosis of pulmonary embolism
Abnormalities in the perfusion scan are checked against a plain chest X-ray; defects on the perfusion scan are not diagnostic if they correspond to radiographic changes. Scans are classified based on the probability of a pulmonary embolism as:
1. Normal—commonly reported as 'low-probability'.
2. High probability.
3. Non-diagnostic.

Non-diagnostic scans include those where patients have obstructive diseases such as asthma or COPD which lead to perfusion and ventilation defects; pulmonary embolus cannot be diagnosed if such a pattern is obtained—other investigations (see below) are then indicated.

## Pulmonary angiography
Pulmonary angiography is the gold standard test for diagnosing pulmonary embolus. Indications are:
- When a ventilation:perfusion scan is inconclusive for pulmonary embolus, but the patient is acutely ill
- Before surgery or thrombolysis for pulmonary embolism.

The test is performed by injection of contrast media through a catheter introduced in the main pulmonary artery using the Seldinger technique. Obstructed vessels or filling defects can be seen clearly and emboli show as filling defects. Despite the accuracy of the test, in practice pulmonary angiography is not often performed because it is invasive and time-consuming. Where ventilation:perfusion scans are inconclusive, and the patient is not acutely ill, it is more common to proceed to lower limb venography or Doppler ultrasound. When angiography is performed, a less invasive test involving computerized tomography (CTPA) is increasingly preferred.

# Computerized tomography

Computerized tomography (CT) is the imaging modality of choice for mediastinal and many pulmonary conditions. CT scans provide detailed cross-sectional images of the thorax. The images can be electronically modified to display different tissues (e.g. by using a bone setting compared with a soft-tissue setting).

The patient passes through a rotating gantry which has X-ray tubes on one side and a set of detectors on the other. Information from the detectors is analysed and displayed as a two-dimensional image on visual display units, then recorded.

CT gives a dose of radiation approximately 100 times that of a standard plain film chest radiograph.

## Applications of computerized tomography
### Detection of pulmonary nodules

CT can evaluate the presence of metastases in a patient with known malignancy; however, it cannot distinguish between benign and malignant masses.

### Mediastinal masses

CT is a useful technique in searching for lymphadenopathy in a person with primary lung carcinoma.

### Carcinoma of the lung

CT can evaluate the size of a lung carcinoma, and detect mediastinal extension and staging.

### Pleural lesions

CT is effective at detecting small pleural effusions and identifying pleural plaques (Fig. 10.27).

### Vascular lesions

Contrast studies allow imaging of vascular lesions (e.g. aortic aneurysms).

# High-resolution computerized tomography

High-resolution CT is useful in imaging diffuse lung disease: thinner sections of 1–2mm show greater lung detail (Fig. 10.28).

**Fig. 10.27** CT scan of a pleural mass. Enhanced CT scan at level of bifurcation of main pulmonary artery. The left lung is surrounded by pleural masses (arrowheads), and the posterior mass is invading the chest wall. The vascular anatomy of the mediastinum is well shown. a = azygos vein; RPA = right pulmonary artery; LPA = left pulmonary artery; AA = ascending aorta; SVC = superior vena cava; DA = descending aorta. (Courtesy of Dr D. Sutton and Dr J.W.R. Young.)

**Fig. 10.28** Technical differences between CT and high-resolution CT (HRCT).

## Applications of high-resolution computerized tomography
### Bronchiectasis

High-resolution CT has replaced bronchography. In dilated bronchi, the technique can show:

- Collapse
- Scarring
- Consolidation.

## Interstitial lung disease

High-resolution CT is more specific than plain film radiography. Disorders that have specific appearances on high-resolution CT include sarcoidosis, occupational lung disease and interstitial pneumonia.

High-resolution CT can be used for biopsy guidance.

## Atypical infections

High-resolution CT provides diagnosis earlier than using plain chest radiography and is useful in monitoring disease and response to treatment. It also provides good delineation of disease activity and destruction.

High-resolution CT is used in imaging of patients with AIDS (e.g. PCP).

## Diagnosis of lymphangitis carcinomatosa

High resolution CT can be used in the diagnosis of lymphagitis carcinomatosa.

## Magnetic resonance imaging (MRI)

MRI uses the magnetic properties of the hydrogen atom to produce images. MRI gives excellent imaging of soft tissues and the heart, but has limited use in the respiratory system. Flowing blood does not provide a signal for MRI imaging, and vascular structures appear as hollow tubes. MRI imaging can be used to differentiate masses around the aorta or in the hilar regions. It has the advantage of not using ionizing radiation.

- Summarize the basic haematological tests performed.
- What key information does arterial blood gas analysis give us?
- What tests can be performed on a sputum sample?
- What is the main use of the histopathology laboratory in diagnosing respiratory disease?
- Describe how to accurately perform a PEFR test.
- List the uses and limitations of the PEFR test.
- How do you test for airway narrowing?
- What is the importance of spirometry in differentiating obstructive from restrictive disorders?
- Describe the differences between obstructive and restrictive lung disease.
- Interpret and draw abnormal flow–volume loops.
- Discuss the implications of an abnormal transfer factor test result.
- How can airway compliance and resistance be calculated?
- When is exercise testing used?
- What are the main uses for ultrasound in respiratory medicine?
- Describe how to read a PA plain film chest radiograph.
- What are the differences between interstitial and alveoli appearances?
- What is the silhouette sign? What are its uses?
- What is an air bronchogram? What are its uses?
- Describe the differences between collapse and consolidation on chest radiographs.
- What are the uses and limitations of CT and MRI imaging in respiratory imaging?

# SELF-ASSESSMENT

## Indicate whether each answer is true or false.

**1.** Nasal cavities and air sinuses:

(a) The maxillary sinus and frontal nasal duct open into the middle meatus.
(b) Consist of three conchae and two air passages opening posteriorly into the choana.
(c) The sphenoethmoidal recess opens between the ethmoid sinus and the middle meatus.
(d) The nasolacrimal duct opens into the inferior meatus.
(e) The upper 2/3 of the nasal cavity is lined by olfactory mucosa.

**2.** Bronchioles:

(a) Contain no smooth muscle in their walls therefore significantly reduce airway resistance.
(b) Differ from bronchi which contain cartilage in their walls.
(c) Contain clara cells which secrete highly proteinaceous fluid.
(d) Contribute to more than 50% of resistance to flow in the lower respiratory tract.
(e) Are a major site of gas exchange.

**3.** Patent ductus arteriosus:

(a) Is a cyanotic heart disease.
(b) Gives a murmur of machinery quality.
(c) Results in blood flowing from the pulmonary artery to the aorta after birth.
(d) May lead to Eisenmenger's syndrome.
(e) Causes delay between radial and femoral pulses.

**4.** Metabolism in the lungs:

(a) The endothelium of the lungs is a major site of production of angiotensin converting enzyme (ACE).
(b) Administration of an ACE inhibitor such as captopril increases the breakdown of bradykinin.
(c) The lungs are involved in the removal of serotonin, prostaglandins and leukotrienes.
(d) Type I pneumocytes produce surfactant.
(e) $PGF_{2\alpha}$ is removed by the lungs.

**5.** Mucociliary clearance:

(a) Cilia within the respiratory bronchioles waft mucus and debris up to the trachea.
(b) Is inhibited in smoking.
(c) Is reduced in Kartagener's syndrome due to highly viscous mucus secretion.
(d) Allows foreign material to be trapped in a sticky mucus film within the bronchi and bronchioles and then transported to the trachea and larynx.
(e) Forms part of the cough reflex.

**6.** In fetal circulation:

(a) Ductus venosus carries oxygenated blood from the umbilical arteries to the inferior vena cava.
(b) Approximately 50% of the blood returning to the right side of the heart passes through the pulmonary circulation and back into the left atrium.
(c) The ductus arteriosus closes within the first 24 hours after birth in response to oxygenated blood.
(d) A patency usually exists between the left and right ventricles covered by the flap-like septum secundum called the foramen ovale.
(e) The umbilical arteries carry oxygenated blood.

**7.** Mucosal associated lymphoid tissue in the respiratory tract:

(a) Is capsulated lymphoid tissue within the walls of the airways.
(b) It is a major site of lymphocytic activation in the airways.
(c) Activated lymphocytes will specifically home back to respiratory mucosa.
(d) Within the upper respiratory tract makes up Waldeyer's ring.
(e) Consists mainly of a distribution of T cells within the lamina propria covered by antigen targeting and transporting cells (M cells).

**8.** Ventilation in the healthy lung:

(a) Dead space comprises both anatomic and physiological space.
(b) Physiological dead space is much greater than anatomic dead space.
(c) Minute ventilation is greater than alveolar minute ventilation.
(d) Ventilation per unit of lung tissue is higher at the top of the lung.
(e) The V/Q ratio is slightly more than 1.

9. **In a normal adult at rest:**

(a) Alveolar ventilation is about 5 L/min.
(b) Pulmonary perfusion is about 5 L/min.
(c) $P_aO_2$ is 4.8–6.0 kPa.
(d) Respiratory rate is less than 12 breaths/min.
(e) Anatomic dead space is about 300 ml.

10. **In quiet breathing:**

(a) Ventilation is brought about by expansion of the chest mainly by the intercostal muscles.
(b) The abdominal muscles relax during inspiration.
(c) The elastic recoil forces of the lung parenchyma are responsible for expiration.
(d) Intrapleural pressure is more negative in expiration than inspiration.
(e) The diaphragm is responsible for approximately 75% of the work of ventilation.

11. **Airway resistance:**

(a) Increases with increasing air flow rate.
(b) Under laminar flow conditions is directly proportional to radius of the airway to the fourth power.
(c) Under laminar flow conditions is described by Poiseuille's law.
(d) Increases with increasing lung volume.
(e) Can be actively altered.

12. **Surfactant:**

(a) Is secreted by type I pneumocytes.
(b) Is not present at birth.
(c) Is soluble in water.
(d) Decreases lung compliance.
(e) Explains hysteresis in pressure–volume curves.

13. **The following questions refer to adult haemoglobin (HbA):**

(a) The concentration of HbA is higher in females than males, usually 13–18 g/dL.
(b) Oxygen binds to iron in the ferric state.
(c) Haemoglobin is a good buffer because of its 38 histidine residues.
(d) Haemoglobin is capable of combining with both carbon dioxide and oxygen.
(e) It has a lower affinity for oxygen than fetal haemoglobin because of its α polypeptide chains.

14. **Concerning sickle-cell anaemia:**

(a) The disorder is autosomal dominant.
(b) The defective haemoglobin is caused by a substitution of valine for glutamate in position 6 of the β polypeptide chain.
(c) It is most prevalent in Caucasians.
(d) Crisis is more likely to occur at high altitude.
(e) Crisis may lead to interpulmonary shunting and bone pain.

15. **The following questions refer to the oxygen dissociation curve:**

(a) Is shifted to the right with increased temperature.
(b) Is shifted to the left with decreased 2,3-DPG.
(c) Is identical for adult and fetal haemoglobin.
(d) The shape of the curve is unaffected by anaemia but the magnitude of the $O_2$ content is.
(e) Describes the variation of saturation of Hb with change in arterial $PO_2$.

16. **On the transfer of gases across the blood–gas barrier:**

(a) The surface area of the membrane is a factor.
(b) Oxygen diffuses more quickly than carbon dioxide.
(c) The greater the molecular weight of a gas, the faster it diffuses.
(d) Solubility is irrelevant when dealing with gases.
(e) The thickness of the membrane is important.

17. **The following statements relate to diffusion within the lungs:**

(a) The rate of diffusion through a membrane is approximated by Fick's law.
(b) A reduced rate of diffusion may be due to oedema of the alveolar capillary wall.
(c) May be decreased due to a reduced overall area of the alveolar capillary membrane.
(d) $O_2$ therapy increases the rate of diffusion by increasing the partial pressure of oxygen in the blood.
(e) The transfer of $N_2O$ across the alveolar capillary membrane is said to be diffusion limited.

18. **The following questions refer to gas diffusion from the lungs to the blood:**

(a) Henry's law describes the solubility of a gas in a liquid.
(b) Carbon monoxide transfer is diffusion limited.
(c) The rate of diffusion of $CO_2$ is 15 times that of $O_2$.
(d) Diffusing capacity is an insensitive test of minor impediments to diffusion.
(e) The diffusion of oxygen from alveolar gas to the blood is dependent on the concentration difference between oxygen in the alveolar gas and oxygen in the blood.

19. **The following are true of $V_A/Q$:**

(a) Ventilation increases towards the apex of the lung.
(b) Perfusion increases towards the base of the lung.
(c) $V_A/Q$ is dependent on lung volume and posture.
(d) $V_A/Q$ is uniform throughout the lung in the healthy patient.
(e) Perfusion is increased to those areas of lung which are under-ventilated.

**20. The following statements relate to the pulmonary circulation:**

(a) The volume of blood is much lower than the systemic circulation.
(b) Alveolar vessels will dilate as the lung expands.
(c) Histamine will increase pulmonary vascular resistance.
(d) Low $P_aO_2$ will cause hypoxic vasoconstriction.
(e) Hydrostatic pressure can recruit more vessels.

**21. The following questions relate to acid–base disturbance:**

(a) Uncomplicated respiratory acidosis results from an increase in $PCO_2$.
(b) Renal compensation returns the blood gases and pH to normal in respiratory acidosis.
(c) Metabolic acidosis may cause respiratory compensation, increasing ventilation and therefore increasing $PCO_2$.
(d) The bicarbonate buffer system is important in the acid–base balance because its pK is very close to physiological pH.
(e) Normal physiological pH range is 7.4–7.45.

**22. During exercise:**

(a) Moderate exercise causes an increased $P_aCO_2$ which drives the ventilatory increase.
(b) Oscillations in $PCO_2$ are similar in amplitude to those at rest due to the fine control achieved by the respiratory system.
(c) The build–up of aerobic metabolites in severe exercise leads to an oxygen debt.
(d) In moderate exercise ventilation is excessive for metabolic demands and the subject hyperventilates.
(e) Exercise may be an important aetiological factor in some asthma.

**23. Pulmonary vascular resistance:**

(a) Is much lower than systemic vascular resistance.
(b) Can be further reduced by extension and recruitment of pulmonary capillaries.
(c) Is increased during exercise.
(d) Is lower than systemic vascular resistance since pulmonary vessels are easily distended.
(e) Is higher at the apex of the lung therefore reducing blood flow to the apex.

**24. Central chemoreceptors:**

(a) Can be found on the ventral surface of the medulla.
(b) Respond to hypoxaemia by increasing ventilation.
(c) Are sensitive to rapid changes in pH.
(d) Have a rapid response to $PCO_2$.
(e) Are responsible for about 10% of the control of ventilation due to short-term changes in $PO_2$.

**25. Peripheral chemoreceptors:**

(a) Are located in the aortic bodies and carotid sinuses.
(b) Are sensitive to hypoxaemia.
(c) Have a relatively low blood flow enabling them to measure small changes in arterial blood gas tensions.
(d) Parasympathetic nerves cause vasoconstriction and reduce blood flow to these receptors.
(e) Are not sensitive to changes in arterial pH.

**26. Ipratropium bromide:**

(a) Is an antimuscarinic agent.
(b) May cause urinary retention.
(c) Increases sputum viscosity.
(d) Causes bronchodilation.
(e) May affect intraocular pressure.

**27. The following drugs are respiratory depressants:**

(a) Barbiturates.
(b) Benzodiazepines.
(c) Alcohol.
(d) Doxapram.
(e) Aminophylline.

**28. The following drugs used in the treatment of asthma have an anti-inflammatory action:**

(a) Glucocorticoids.
(b) Salmeterol.
(c) Theobromine.
(d) Sodium cromoglicate.
(e) Terfenadine.

**29. Salbutamol:**

(a) Is an $\alpha$ agonist.
(b) May produce a tremor.
(c) Is usually administered sublingually.
(d) May cause hyperkalaemia with high doses.
(e) May cause peripheral vasoconstriction.

**30. Doxapram:**

(a) Is a respiratory depressant.
(b) May be given orally.
(c) May cause hypertension.
(d) Is contraindicated in coronary artery disease.
(e) Is used to treat asthma.

**31. Features of acclimatization include:**

(a) Polycythaemia.
(b) Increased fluid in the interstitium.
(c) Hyperventilation.
(d) Right shift of the oxyhaemoglobin dissociation curve.
(e) An increase in oxidative enzymes.

**32. The following relate to respiratory support:**

(a) Oxygen therapy corrects hypoxaemia in right to left shunt.
(b) High dose oxygen is useful in type II respiratory failure.
(c) Patients on BiPAP are at risk of aspiration pneumonia.
(d) LTOT is only beneficial when used for 19 hours/day.
(e) Ventilatory support is usually delivered at a positive pressure.

**33. The following relate to long-term oxygen therapy (LTOT) in patients with COPD:**

(a) It should be given for no more than 8 hours a day, or oxygen toxicity is likely.
(b) The newer systems can safely be used in smokers.
(c) Oxygen should be given through a mask.
(d) Has an effect after 6 months and can then be withdrawn.
(e) Arterial saturation should be at least 90%.

**34. In emphysema:**

(a) The distance for diffusion of $O_2$ is decreased due to destruction of the lung parenchyma.
(b) Over 10% of cases have $\alpha_1$ antitrypsin deficiency.
(c) The overall surface area for gas exchange is decreased despite the increase in alveolar size.
(d) Patients develop stiff fibrotic lungs.
(e) Radial traction is increased therefore reducing airway resistance.

**35. Typical features of bronchiectasis are:**

(a) Cough with small amounts of sputum.
(b) Lower lobes are less affected.
(c) Empyema.
(d) Haemoptysis.
(e) Coarse crepitations on auscultation.

**36. Referring to $\alpha_1$ antitrypsin:**

(a) Deficiency results in increased breakdown of lung parenchyma due to the action of proteolytic enzymes.
(b) Is inhibited by aspirin.
(c) Deficiency accounts for approximately 2% of cases of emphysema.
(d) Deficiency is caused by smoking.
(e) Is important in the metabolism of angiotensin II to inactive peptides.

**37. In asthma:**

(a) The peak expiratory flow rate is increased.
(b) There is constriction of smooth muscle in bronchioles.
(c) There is mucosal oedema in the airways.
(d) Mucus secretion is decreased.
(e) House dust may be an allergen.

**38. Pulmonary embolism:**

(a) Is usually accompanied by lung infarction.
(b) Usually arises from the deep veins of the legs and pelvis.
(c) May cause sudden death.
(d) Is treated with anticoagulants.
(e) Is one of the most frequent causes of postoperative death.

**39. Chronic bronchitis:**

(a) Is associated with hypoplasia of bronchial mucus glands.
(b) Is defined as a productive cough for at least 3 months in 2 consecutive years.
(c) Is associated with *Haemophilus influenzae* infection.
(d) Usually coexists with emphysema.
(e) Is associated with cigarette smoking.

**40. COPD:**

(a) Steroids are the mainstay of treatment.
(b) Causes some 3000 deaths each year in the UK.
(c) May be complicated by pneumothorax.
(d) Exacerbations are often caused by *H. influenzae*.
(e) Is often caused by a genetic defect.

**41. COPD and asthma:**

(a) $T_LCO$ is reduced in both.
(b) Both may present with cough.
(c) Cough is typically worse in the morning in asthma.
(d) Wheeze is only present in asthma.
(e) Air trapping is a feature of both disorders.

**42. Coal worker's pneumoconiosis:**

(a) Is caused by asbestos fibres.
(b) May cause respiratory failure.
(c) Is accompanied by focal emphysema.
(d) Has positive association with mesothelioma.
(e) May be caused by very low exposure to coal dust.

**43. Small-cell carcinoma of the lung:**

(a) Is usually treated by surgical resection.
(b) Shows keratin production on histological examination.
(c) Rarely metastasizes.
(d) Has a positive association with asbestos exposure.
(e) Usually arises in the periphery of the lung.

**44. Malignant mesothelioma:**

(a) Has a positive association with asbestos exposure.
(b) Has usually metastasized by the time of presentation.
(c) May cause death by respiratory failure.
(d) May cause cardiac tamponade.
(e) Is an epithelial tumour.

**45. Squamous cell carcinoma of the lung:**

(a) Is associated with cigarette smoking.
(b) Shows mucin production on histological examination.
(c) May be treated by surgical resection.
(d) May produce ectopic hormones.
(e) May respond to radiotherapy.

**46. Emphysema:**

(a) Is associated with $\alpha_1$ antitrypsin deficiency.
(b) Is defined as enlargement of airspaces distal to the terminal bronchiole with destruction of the alveolar walls.
(c) Causes decreased alveolar surface area.
(d) May cause respiratory failure.
(e) Is always associated with chronic bronchitis.

**47. The following definitions are correct:**

(a) Haemothorax—collection of blood in the pleural cavity.
(b) Pyothorax—collection of lymph in the pleural cavity.
(c) Pneumothorax—collection of air in the pleural cavity.
(d) Chylothorax—collection of pus in the pleural cavity.
(e) Hydrothorax—collection of fluid in the pleural cavity.

**48. The following factors have a positive association with the development of lung carcinoma:**

(a) Coal mining.
(b) Haematite mining.
(c) Asbestos exposure.
(d) Diffuse pulmonary fibrosis.
(e) Woodworking with hardwoods.

**49. Fibrosing alveolitis:**

(a) Usually occurs in young people.
(b) Is usually caused by inhaled dust.
(c) May result in 'honeycomb' lung.
(d) Gives an obstructive pattern of deficit on pulmonary function tests.
(e) Histologically shows proliferation of type II pneumocytes.

**50. Atopic asthma:**

(a) Is mediated by a type III hypersensitivity reaction.
(b) Is associated with hay fever.
(c) Is associated with eczema.
(d) Is associated with hypoplasia of bronchial wall smooth muscle.
(e) May be treated with $\beta_2$ agonists.

**51. In asthma:**

(a) Peak expiratory flow rate during an acute attack is usually decreased.
(b) The disease results from the destruction of lung parenchyma caused by smoking.
(c) An acute attack is characterized by bronchoconstriction which is not usually reversible.
(d) Acute asthma can be treated by using ipratropium bromide.
(e) Sodium cromoglycate inhibits phosphodiesterase therfore increasing cAMP which leads to bronchodilatation.

**52. Acute severe asthma is characterized by:**

(a) PEFR <33% predicted or best.
(b) Pulse of >100 beats/min.
(c) Silent chest and cyanosis.
(d) Urea >7mmol/L.
(e) Inability to speak in one breath.

**53. Cor pulmonale:**

(a) Is failure of left heart.
(b) Is seen in COPD.
(c) Is characterized by oedema and raised JVP.
(d) Is associated with pulmonary hypertension.
(e) Has a good prognosis.

**54. Occupational causes of asthma include:**

(a) Asbestos.
(b) Isocyanates.
(c) Flour.
(d) Seafoods.
(e) Dyes.

**55. The following relate to sleep apnoea:**

(a) It is associated with hypertension.
(b) Obesity is a risk factor.
(c) Women are more often affected than men.
(d) It can often be treated conservatively.
(e) Patients have an increased risk of road traffic accidents.

**56. Lung cancer can metastasize to the:**

(a) Ovary.
(b) Bone.
(c) Breast.
(d) Prostate.
(e) Kidney.

**57. Tuberculosis:**

(a) Is decreasing in developing countries.
(b) May be an incidental finding on CXR.
(c) Is always asymptomatic in the primary type.
(d) May be present with pneumonia.
(e) Is not seen in immunized individuals.

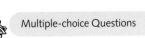 

**58. Interstitial lung diseases:**

(a) Cause a restrictive pattern of disease.
(b) Are sometimes caused by drugs.
(c) Invariably cause finger clubbing.
(d) May present first with haemoptysis.
(e) May coexist with renal disease.

**59. Extrinsic allergic alveolitis:**

(a) Is immunologically mediated.
(b) May affect farmers.
(c) Causes symptoms related to extent of exposure to antigen.
(d) Honeycomb lung may be a feature.
(e) There are increased lymphocytes in BAL fluid.

**60. Tuberculosis in the immunocompromised:**

(a) May be caused by MAC.
(b) May present with progressive anaemia.
(c) Treatment with steroids should be commenced immediately.
(d) Is associated with bronchiectasis.
(e) May require a pleural biopsy for diagnosis.

**61. Prognosis is poor in severe pneumonia when:**

(a) Urea <7 mmol/L.
(b) Respiratory rate <20 min.
(c) The patient is confused.
(d) The patient is hypertensive.
(e) Hypoxaemia is present.

**62. Causes of transudate include:**

(a) Hypothyroidism.
(b) Pneumonia.
(c) Heart failure.
(d) Liver failure.
(e) Bronchial carcinoma.

**63. Occupational lung diseases:**

(a) There may be a latency period in nonallergic asthma.
(b) Caplan's syndome is associated with asbestosis.
(c) Patients may be eligible for compensation.
(d) Can affect workers in animal laboratories.
(e) Symptoms may improve at weekends.

**64. Surgery is contraindicated in:**

(a) Lung carcinoma with mediastinal nodes >2 cm diameter.
(b) Cystic fibrosis if both lungs are affected.
(c) Lung carcinoma if $FEV_1$ is <0.8 L.
(d) Respiratory failure.
(e) Most cases of small-cell lung cancer.

**65. Features of mycoplasmal pneumonia include:**

(a) Epidemics typically occur every 10 years.
(b) Cold agglutinins are a feature in almost all patients.
(c) It is found in water cooling towers.
(d) It is treated effectively with penicillin.
(e) Institutional outbreaks amongst the elderly.

**66. *Legionella pneumophila*:**

(a) Is a Gram +ve organism.
(b) Causes a pneumonia with a high mortality rate.
(c) Antigen may help diagnosis.
(d) A vaccine is available.
(e) Is ubiquitous in water.

**67. Pneumonia may present with:**

(a) Pleuritic pain.
(b) Headache.
(c) Haemoptysis.
(d) Diarrhoea.
(e) Urinary symptoms.

**68. Pulmonary embolism:**

(a) Thrombolysis is indicated in most patients.
(b) Heparin is the mainstay of treatment.
(c) Anticoagulants should be continued for a week after the event.
(d) Can be excluded when a CXR is normal.
(e) Is a common finding at autopsy.

**69. Small-cell lung cancers:**

(a) Are treated with chemotherapy with intent to cure.
(b) Are the most common type of lung cancer.
(c) Have a particularly poor prognosis.
(d) Are staged with the TNM classification.
(e) Arise from endocrine cells.

**70. Bronchial adenocarcinoma:**

(a) Is more common in women than men.
(b) Is strongly associated with smoking.
(c) Stains for keratin histologically.
(d) Is often a central tumour.
(e) Commonly causes obstructive symptoms.

**71. Cavitating lesions in the lung are seen in:**

(a) Rheumatoid arthritis .
(b) TB.
(c) COPD.
(d) Coal worker's pneumoconiosis.
(e) Idiopathic pulmonary haemosiderosis.

**72. Features of idiopathic fibrosing alveolitis include:**

(a) Productive cough.
(b) Reduced chest expansion.
(c) Wheeze.
(d) Weight loss.
(e) Pulmonary hypertension.

**73. Published guidelines on pulmonary embolism (PE) state:**

(a) Recent fractures are a lesser risk factor.
(b) Obesity is not a proven risk factor.
(c) Anticoagulation reduces the risk of fatal recurrent embolism.
(d) Serious underlying disease often coexists with PE.
(e) Lung scans may be misleading in patients with COPD.

**74. Published guidelines on asthma state:**

(a) Inhaled steroids are always indicated.
(b) It is unwise to step down treatment.
(c) Avoidance of provoking factors is advised.
(d) Bronchodilators may be used twice a day before moving to Step 2.
(e) High-dose steroids are contraindicated in children.

**75. Sarcoidosis:**

(a) May be diagnosed using the Schick test.
(b) Is characterized histologically by caseous granulomas.
(c) Affects the terminal ileum most frequently.
(d) May cause interstitial lung fibrosis.
(e) May cause hilar lymphadenopathy.

**76. Adult respiratory distress syndrome (ARDS):**

(a) Is associated with inhalation of sulphur dioxide.
(b) Is characterized by proliferation of type I pneumocytes.
(c) Is characterized by formation of hyaline membranes in the alveoli.
(d) Is rarely fatal.
(e) Is associated with endotoxic shock.

**77. Cystic fibrosis:**

(a) Is an autosomal dominant genetic condition.
(b) Is associated with meconium ileus in infants.
(c) May be confirmed by measuring sodium concentration in sweat.
(d) Is associated with bronchiectasis.
(e) Is associated with infertility in females.

**78. Community acquired pneumonia:**

(a) Is commonly caused by Gram-negative organisms.
(b) Is more common in smokers.
(c) May be complicated by empyema.
(d) Is more often viral in adults.
(e) Has a poorer prognosis if the patient is confused on admission.

**79. Carcinoma of the larynx:**

(a) Is usually of adenocarcinomatous differentiation.
(b) Usually affects subjects below 40 years of age.
(c) Affects females more commonly than males.
(d) Is associated with cigarette smoking.
(e) May produce dysphagia.

**80. Wegener's granulomatosis:**

(a) Is a necrotizing vasculitis.
(b) Affects mainly elastic arteries.
(c) Is caused by an anti-glomerular basement membrane antibody.
(d) Causes a necrotizing glomerulonephritis.
(e) Causes lung necrosis.

**81. Bronchiectasis:**

(a) Is associated with Kartagener's syndrome.
(b) Usually affects the upper lobes most prominently.
(c) May be complicated by amyloid formation.
(d) Is characterized by bronchial constriction.
(e) May be complicated by metastatic cerebral abscesses.

**82. Causes of a chronic recurrent cough include:**

(a) Asthma.
(b) COPD.
(c) Gastro-oesophageal reflux.
(d) Chronic sinusitis.
(e) ACE inhibitors.

**83. Haemoptysis:**

(a) May be caused by TB.
(b) Is sometimes fatal.
(c) May lead to malaena.
(d) Is commonly sputum streaked with blood in lung cancer.
(e) May be due to acute bronchitis.

**84. Concerning type I respiratory failure:**

(a) $PO_2$ <8kPa.
(b) Tolerance to high arterial oxygen tension develops.
(c) It must be treated effectively with low-dose oxygen.
(d) It differs from type II because it is of pulmonary vascular origin.
(e) It may be caused by spontaneous pneumothorax.

**85. The following relate to respiratory failure:**

(a) It is often caused by ventilation:perfusion mismatching.
(b) The most important investigation is a CXR.
(c) Type I is classically caused by pump failure.
(d) Arterial blood gases may be normal.
(e) Renal compensation frequently occurs in both types.

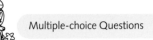
**86. Features of hypercapnia include**

(a) Flapping tremor.
(b) Peripheral vasoconstriction.
(c) Coma.
(d) Headache.
(e) Papilloedema.

**87. Signs of COPD on examination include:**

(a) Pursed lip breathing.
(b) Tracheal tug.
(c) Hoover's sign.
(d) Wheeze.
(e) Hyperinflation.

**88. Finger clubbing is seen in:**

(a) Bronchiectasis.
(b) Asthma.
(c) Chronic bronchitis.
(d) Pulmonary fibrosis.
(e) Cyanotic heart disease.

**89. Signs found on respiratory examination may include:**

(a) Mediastinal shift in a simple pneumothorax.
(b) Hyperresonant lung fields on percussion in pleural effusion.
(c) Decreased vocal resonance in pneumonia.
(d) Decreased chest expansion in lung collapse.
(e) Coarse crackles in pneumonia.

**90. The following relate to lung function tests:**

(a) Transfer factor corrects for lost lung volume.
(b) Normal PEFR is 100–200 in adults.
(c) Closing volume is decreased with air trapping.
(d) Fowler's method measures physiological dead space.
(e) Body plethysmography measures lung compliance.

**91. Features of consolidation on a CXR:**

(a) Fissures are displaced.
(b) May be in a bat's wing distribution.
(c) Silhouette sign is seen.
(d) Air bronchograms are unlikely to be present.
(e) Peripheral lung fields may be spared.

**92. Diffusing capacity ($T_L$CO):**

(a) Is equivalent to transfer factor.
(b) Corrects for lost lung volume.
(c) Is reduced by exercise.
(d) Is a sensitive test.
(e) Is a specific test.

**93. The following statements relate to lung volumes:**

(a) Functional residual capacity is that amount of air left within the lung following a maximal expiration.
(b) Vital capacity is usually about 4800 mL in the upright 70 kg male subject.
(c) Tidal volume can be measured by spirometry.
(d) Total lung volume is normally increased in fibrosing alveolitis.
(e) The ratio of $FEV_1$/FVC is usually greater than 80% in asthmatics.

**94. Peak expiratory flow rate:**

(a) Records the volume of a forced expiration in one second.
(b) Detects restrictive lung defects.
(c) Is higher in the morning in asthma.
(d) Is dependent on age, gender and height.
(e) Is more accurate than plethysmography in measuring true airflow resistance.

**95. Radioisotope lung scanning:**

(a) With ventilation:perfusion scans can detect pulmonary embolism.
(b) Uses microaggregated human albumin to detect ventilation.
(c) Is the gold standard test for detecting pulmonary emboli.
(d) Is used less often than pulmonary angiograms.
(e) Is the basis for the single-breath nitrogen test.

**96. Collapse of the lung:**

(a) Will show the trachea deviated to the opposite side on CXR.
(b) Gives an irregular, 'bitty' whiteness on CXR.
(c) May occur at birth.
(d) May lead to fibrosis.
(e) May show a displaced horizontal fissure on CXR.

**97. The following relate to bronchoscopy:**

(a) Rigid bronchoscopy is used more often than fibreoptic.
(b) Haemoptysis is a key indication for bronchoscopy.
(c) It can be used to sample bronchial secretions.
(e) Is used to diagnose mediastinal tumours.
(e) In fibreoptic bronchoscopy patients are not sedated.

**98. The following are recognised, appropriate investigations:**

(a) Multiple inert gas procedure for pulmonary embolism.
(b) Bronchoscopy in a smoker with a persistent monophonic wheeze.
(c) Ultrasound for pleural effusion.
(d) Transbronchial biopsy in pulmonary fibrosis.
(e) MRI scan in tension pneumothorax.

**99. Lung function tests in COPD show:**

(a) A decrease in gas transfer.
(b) A decrease in $FEV_1$.
(c) A decrease in functional residual capacity.
(d) An increase in closing volume.
(e) An increase in $FEV_1$:FVC ratio.

**100. Investigations in asthma:**

(a) Bronchial provocation tests are essential for diagnosis.
(b) $FEV_1$ improves after bronchodilation.
(c) $T_L CO$ is decreased.
(d) Residual volume may be increased.
(e) Skin prick tests are usually negative in extrinsic asthma.

# Short-answer Questions (SAQs)

1. What is a surfactant? Describe its functions within the lung.

2. Give the normal values for haemoglobin concentration in the blood. Draw the oxyhaemoglobin dissociation curve, giving arterial and venous $PO_2$.

3. Define the term venous admixture. If a patient presents with a pulmonary embolus how may their blood gases show a low $PO_2$ but a normal or lowered $PCO_2$?

4. Define airway resistance. How is calibre of the airway related to airway resistance under laminar flow conditions and what factors influence smooth muscle tone of the airways?

5. Write short notes on lung carcinoma.

6. Write short notes on bronchial asthma.

7. Write short notes on bronchiectasis.

8. Write short notes on adult respiratory distress syndrome.

9. Write short notes on malignant mesothelioma.

10. Write short notes on cystic fibrosis.

11. Write short notes on pneumonia in the immunocompromised.

12. A 62-year-old woman, with a diagnosis of breast carcinoma, presents to A&E in an anxious state, complaining of shortness of breath and chest pain that is worse on breathing in. She mentions that she has just coughed up a small amount of bright red blood.
    (a) What other information should you elicit from the history?
    (b) What are the main risk factors for pulmonary embolism?
    (c) What investigations should you perform?
    (d) How would you manage the patient?

13. A 58-year-old man consults his GP, complaining of increasing shortness of breath. He has been getting progressively more breathless for the last 3 years and now cannot walk upstairs in his home without stopping once or twice. The cough that used to be a feature of the winter months now seems to be present all year round. He has smoked since he was 15 years old and although he has tried to give up several times he has averaged a pack a day over most of this period. His GP sends him for a chest X-ray and some lung function tests.
    (a) What lung function tests are indicated and what are they likely to show?
    (b) The patient's smoking history equates to how many pack years? What help could his GP give him in his attempts to stop smoking?
    (c) How might the patient be treated?
    (d) How does smoking cause the symptoms seen in this patient?

14. A 64-year-old chronic smoker presents to A&E with acute dyspnoea and a cough productive of green sputum. On analysis, his blood gases are:

    | | |
    |---|---|
    | pH | 7.22 |
    | $P_aO_2$ | 4.8 |
    | $P_aCO_2$ | 8.3 |
    | $HCO_3^-$ | 35 |

    (a) Is the patient in respiratory failure?
    (b) If respiratory failure is present, is it type I or type II?
    (c) Comment on his acid–base status.
    (d) What treatment would you give the patient?

15. A 33-year-old woman with a known history of asthma presents to A&E with acute shortness of breath. Her asthma has been well controlled with bronchodilators and regular inhaled steroids. The patient woke today with severe breathlessness which has worsened throughout the day. Her inhaled bronchodilators seemed to have little effect on her symptoms. On evaluation she is found to be in respiratory distress, unable to speak in full sentences and with a pulse rate of 110 b.p.m. and using accessory muscles.
    (a) What other signs might you notice on examination?
    (b) How is acute severe asthma defined?
    (c) Comment on the pathogenesis of asthma; why might her bronchodilators not be working?
    (d) What treatment would you instigate?

**16.** A 23-year-old man presents to his GP complaining of breathlessness and wheeze. He has had a non-productive cough for about 4 days. This is worse at night and he been kept awake coughing. On enquiry his family history was notable for eczema and hayfever on his father's side. He has no pets but mentions that his girlfriend has recently acquired a cat.
 (a) What is the likely diagnosis?
 (b) How might this be confirmed?
 (c) What are the common precipitants of asthma?
 (d) What occupations are associated with an increased incidence of asthma?

**17.** A 65-year-old obese man attends his local GP's surgery after his wife 'insisted that he do something about his snoring'. Although he is not aware of sleeping badly, he awakes unrefreshed and is always tired during the day; he has recently fallen asleep during a meeting at work, which caused much embarrassment. His wife is, however, aware that his sleep is disturbed; she notices that he jolts awake several times each night particularly if he has been to the pub.
 (a) What tests might the GP perform to diagnose this man's disorder?
 (b) How might his condition be managed (i) conservatively; (ii) more aggressively?
 (c) What are the complications of sleep apnoea?
 (d) Why else might it be important to manage this patient's condition?

**18.** A 60-year-old man presents to his GP with a 4-month history of a cough which is sometimes tinged with blood. He has also noticed that he has lost about 10lb in weight over the past 6 months or so. He has smoked heavily for about 40 years and is very worried that his symptoms may be due to 'something sinister'. On examination the patient appeared anxious but there were no signs to confirm his fears. A CXR was normal but flow–volume loop showed a truncated expiratory loop.
 (a) What are the main causes of haemoptysis?
 (b) Given the patient's history what signs would the GP be looking for?
 (c) What would be an appropriate investigation to perform next?
 (d) Describe the significance of the flow–volume result? What disorders are likely to generate this pattern?

**19.** A 78-year-old man is admitted to hospital as an emergency after a home visit from his GP. The patient had a history of recent upper respiratory tract infection, with a sore throat which persisted. Over the course of two or three days he began to feel increasingly unwell with fever, anorexia and pain in his chest which was worse on coughing. On the day that he was admitted his daughter had visited and found him delirious and confused; she immediately called his GP.
 (a) What are the core adverse prognostic factors in severe community acquired pneumonia?
 (b) What signs might this patient demonstrate on examination?
 (c) If he went on to develop a complication of pneumonia such as pleural effusion, how might this be treated?
 (d) Which are the common pathogens in community acquired pneumonia?

**20.** A 22-year-old student presented to A&E with breathlessness and chest pain. The breathlessness had come on suddenly whilst he was cycling home from a lecture and the pain was over one side of his chest and worse on breathing and coughing. Examination revealed a tall thin young man with reduced chest expansion. There was hyperresonance to percussion on the right. Breath sounds were diminished and tactile fremitus decreased over the affected side. The trachea was not deviated. On the basis of the clinical findings and a CXR, a diagnosis of spontaneous pneumothorax was made.
 (a) What is spontaneous pneumothorax and how does it occur?
 (b) How might a pneumothorax appear on CXR?
 (c) What procedure might be undertaken in recurrent pneumothoraces?
 (d) How should a tension pneumothorax be managed?

# Essay Questions

1. Write an account of ventilation and perfusion matching in the normal lung and in disease.

2. Describe the underlying pathology of pulmonary fibrosis and comment on how fibrosis might affect the results of common lung function tests.

3. Write an account of the development of the lower respiratory tract.

4. Describe three ways in which breathing is controlled.

5. Discuss the mechanism of action of steroids and their use in managing respiratory disease.

6. What is meant by the term, paraneoplastic syndrome? Describe how paraneoplastic syndromes might present in lung cancer.

7. What diseases can affect the pleura? With reference to at least two conditions, discuss how pleural disease might present.

8. What is an obstructive disease? Which are the primary tests used to diagnose an obstructive disease?

9. What is ARDS? What are the underlying mechanisms and how does it present?

10. List the three main types of lung cancer and discuss the possible treatments in each.

11. With the aid of a graph, describe lung compliance. How might it be affected by disease?

12. Discuss the drugs used to treat tuberculosis and their side effects.

13. How does the fetal circulation differ from the adult circulation? Describe one form of congenital defect that can affect the lungs.

14. Describe the mechanism of action of theophylline and list the factors that increase and decrease clearance.

15. What is bronchiectasis and what can cause the disorder? How is it treated?

16. Give a short account of the defence mechanisms of the respiratory system.

17. With the aid of a diagram, describe the paranasal sinuses and comment on the pathology of sinusitis.

18. Discuss the stepwise approach to treating asthma, briefly indicating how each type of drug works.

19. Give an account of the different types of mechanical ventilation, indicating their uses.

20. What are the industrial dust diseases? How do they commonly present?

# MCQ Answers

1.
(a) T—The anterior and middle ethmoid sinuses also open into the middle meatus
(b) F—Open anteriorly into the choanae
(c) F—The sphenoethmoidal recess is the opening of the sphenoid sinus
(d) T—
(e) F—The upper third is lined by olfactory mucosa

2.
(a) F—Bronchioles have no cartilage, but they do have smooth muscle
(b) T—See above
(c) T—Clara cells are present within the bronchiole walls
(d) F—The upper airways contribute about one half of total resistance
(e) F—Alveoli are the major site of gas exchange

3.
(a) F—It is a left-to-right shunt
(b) T—Murmur extends throughout cardiac cycle
(c) F—From the aorta to pulmonary artery
(d) T—If pulmonary hypertension and shunt reversal occur
(e) F—Coarctation of the aorta causes radio-femoral delay

4.
(a) T—Vascular endothelial cells produce this important enzyme
(b) F—Inhibits breakdown of bradykinin
(c) T—The lungs can both produce and remove arachidonic acid metabolites
(d) F—Type II produce surfactant
(e) T—During arachidonic acid removal

5.
(a) F—Goblet cells are absent in the respiratory bronchioles
(b) T—Plus cold air, drugs, sulphur and nitrogen oxides
(c) F—Reduced due to abnormal motility of cilia
(d) T—An important defence mechanism
(e) F—Separate mechanism, ejecting unwanted material

6.
(a) F—From the umbilical vein to IVC
(b) F—The majority bypasses pulmonary circulation
(c) T—Failure to close leads to patent ductus arteriosus
(d) F—The foramen ovale usually closes following birth
(e) F—Umbilical veins, not arteries carry oxygenated blood

7.
(a) F—Non-capsulated lymphoid tissue
(b) T—It plays an important role in immunological protection
(c) T—Although MALT also exists in the gastrointestinal and urogenital tracts
(d) T—Comprises nasopharyngeal tonsil, palatine tonsil and lymphoid tissue on dorsum of tongue
(e) F—They are mostly B lymphocytes

8.
(a) T—Dead space is the sum of the two
(b) F—In health, physiological dead space is low
(c) T—Due to 'wasted' ventilation
(d) F—Higher at the base
(e) F—Slightly less than 1

9.
(a) T—Similar to pulmonary perfusion
(b) T—Ratio of V/Q is slightly less than 1
(c) F—Normal range for $O_2$ is >10.6
(d) F—12–20 breaths/min
(e) F—About 150mL

10.
(a) F—Diaphragm is the main muscle of quiet breathing
(b) T—To allow the abdominal contents to be displaced
(c) T—Elastic recoil drives air out of the lungs
(d) F—Inspiration increases lung volume, making pressure more negative
(e) T—

11.
(a) T—High flows induce turbulence and increase resistance
(b) F—Directly related to the pressure drop between two ends and fourth power of radius
(c) T—Poiseuille's Law describes laminar, not turbulent flow
(d) F—Decreased airway resistance at high volumes
(e) T—For example by mouth breathing

12.
(a) F—Type II pneumocytes
(b) F—After week 32 sufficient surfactant is present
(c) F—Insoluble; it floats on surface of alveolar lining fluid
(d) F—Increases compliance by reducing surface tension
(e) T—Allows surface area to vary with volume

13.
(a) F—Lower in females (11.5–16g/dL)
(b) F—The iron remains in the ferrous form
(c) T—The imidazole groups dissociate less readily in the deoxygenated form.
(d) T—Transports $CO_2$ as carbamino compounds
(e) F—Because of the beta chains

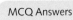

14. (a) F—It is an autosomal recessive disorder
    (b) T—Results in the production of HbS rather than HbA
    (c) F—Common in black Africans and their descendents
    (d) T—Crises can be precipitated by cold, ischaemia etc.
    (e) T—May also cause abdominal pain

15. (a) T—Plus decreased pH and increase in 2,3-DPG
    (b) T—2,3-DPG binds to the β chains
    (c) F—Fetal haemoglobin has a higher affinity for oxygen
    (d) T—Percentage saturation is unaffected by anaemia
    (e) T—Under specific conditions, e.g. pH 7.4, etc.

16. (a) T—According to Fick's law
    (b) F—Carbon dioxide diffuses $20 \times$ faster
    (c) F—Higher molecular weight gases diffuse more slowly
    (d) F—Fick's law
    (e) T—The rate of diffusion is inversely proportional to the membrane thickness

17. (a) T—Fick first described diffusion through a membrane
    (b) T—Other causes include reduced alveolar surface area, reduced partial pressure of $O_2$
    (c) T—See above
    (d) F—Increases the partial pressure of oxygen in the alveoli
    (e) F—Perfusion limited

18. (a) T—Amount of dissolved gas is proportional to the partial pressure of the gas and its solubility
    (b) T—Taken up very quickly so rarely diffusion limited
    (c) F—About 20 times
    (d) F—Sensitive but not specific
    (e) F—Reaches equilibrium about one-third of the way along the capillary

19. (a) F—Greater at base due to gravity
    (b) T—See above
    (c) T—Changes in posture after the ventilation:perfusion ratio
    (d) F—Inequalities exist even in health
    (e) F—Perfusion is decreased (hypoxic vasoconstriction)

20. (a) F—It is only slightly lower
    (b) F—Extra-alveolar vessels dilate with increased volume
    (c) T—It causes vasoconstriction
    (d) F—Low alveolar levels cause vasoconstriction
    (e) T—As occurs in exercise

21. (a) T—$CO_2$ is an acidic gas, an uncompensated increase causes acidosis
    (b) F—Returns them towards normal but cannot completely correct
    (c) F—Increasing ventilation decreases $PCO_2$
    (d) F—pK is low relative to pH of the blood
    (e) F—7.35–7.45

22. (a) F—Reduces $PaCO_2$ ($CO_2$ is blown off)
    (b) F—Oscillations during exercise stimulate changes in ventilation
    (c) F—Anaerobic metabolism takes place, not aerobic
    (d) F—It causes hyperpnoea not hyperventilation
    (e) T—Exercise induced asthma is a recognized sub-group

23. (a) T—Low pressure, low resistance system
    (b) T—As in exercise
    (c) F—Decreased as more capillaries are recruited
    (d) T—The pulmonary circulation offers lower resistance
    (e) T—Hydrostatic pressure is lower at apex

24. (a) T—Close to the exits of cranial nerves IX and X
    (b) F—Respond to hydrogen in concentration
    (c) F—But response is rapid to $PCO_2$
    (d) T—See above
    (e) F—They are responsible for about 80% of ventilatory drive

25. (a) F—They are situated in the carotid and aortic bodies
    (b) T—The carotic bodies are stimulated by hypoxaemia
    (c) F—There is a rich supply of blood to the peripheral chemoreceptors
    (d) F—Parasympathetic nerves cause vasodilation
    (e) F—They are sensitive to pH, $P_aO_2$, $P_aCO_2$ etc.

26. (a) T—An antimuscarinic bronchodilator
    (b) T—Other side effects include dry mouth and constipation
    (c) F—Reduces mucous secretions
    (d) T—Hence it is used in COPD
    (e) T—Acute angle-closure glaucoma has been reported with nebulised ipratropium

27. (a) T—Depresses central chemoreceptors
    (b) T—It is a respiratory depressant
    (c) T—It is a respiratory depressant
    (d) F—It is a respiratory stimulant
    (e) F—It is a respiratory stimulant

28. (a) T—Hence their key role in asthma
    (b) F—Bronchodilator acts on smooth muscle
    (c) F—Unlike theophylline
    (d) T—Acts to stabilize mast cells—mainly used to treat children
    (e) T—An antihistamine

29. (a) F—$\beta_2$ agonist
    (b) T—Classic fine tremor seen in inhaled bronchodilators
    (c) F—Usually inhaled (aerosol or nebulized solution)
    (d) F—May cause hypokalaemia
    (e) F—Peripheral vasodilation

30. (a) F—Respiratory stimulant
    (b) F—Given by continuous intravenous infusion
    (c) T—Hypertension is contraindication of the drug
    (d) T—And in epilepsy, hypertension and hyperthyroidism
    (e) F—Used in respiratory failure

31. (a) T—Mitigates the effect of low oxygen saturation
    (b) F—A feature of pulmonary oedema not acclimatization
    (c) T—Stimulation of peripheral chemoreceptors by hypoxaemia
    (d) T—Right shift to aid unloading of $O_2$
    (e) T—Oxidative enzymes increase

32. (a) F—Blood is not exposed to the $O_2$
    (b) F—Hypoxic drive can make high doses dangerous
    (c) F—BiPAP avoids intubation
    (d) F—Beneficial at 15h/day
    (e) T—As in Positive Pressure Ventilation (PPV)

33. (a) F—19 hours necessary to improve prognosis
    (b) F—Oxygen should not be prescribed to smokers
    (c) F—Nasal cannulae
    (d) F—Patients require life-long therapy
    (e) T—Minimum recommended saturation

34. (a) T—Air spaces are enlarged and their walls destroyed
    (b) F—Only about 2%
    (c) T—Due to loss of lung parenchyma
    (d) F—Compliance is increased
    (e) F—Radial traction is decreased as supporting architecture is destroyed

35. (a) F—Frequently copious amounts
    (b) F—Dependent lobes more affected due to gravity
    (c) T—May complicate pneumonia
    (d) T—May be long-standing
    (e) T—Due to secretions

36. (a) T—Lack of antiprotease causes increased destruction
    (b) T—Also inhibited by Oxygen radicals released by leucocytes
    (c) T—Vast majority of cases linked to smoking
    (d) F—Inherited as an autosomal dominant condition
    (e) F—Plays no role in angiotension conversion

37. (a) F—PEFR is reduced
    (b) T—Inflammatory mediators cause bronchoconstriction
    (c) T—Due to inflammation
    (d) F—Goblet cell hyperplasia increases secretion
    (e) T—Common allergen

38. (a) F—Less than 10% of pulmonary emboli cause infarction
    (b) T—Hence risks associated with surgery or fractures to pelvis or lower limb
    (c) T—Massive pulmonary embolism may be rapidly fatal
    (d) T—Prophylactic measures (TEDS etc.) are also important
    (e) T—Hence prophylactic anticoagulation

39. (a) F—Hyperplasia and hypertrophy
    (b) T—Careful history taking is necessary to establish time frame
    (c) T—Frequent cause of exacerbations
    (d) T—COPD is chronic bronchitis and emphysema
    (e) T—Smoking is the major aetiological factor

40. (a) F—Only of use if reversibility demonstrated by spirometry
    (b) F—30000 deaths p.a.
    (c) T—Due to rupture of bullae
    (d) T—Common pathogen seen in COPD
    (e) F—Only about 2%

41. (a) F—Only reduced in COPD
    (b) T—Very common presentations
    (c) F—Typically worse at night; COPD is worse in morning
    (d) F—Wheeze is a feature of both disorders
    (e) T—Although, more so of COPD

42. (a) F—Caused by coal dusts
    (b) T—In advanced disease
    (c) T—Due to inflammatory reaction and protease activity
    (d) F—Mesothelioma is caused by asbestos exposure
    (e) F—Low exposure does not lead to disease.

43. (a) F—Usually treated with chemotherapy
    (b) F—Squamous cell shows keratin
    (c) F—Metastases are very common
    (d) T—Relative risk rises to 5 with exposure
    (e) F—Mostly originate in large bronchi

44. (a) T—Strong association, especially with small fibres
    (b) F—Rarely metastasizes
    (c) T—Death is usually due to infection, vascular compromise or pulmonary embolism
    (d) T—Plus recurrent pleural effusions
    (e) F—Mesothelial tumour

45. (a) T—Very strong association
    (b) F—Adenocarcinomas show mucin production
    (c) T—Only treatment of value but tumours rarely operable
    (d) T—For example PTH production causing hypercalcaemia
    (e) T—Used for inoperable tumours

46. (a) T—Panacinar (panlobular) emphysema is associated with $\alpha_1$ antitrypsin deficiency
    (b) T—Enlargement of airspaces is permanent
    (c) T—Due to destruction of alveolar walls
    (d) T—Either Type I or Type II respiratory failure
    (e) F—Panacinar is not usually associated with chronic bronchitis

47. (a) T—Common in chest injuries
    (b) F—Collection of pus in the pleural cavity
    (c) T—May occur spontaneously or after trauma
    (d) F—Collection of lymph in the pleural cavity
    (e) T—A common feature of congestive heart failure

48. (a) F—No association
    (b) T—Associated with occupational exposure to carcinogens
    (c) T—Especially crocidolite and amiosite (mesothelioma)
    (d) T—Relative risk is ×5
    (e) F—Associated with nasal carcinoma

49. (a) F—Peak incidence at age 45–65
    (b) F—Idiopathic
    (c) T—Indicates extensive destruction of tissue
    (d) F—Restrictive pattern
    (e) T—Increased number of neutrophils are also seen

50. (a) F—Type I hypersensitivity reaction
    (b) T—Hayfever and eczema
    (c) T—See above
    (d) F—Hypertrophy of smooth muscle
    (e) T—$\beta_2$ agonists ('relievers') cause bronchodilation

51. (a) T—Due to airway narrowing
    (b) F—This describes emphysema rather than asthma
    (c) F—Bronchoconstriction is usually reversible
    (d) T—Ipratropium bromide is an anticholinergic drug
    (e) F—Xanthines work in this way

52. (a) F—<50%
    (b) F—>110 b.p.m.
    (c) F—Feature of life-threatening asthma
    (d) F—Prognostic factor for pneumonia
    (e) T—A marker of severe airflow restriction

53. (a) F—Right heart failure associated with lung disease
    (b) T—Chronic lung disease in general is a cause
    (c) T—Signs include oedema, cyanosis, tachycardia and raised JVP
    (d) T—Pulmonary hypertension leads to right heart failure
    (e) F—Prognosis is poor, 50% die within 5 years

54. (a) F—Cause of asbestosis
    (b) T—A common cause
    (c) T—Bakers, millers
    (d) T—Seafood processors
    (e) T—For example textile workers

55. (a) T—Blood pressure surges during each arousal
    (b) T—Plus male sex
    (c) F—See above (also common in post-menopausal women)
    (d) F—Rarely. Patients frequently require CPAP at night
    (e) T—Loss of concentration or falling asleep at the wheel

56. (a) T—All possible sites for metastases
    (b) T—All possible sites for metastases
    (c) T—All possible sites for metastases
    (d) T—All possible sites for metastases
    (e) T—All possible sites for metastases

57. (a) F—Incidence is increasing due to HIV and intercontinental travel
    (b) T—In asymptomatic patients
    (c) F—Commonly asymptomatic, but sometimes febrile illness
    (d) T—Or pleural effusion
    (e) F—Although immunization reduces risk by 70%

58. (a) T—Due to fibrosis
    (b) T—For example bleomycin, methotrexate
    (c) F—Asbestosis and idiopathic fibrosing alveolitis
    (d) T—For example in Goodpastures
    (e) T—See above

59. (a) T—Immune reaction to antigen
    (b) T—As in farmer's lung
    (c) T—Concentrated, short exposure causes acute, severe symptoms
    (d) T—
    (e) T—Inflammatory marker

60. (a) T—Opportunistic pathogen
    (b) T—A feature of TB caused by MAC
    (c) F—Further immunosuppression would probably be fatal
    (d) T—Post-infection bronchiectasis
    (e) T—TB in any host

61. (a) F—>7mmol/L
    (b) F—>30 breaths/min
    (c) T—New confusion
    (d) F—Hypotension (diastolic <60)
    (e) F—May be present in mild pneumonia

62. (a) T—May also cause pericardial effusions
    (b) F—Exudate
    (c) T—Left heart failure
    (d) T—Cirrhosis
    (e) F—Exudate

63. (a) F—Latency period in allergic form of occupational asthma
    (b) F—Coal worker's pneumoconiosis and rheumatoid arthritis
    (c) T—In certain diseases (e.g. mesothelioma, asbestosis) within a specified time-frame
    (d) F—For example in occupational asthma
    (e) T—And during holidays

64. (a) F—Size alone is not an indication of metastasis
    (b) T—Only indicated in young patients with sufficient respiratory reserve and confined disease
    (c) T—Lung function tests are important in assessment
    (d) T—Oxygen and/or assisted ventilation to correct hypoxia are more appropriate
    (e) T—Has mostly metastasized early

65. (a) T—About every 3–4 years
    (b) F—In 50% of patients
    (c) F—Legionella is found in cooling towers
    (d) F—No bacterial cell wall so penicillin is ineffective—treated with erythromycin
    (e) F—Institutional outbreaks amongst young people

66. (a) F—Gram-negative organism
    (b) T—Very severe pneumonia
    (c) T—Test include stypical serology
    (d) F—No vaccine is available
    (e) T—Found in cooling towers and air-conditioning

67. (a) T—In about 60% of patients
    (b) T—Frequently in Chlamydia pneumoniae
    (c) T—In about 15%, classically rusty with S. pneumoniae
    (d) T—In about 25% of patients
    (e) T—Not uncommon

68. (a) F—In those who are haemodynamically unstable
    (b) T—Anticoagulation is essential
    (c) T—Warfarin should be taken for a minimum of 3 months
    (d) F—CXR commonly normal
    (e) T—Incidence at autopsy of about 12%

69. (a) F—Not undertaken with intent to cure
    (b) F—Non-small-cell (70%)
    (c) T—Most aggressive type of lung cancer
    (d) F—Staged as limited or extensive
    (e) T—From Kulchitsky cells

70. (a) T—Commonest in non-smoking elderly women
    (b) F—See above
    (c) F—Stains for mucin
    (d) F—Usually peripheral
    (e) F—May be clinically silent

71. (a) T—Cavitating rheumatoid nodules
    (b) T—Cavitation may be seen on chest X-ray
    (c) F—Does not cause cavitation
    (d) T—May rupture producing black sputum
    (e) F—Does not cause cavitation

72. (a) F—Typically dry cough
    (b) T—As in all restrictive diseases
    (c) F—Wheeze classically absent
    (d) T—Often marked
    (e) T—Progression over time

73. (a) F—Major risk factor
    (b) F—Confirmed as an independent risk factor
    (c) T—Anticoagulation usually recommended for 6 weeks to 3 months after PE
    (d) T—Maligancy, heart disease, chronic lung disease
    (e) T—Due to local variations in ventilation and damaged vascular bed

74. (a) F—Occasional symptoms may be controlled with bronchodilators
    (b) F—Treatment may be stepped down at any time
    (c) T—Patients are advised to avoid provoking factors such as cat dander
    (d) F—If more than daily, move to Step 2
    (e) F—But children requiring high doses should be referred to a specialist

75. (a) F—Kveim test (used in past) or tuberculin test
    (b) F—Widespread non-caseating granulomas are present
    (c) F—Affects lymphatics and walls of airways and blood vessels
    (d) T—In progressive sarcoidosis
    (e) T—Classical radiological sign

76. (a) T—Associated with inhalation of toxic gases and smoke
    (b) F—Hyperplasia of type 2 pneumocytes
    (c) T—Alveolar exudate promotes formation
    (d) F—Mortality generally greater than 50%
    (e) T—Gram-negative septicaemia

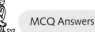 

77. (a) F—Autosomal recessive
    (b) T—Plus malabsorption and failure to thrive
    (c) T—CF sweat test
    (d) T—Associated with recurrent infections and bronchiectasis
    (e) F—Associated with infertility in males due to immotile sperm

78. (a) F—Hospital acquired pneumonia is mainly Gram-negative
    (b) T—Due to destruction of cilia
    (c) T—Or pleural effusion
    (d) F—More often bacterial
    (e) T—One of the BTS prognostic factors

79. (a) F—Usually squamous cell carcinoma
    (b) F—Peak incidence 60–70 years
    (c) F—M : F = 5 : 1
    (d) T—Very rare in non-smokers
    (e) T—Commonly present first with hoarseness

80. (a) T—Rare necrotizing vasculitis
    (b) F—Affects small arteries and veins
    (c) F—Aetiology is unknown
    (d) T—Leading to renal failure
    (e) T—Mucosal thickening and ulceration

81. (a) T—Rare cause of bronchiectasis
    (b) F—Dependent lobes are affected
    (c) T—Kidneys are sometimes affected by amyloid deposits
    (d) F—Permanent bronchial dilatation
    (e) T—Complications include pneumonia, pneumothorax, empyema and meningitis

82. (a) T—Common presentation of asthma
    (b) T—Productive of sputum
    (c) T—A common cause of cough in non-smoking adults
    (d) T—From postnasal drip
    (e) T—A well-known side-effect

83. (a) T—An important cause of haemoptysis
    (b) T—Massive haemoptysis
    (c) T—If blood is swallowed
    (d) T—Frequent and blood streaked
    (e) T—Simple cause of a sinister sign

84. (a) T—This is the definition of respiratory failure
    (b) F—Tolerance to increased $P_aCO_2$ may develop in Type II
    (c) F—High-dose oxygen used in type I
    (d) F—Differs due to absence of hypercapnia
    (e) T—Or any disease which causes severe V/Q mismatch

85. (a) T—Key cause
    (b) F—Arterial blood gas analysis
    (c) F—Type II: ventilatory or pump failure
    (d) F—Defined by a $P_aO_2 < 8\,kPa$
    (e) F—Renal compensation is common in type II failure (acute-on-chronic)

86. (a) T—Flapping tremor is a standard test for $CO_2$ retention
    (b) F—Vasodilation leads to warm peripheries
    (c) T—In severe cases
    (d) T—Often headache occurs on waking
    (e) T—Swelling of the optic disk is sometimes seen

87. (a) T—An attempt to reduce expiratory pressure
    (b) T—Due to flattened diaphragm (air trapping)
    (c) T—Due to flattened diaphragm (air trapping)
    (d) T—Airways obstruction
    (e) T—Due to air trapping

88. (a) T—And in other pyogenic lung diseases, e.g. empyema and abcess
    (b) F—Asthma does not cause clubbing
    (c) F—Chronic bronchitis never causes clubbing
    (d) T—In, for example, fibrosing alveolitis
    (e) T—Due to shunt mechanism

89. (a) F—Tension pneumothorax
    (b) F—Classically stony dull
    (c) F—Increased
    (d) T—Decreased on affected side
    (e) T—Changed by coughing

90. (a) F—$KCO$ (transfer coefficient) corrects for lost volume
    (b) F—400–650 L/min
    (c) F—Increased with air trapping
    (d) F—Measures anatomical dead space
    (e) F—Airway resistance

91. (a) F—Displaced in collapse
    (b) T—Or segmental distribution
    (c) F—Silhouette of mediastinum against aerated lung
    (d) F—Bronchi containing air shown against consolidated lung
    (e) T—Common in pulmonary oedema

92. (a) T—They are synonymous
    (b) F—$KCO$ corrects for lost volume
    (c) F—Increased by exercise
    (d) T—Will highlight even limited disease
    (e) F—Many causes of reduced $T_LCO$

93. (a) F—At the end of a normal expiration
    (b) T—Approximately 5 L
    (c) T—Only RV, FRC and TLC cannot be measured by spirometry
    (d) F—Lung volumes normally decreased
    (e) F—Obstructive disorder: <80%

94. (a) F—Records the maximum expiratory rate in first 10 ms
    (b) F—Detects airway resistance (i.e. obstructive defects)
    (c) F—Lower due to morning dipping
    (d) T—Patient results are assessed against normal values, matched for age, gender and height
    (e) F—Less accurate but more practical

95.   (a)  T—This is its primary role
     (b)  F—To detect perfusion
     (c)  F—Pulmonary angiography is the gold standard
     (d)  F—Less invasive; used more often
     (e)  F—Radioisotopes not used in this test

96.   (a)  F—Trachea deviated to the affected side
     (b)  F—Homogeneous whiteness is seen
     (c)  T—Congenital atelectasis where lungs fail to expand
     (d)  T—Fibrosis is a recognized complication
     (e)  T—Displaced fissures is a useful sign in differentiating collapse and consolidation

97.   (a)  F—Fibreoptic used more often (does not require general anaesthetic)
     (b)  T—Especially in a smoker
     (c)  T—Bronchial alveolar lavage
     (d)  F—Cannot be reached by bronchoscope
     (e)  F—Light sedation may be used to suppress cough and reduce anxiety

98.   (a)  F—Ventilation:perfusions scans and pulmonary angiography
     (b)  T—Also used in staging lung cancers
     (c)  T—May detect small effusions not seen on CXR
     (d)  T—May require open biopsy
     (e)  F—Medical emergency; aspiration required before investigations

99.   (a)  T—Due to destruction of lung parenchyma
     (b)  T—A measure of airway narrowing
     (c)  F—Increased through air trapping
     (d)  T—Due to air trapping
     (e)  F—Classically reduced in obstructive diseases

100.  (a)  F—Rarely performed; only if diagnosis is in doubt
     (b)  T—Should improve by 15% or more
     (c)  F—No change in $T_L\text{CO}$
     (d)  T—Due to air trapping
     (e)  F—Identifies allergens (i.e. extrinsic causes)

# SAQ Answers

1. Surfactant.

Surfactant is a substance secreted by type II pneumocytes in the alveolus and contains phospholipid (dipalmitoyl phosphatidylcholine, DPC) which reduces the surface tension (ST) of the alveolar lining fluid. It therefore increases lung compliance. Surface tension of surfactant shows hysteresis, i.e. its surface tension is greater on expansion than on compression.

The function of surfactant in the lung:
- Reduce the work of breathing (P$\alpha$ $T$—Laplace's law).
- Maintain alveolar stability (P$\alpha$ 1/$R$—Laplace's law).
- Prevent transudation of fluid into the alveoli.

Alveoli vary in size, but because of surfactant the ST of the fluid that lines them is proportional to the surface area and so the $T{:}R$ ratio remains constant. Thus all the alveoli can be inflated by the same pressure. This prevents collapse of small alveoli and overinflation of large ones.

Surfactant reduces the hydrostatic pressure gradient across the capillary wall (by making tissue pressure less negative), so decreasing the ultrafiltration forces.

2. Normal values for Hb concentration:

Male:    13.5–18.0 g/dL.
Female:    11.5–16.0 g/dL.
See Fig. 5.22 Oxyhaemoglobin dissociation curve.
Arterial $PO_2$ = 100 mmHg (13.3 kPa).
Venous $PO_2$ = 40 mmHg (5.3 kPa).

3. Venous admixture.

The venous admixture is that blood entering the systemic circulation that has bypassed gas exchange in the lungs. It will not have taken up oxygen or released its carbon dioxide, therefore its levels of $PO_2$ and $PCO_2$ are venous levels and for this reason it is termed venous admixture.

In a patient presenting with a pulmonary embolus, some of the pulmonary capillaries of the patient's lung will not be perfused with blood. The blood will not undergo gas exchange. This can be considered as a right-to-left shunt.

This initially causes a rise in arterial $PCO_2$ and a fall in $PO_2$. The rise in $PCO_2$ causes an increase in ventilation.

This allows those areas of lung that are well perfused and ventilated to lower the $PCO_2$ since a significant proportion (approximately 10%) of $CO_2$ is dissolved in the blood and is released in the alveoli.

Due to the shape of the oxyhaemoglobin dissociation curve any increase in ventilation doesn't increase $O_2$ carriage significantly and increases the dissolved $O_2$ by only a small amount (due to the low solubility of oxygen in the blood).

This non-shunted blood returning to the systemic circulation has a higher $PO_2$ and a small amount of additional $O_2$ carriage (in dissolved form) but on mixing with shunted blood this additional dissolved $O_2$ quickly combines with the unsaturated Hb of the shunted blood and the $PO_2$ is lowered.

Thus overventilating those areas which are well perfused allows the $PCO_2$ of arterial blood to be normal or lowered but arterial $PO_2$ cannot be increased to normal.

4. Airway resistance.

The resistance to flow of a gas within the airways of the lung, i.e. the resistance presented by the airways themselves, is represented by the equation below:

$$\text{Airway resistance} = \frac{\text{mouth pressure} - \text{alveolar pressure}}{\text{air flow rate}}$$

~0.5 – 1.5 cmH$_2$O

In laminar flow, the flow of a fluid is in streamlines or laminae (parallel to the walls of the tube). The layer closest to the tube wall is believed to be stationary and therefore the resistance to flow is independent of roughness of the tube.

The resistance to flow is dependent on the viscosity of the fluid and the dimensions of the tube.

Poiseuille's law describes the resistance to flow under laminar flow conditions.

$$\text{Resistance} = 8\eta l/\pi r^4$$

$l$ = length of tube, $r$ = radius of tube, $\eta$ = viscosity of fluid.

Thus the resistance to flow is inversely proportional to the radius of the tube to the fourth power.

Factors affecting smooth muscle tone of the airways.
- Nervous factors

Parasympathetic (vagus) $\Rightarrow$ bronchoconstriction. Acetylcholine (Ach) acting on muscarinic receptors. Major importance in control of bronchomotor tone

Sympathetic $\Rightarrow$ bronchodilation. Noradrenaline acts via $\beta_2$ receptors. Not of major importance in controlling smooth muscle tone in man, but important in the treatment of asthma.

NANC (vagus) $\Rightarrow$ bronchodilation. It is believed that nitric oxide (NO) is the neurotransmitter responsible. Only effective neural bronchodilator pathway in man.

- Chemical factors
  Constriction caused by:
  Histamine via $H_1$ receptors
  Prostaglandins
  Leukotrienes
  Bradykinin
  5-HT via 5-$HT_2$ receptors
  Irritants
  Cold air
  Increased $PCO_2$ via central chemoreceptors
  Decreased $PO_2$ via peripheral chemoreceptors

Dilation caused by:
  Adrenaline via $\beta_2$ receptors
  NO

See Fig. 4.33

5. Lung carcinoma
   - Incidence—most common malignant tumour in Britain.
   - Age distribution—middle to old age.
   - Sex distribution—males > females at present but incidence increasing in females.
   - Predisposing factors—cigarette smoking; asbestos exposure; haematite mining; radon and other radioactive gases; chemical exposure: nickel, chromates, mustard gas, arsenic, coal-tar distillates; diffuse pulmonary fibrosis.
   - Macroscopic appearances—tumour, usually central (squamous cell, small-cell and large-cell undifferentiated), sometimes peripheral (mainly adenocarcinoma).
   - Microscopic appearances—squamous cell, small-cell, adenocarcinoma, large-cell undifferentiated.
   - Spread—direct to pleural membranes, lymphatics to hilar lymph nodes includes subcarinal node, blood to anywhere in systemic circulation if erodes into a pulmonary vein, transcoelomic across pleural cavities.
   - Prognosis—related to type (worse with small-cell) and stage (some squamous cell and adenocarcinomas may be surgically resectable) but overall 5-year survival rate 4–7%.

6. Bronchial asthma
   - Definition—reversible airways obstruction due to increased irritability of bronchial tree.
   - Types—atopic, non-atopic, aspirin-induced, occupation, allergic bronchopulmonary aspergillosis.
   - Mechanisms—type I, type II, type III, or mixture of hypersensitivity reactions. Immediate early response due to mast cell degranulation and release of histamine and leukotrienes. The late asthmatic response is due to recruitment and activation of inflammatory cells within the airway and the release of cytokines and other mediators.
   - Consequences—bronchial obstruction with distal overinflation, mucus plugging of bronchi, mucous gland hypertrophy, bronchial wall smooth muscle hypertrophy, inflammation extending into bronchioles, possible centrilobular emphysema.
   - Treatment—$\beta_2$ adrenoceptor agonists (short and long acting), corticosteroids, sodium chromoglycate and aminophylline.

7. Bronchiectasis
   - Definition—permanent dilatation of bronchi and bronchioles.
   - Causes—bronchial obstruction and severe inflammation, e.g. measles, cystic fibrosis, chronic bronchitis, immotile cilia syndromes.
   - Features—dilatation of bronchi and bronchioles, destruction of alveolar walls, pulmonary fibrosis.
   - Complications—pneumonia, empyema, septicaemia, meningitis, metastatic abscesses, amyloid formation.
   - Treatment—symptomatically, treat active infections, surgical resection of localized areas of bronchiectasis.

8. ARDS
   - Definition—diffuse alveolar damage with hyaline membrane formation.
   - Causes—shock (haemorrhagic, cardiogenic, septic, anaphylactic, endotoxic), trauma (direct lung trauma, multisystem trauma), viral or bacterial pneumonia, gas inhalation (nitrogen dioxide, sulphur dioxide, chlorine), narcotic abuse, ionizing radiation, gastric aspiration, disseminated intravascular coagulation, oxygen toxicity.
   - Pathogenesis—diffuse alveolar damage +/− oxygen toxicity.
   - Histological appearances—hyaline membranes, oedema, red cells, proliferation type II pneumocytes.
   - Prognosis—50% mortality rate.

9. Malignant mesothelioma
   - Definition—malignant tumour derived from mesothelial cells.
   - Site—usually pleural, sometimes peritoneal.
   - Causes—asbestos especially blue asbestos, long latent period (20–30 years).
   - Macroscopic appearances—malignant tumour, often spindle-celled, distinguished from diffuse adenocarcinoma.
   - Spread—locally through pleural cavities, distant spread less common.
   - Prognosis—poor, may remain localized for years but universally fatal.

10. Cystic fibrosis
    - Definition—autosomal recessive genetic condition affecting production of exocrine secretions.
    - Pathogenesis—deletion in cystic fibrosis transmembrane conductance regulator leading to unresponsiveness to cAMP control and defective transport of chloride ions and water across epithelial cell membranes.
    - Diagnosis—genetic or sweat test (increased sodium concentration).
    - Features—meconium ileus in infants, failure to thrive, recurrent lung infections, bronchiectasis, chronic pancreatitis, malabsorption, male infertility.

11. Pneumonia in the immonocompromised
    - Causes of immunosuppression—human immunodefiency virus–acquired immune deficiency syndrome (AIDS), severe combined

immunodeficiency (SCID), intensive chemotherapy and/or radiotherapy for disseminated malignancy.

- *Pneumocystis carinii* pneumonia—common in AIDS, protozoan, diffuse radiographic shadowing.
- Cytomegalovirus—common in AIDS, reactivation of dormant infection or acquisition through blood products, owl's eye nuclei.
- Aspergillus—any immunodeficiency state, fungus, diagnosis from bronchial washings.
- Cryptococcus—fungus, diagnosis by serology or direct examination of bronchial washings.
- Varicella zoster virus.
- Lymphoma—neoplastic but can give a pneumonic pattern on radiography.
- Kaposi's sarcoma—neoplastic but can give a pneumonic pattern on radiography.

12. (a) Any other symptoms (e.g. syncope, calf swelling)? Was haemoptysis a solitary event? Explore risk factors: recent surgery etc. Is there a family history of DVT or PE? Is she a smoker?
 (b) Malignancy (as seen here), recent surgery, fractures, recent stroke/MI; pregnancy; immobility; clotting disorders.
 (c) CXR, V/Q scan—depending on results and her status possibly Doppler/CTPA.
 (d) Anticoagulation—heparin and then overlap with warfarin. Warfarin to be continued for at least 3 months. Measure INR to assess response—aim for INR of 2–3. Also other prophylaxis, e.g. TED stockings.

13. (a) Spirometry is the most useful test here; likely to demonstrate decrease in $FEV_1$ and reduction in $FEV_1/FVC$. Also test of bronchodilator response. Exercise testing would assess level of disability. Progressive exercise test likely to show decreased uptake of oxygen against predicted; shuttle test should also show reduced exercise capacity.
 (b) Approx. 40 pack years. This would be consistent with a diagnosis of COPD (patients normally >20 pack years. GP could give him information (advice, Quitline, contact details for support groups etc.) and drugs, e.g. nicotine replacement patches.
 (c) As per BTS guidelines. Strongly encouraged to stop smoking to reduce further damage. Encouraged to exercise. Drug treatment in mild cases: short-acting $\beta_2$ agonists or ipratropium p.r.n. Corticosteroids if subject has concomitant asthma.
 (d) Cough and sputum due to chronic bronchitis: cilia have been damaged by smoke which also causes inflammation, hypertrophy of mucus glands etc. Elastic tissue of lung parenchyma is destroyed as granulocytes release large amounts of protease. Loss of compliance causes early airway collapse and air trapping.

14. (a) The patient is hypoxaemic with $P_aO_2 < 8$ kPa—i.e. respiratory failure.
 (b) Type II respiratory failure as the patient is hypercapnic with $P_aCO_2 > 6.5$ kPa. He is hypoventilating and the $CO_2$ in the blood cannot be blown off in the lungs.

(Type I respiratory failure is defined as a $P_aCO_2$ <6.5 kPa. This is a ventilation:perfusion mismatch.)
 (c) pH is below the normal range i.e. there is an acidosis. This can be explained by rise in $CO_2$—it is a *respiratory* acidosis. Looking at bicarbonate levels (and using the Henderson–Hasselbalch equation) we see that $[HCO_3^-]$ has risen in order to compensate for the rise in $CO_2$; renal compensation has occurred in order to bring pH towards normal. This is typical of the acute-on-chronic situation where long-standing disease allows the renal system time to compensate, but an acute exacerbation (e.g. infection) tips the patient into respiratory failure.
 (d) Treat underlying cause of respiratory failure (i.e. antibiotics for infection). Give nebulized bronchodilators. Give oxygen, but in type II respiratory failure limit the concentration to 24% at first using a controlled-flow mask. Tolerance to high levels of $PCO_2$ may have built up over a long period of time in this patient, reducing the central chemoreceptor drive. Hypoxic drive (low $PO_2$) from the peripheral chemoreceptors then becomes vital. This is significant clinically because if these patients are given high levels of oxygen, this raises the $PO_2$ reducing the drive for ventilation. The patient may therefore stop breathing and die. If, despite treatment, $P_aCO_2$ continues to rise, or a safe $P_aO_2$ cannot be achieved, consider mechanical ventilation.

15. (a) On inspection: cyanosis, hyperinflated lungs, tachypnoea (possibly >25).
 On palpation: pulsus paradoxus.
 On percussion: hyperflation (hyperresonant lungs).
 On auscultation: polyphonic wheeze.
 (b) See BTS guidelines: pulse > 110; respiratory rate >25; inability to complete sentences; PEFR < 50% predicted/best.
 (c) Mention pro-inflammatory components, pre-formed and rapidly generated mediators. Early and late phases; cytokines etc., promotion of inflammatory response is underway and bronchodilators will do little to mitigate airway narrowing.
 (d) Test blood gases. Immediate treatment with high-dose oxygen, nebulized salbutamol. Hydrocortisone IV or prednisolone PO. Then assess.

16. (a) Extrinsic asthma—probably triggered by cat dander (evidence of atopy in family). IgE-specific antibodies produced, leading to inflammatory cascade and airway hyperresponsiveness.
 (b) Could be confirmed by skin prick test to cat dander showing weal.
 (c) Cold air, exercise, stress, allergens (pollen, animal fur/dander, house dust mites), drugs (NSAIDs, β-blockers), infection.
 (d) Many different occupations (see Chapter 9); includes animal laboratory workers, shellfish processors, spray painters, health professionals (latex or drugs). Establish whether symptoms are better at weekends/holidays.

17. (a) Pulse oximetry, video recordings or referral to sleep laboratory for full testing (full monitoring during sleep). Fifteen apnoeas/hypoapnoeas during 1 hour of sleep is diagnostic.
    (b) Weight loss, avoidance of alcohol and tobacco. Or more likely, CPAP via nasal mask during sleep. In very rare cases (where anatomy of jaw is abnormal) surgery to relieve obstruction.
    (c) Consequences for him and his wife: reduced quality of life, daytime sleepiness, morning headache, decreased libido, depression is common. Also blood pressure surges during arousal, may lead to hypertension. Serious complications: pulmonary hypertension and type II respiratory failure.
    (d) Also much higher risk of RTA due to lapses of concentration or falling asleep at the wheel.

18. (a) Bronchial carcinoma, TB, PE. Haemoptysis over years can sometimes occur in bronchiectasis.
    (b) Cachexia, finger clubbing, HPOA, lymphadenopathy. Signs of SVC syndrome etc. Chest may be normal on examination, or signs of obstruction (e.g. monophonic wheeze).
    (c) Given history and abnormal test, flexible fibreoptic bronchoscopy would be next investigation.
    (d) Flow–volume loop showed truncated expiratory limb, indicating there is an intrathoracic obstruction.

19. (a) Adverse prognostic factors: new mental confusion; urea >7 mmol/L; tachypnoea >30 breaths/min; hypotension—diastolic < 60 mmHg.

    (b) Fever, confusion, cyanosis, hypotension, tachycardia, tachypnoea. Chest examination: may be signs of consolidation (dull to percussion, decreased expansion, increased vocal resonance, crackles/bronchial breathing), pleural rub.
    (c) If effusion is large and patient is symptomatic, drainage is indicated. Drain slowly (<2L/h). If bacteriology shows aspirate is infected—empyema—then further antibiotics. A loculated empyema may require intrapleural streptokinase. If persists, surgery is indicated.
    (d) CAP: *S. pneumoniae* most common, also *Haemophilus influenzae* and *Mycoplasma pneumoniae*.

20. (a) Not traumatic; may be primary spontaneous (no underlying disease) or secondary to pre-existing disease such as COPD. Primary spontaneous is common in tall, thin young men due to rupture of subpleural blebs at apices.
    (b) May be able to see reflection of pleura; lung collapsed towards heart border; in tension pneumothorax the trachea is deviated from the affected side (NB a medical emergency—CXR should not be performed, treatment should be started immediately.)
    (c) Recurrent pneumothoraces: pleurodesis is indicated. Irritating agent is introduced into pleural space so that inflammatory reaction causes adhesion of parietal and visceral pleura.
    (d) Air removed with large-bore syringe partially filled with saline (in 2nd intercostal space midclavicular line). Air is allowed to bubble through the syringe.

# Index